D1124593

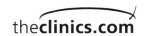
theclinics.com

PSYCHIATRIC CLINICS

OF NORTH AMERICA

Psychosomatic Medicine

GUEST EDITORS
James L. Levenson, MD
David F. Gitlin, MD, and
Cathy Crone, MD

December 2007 • Volume 30 • Number 4

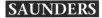

An Imprint of Elsevier, Inc.
PHILADELPHIA   LONDON   TORONTO   MONTREAL   SYDNEY   TOKYO

W.B. SAUNDERS COMPANY
A Division of Elsevier Inc.

1600 John F. Kennedy Boulevard • Suite 1800 • Philadelphia, PA 19103-2899

http://www.theclinics.com

PSYCHIATRIC CLINICS OF NORTH AMERICA   Volume 30, Number 4
December 2007   ISSN 0193-953X
Editor: Sarah E. Barth   ISBN-13: 978-1-4160-5327-9
                                                                  ISBN-10: 1-4160-5327-1

Copyright © 2007 Elsevier Inc. All rights reserved. No part of this publication may be reproduced or transmitted in any form or by any means, electronic or mechanical, including photocopy, recording, or any information retrieval system, without written permission from the Publisher.

Single photocopies of single articles may be made for personal use as allowed by national copyright laws. Permission of the Publisher and payment of a fee is required for all other photocopying, including multiple or systematic copying, copying for advertising or promotional purposes, resale, and all forms of document delivery. Special rates are available for educational institutions that wish to make photocopies for non-profit educational classroom use. Permissions may be sought directly from Elsevier's Global Rights Department in Oxford, UK: phone 215-239-3804 or +44 (0) 1865 843830, fax +44 (0) 1865 853333, e-mail: healthpermissions@elsevier.com. Requests may also be completed on-line via the Elsevier homepage (http://www.elsevier.com/permissions). In the USA, users may clear permissions and make payments through the Copyright Clearance Center, Inc., 222 Rosewood Drive, Danvers, MA 01923, USA; phone: (978) 750-8400, fax: (978) 750-4744, and in the UK through the Copyright Licensing Agency Rapid Clearance Service (CLARCS), 90 Tottenham Court Road, London W1P 0LP, UK; phone: (+44) 171 436 5931; fax: (+44) 171 436 3986. Other countries may have a local reprographic rights agency for payments.

Reprints. For copies of 100 or more, of articles in this publication, please contact the Commercial Reprints Department, Elsevier Inc., 360 Park Avenue South, New York, New York 10010-1710. Tel.: (212) 633-3813, Fax: (212) 462-1935, e-mail: reprints@elsevier.com.

The ideas and opinions expressed in *Psychiatric Clinics of North America* do not necessarily reflect those of the Publisher. The Publisher does not assume any responsibility for any injury and/or damage to persons or property arising out of or related to any use of the material contained in this periodical. The reader is advised to check the appropriate medical literature and the product information currently provided by the manufacturer of each drug to be administered, to verify the dosage, the method and duration of administration, or contraindications. It is the responsibility of the treating physician or other health care professional, relying on independent experience and knowledge of the patient, to determine drug dosages and the best treatment for the patient. Mention of any product in this issue should not be construed as endorsement by the contributors, editors, or the Publisher of the product or manufacturers' claims.

Psychiatric Clinics of North America (ISSN 0193-953X) is published quarterly by Elsevier Inc., 360 Park Avenue South, New York, NY 10010-1710. Months of issue are March, June, September, and December. Business and Editorial Offices: 1600 John F. Kennedy Blvd., Suite 1800, Philadelphia, PA 19103-2899. Customer Service Office: 6277 Sea Harbor Drive, Orlando, FL 32887-4800 Periodicals postage paid at New York, NY and additional mailing offices. Subscription prices are $213.00 per year (US individuals), $362.00 per year (US institutions), $107.00 per year (US students/residents), $255.00 per year (Canadian individuals), $440.00 per year (Canadian Institutions), $297.00 per year (foreign individuals), $440.00 per year (foreign institutions), and $149.00 per year (international & Canadian students/residents). Foreign air speed delivery is included in all *Clinics'* subscription prices. All prices are subject to change without notice. **POSTMASTER:** Send address changes to *Psychiatric Clinics of North America*, Elsevier Periodicals Customer Service, 6277 Sea Harbor Drive, Orlando, FL 32887-4800. Customer Service: 1-800-654-2452 (US). From outside of the US, call 1-407-345-4000.

Psychiatric Clinics of North America is covered in *Index Medicus, Current Contents/Social and Behavioral Sciences, Social Science Citation Index, Embase/Excerpta Medica,* and PsycINFO.

Printed in the United States of America.

PSYCHIATRIC CLINICS
OF NORTH AMERICA

Psychosomatic Medicine

GUEST EDITORS

JAMES L. LEVENSON, MD, Professor of Psychiatry, Medicine, and Surgery, Virginia Commonwealth University School of Medicine, Richmond, Virginia

DAVID F. GITLIN, MD, Director, Division of Medical Psychiatry, Brigham and Women's/Faulkner Hospitals; and Assistant Professor of Psychiatry, Harvard Medical School, Boston, Massachusetts

CATHY CRONE, MD, Associate Professor of Psychiatry, George Washington University School of Medicine, Washington, District of Columbia; Vice Chairperson, Department of Psychiatry, Inova Fairfax Hospital, Falls Church, Virginia

CONTRIBUTORS

LESLEY A. ALLEN, PhD, Department of Psychiatry, Robert Wood Johnson Medical School-UMDNJ, Piscataway, New Jersey

DAVID J. AXELROD, MD, JD, Instructor, Department of Internal Medicine, Thomas Jefferson University; and Clinical Director, Thomas Jefferson University Hospital Sickle Cell Program, Philadelphia, Pennsylvania

MADELEINE BECKER, MD, Instructor, Department of Psychiatry, Thomas Jefferson University, Philadelphia, Pennsylvania

SUMIT BHUTANI, MD, Division of Allergy and Immunology, Department of Internal Medicine, University of Texas Southwestern Medical Center, Dallas, Texas

J. MICHAEL BOSTWICK, MD, Consultant, Department of Psychiatry and Psychology, Mayo Clinic; and Associate Professor of Psychiatry, Mayo Clinic College of Medicine, Rochester, Minnesota

REBECCA W. BRENDEL, MD, JD, Instructor in Psychiatry, Harvard Medical School; and Clinical Assistant in Psychiatry, Massachusetts General Hospital Psychiatry Consultation Service and Law and Psychiatry Service, Boston, Massachusetts

E. SHERWOOD BROWN, MD, PhD, Department of Psychiatry, University of Texas Southwestern Medical Center, Dallas, Texas

JAMES S. BROWN, Jr, MD, MPH, Assistant Professor of Psychiatry, Department of Psychiatry, Virginia Commonwealth University School of Medicine, Richmond; and Consulting Psychiatrist, Clinical Services, Crossroads Community Services Board, Farmville, Virginia

LINDA HAMMER BURNS, PhD, Associate Professor, Department of Obstetrics, Gynecology and Women's Health, University of Minnesota; and Reproductive Medicine Center, Minneapolis, Minnesota

LYDIA A. CHWASTIAK, MD, MPH, Assistant Professor, Departments of Psychiatry and Medicine, Yale University School of Medicine, Yale New Haven Psychiatric Hospital, New Haven, Connecticut

DAWN M. EHDE, PhD, Associate Professor of Rehabilitation Medicine, Department of Rehabilitation Medicine, University of Washington School of Medicine, Harborview Medical Center; and University of Washington Multiple Sclerosis Rehabilitation Research and Training Center, Seattle, Washington

MARC D. FELDMAN, MD, Clinical Professor of Psychiatry, The University of Alabama, Tuscaloosa, Alabama

DAVID A. KHAN, MD, Division of Allergy and Immunology, Department of Internal Medicine, University of Texas Southwestern Medical Center, Dallas, Texas

KURT KROENKE, MD, Professor of Medicine, Indiana University School of Medicine; and Research Scientist, Regenstrief Institute, Indianapolis, Indiana

ELISABETH J. SHAKIN KUNKEL, MD, Professor, Department of Psychiatry, Thomas Jefferson University, Philadelphia, Pennsylvania

MICHAEL J. MARCANGELO, MD, Assistant Professor of Psychiatry, Department of Psychiatry and Behavioral Medicine, Medical College of Wisconsin, Milwaukee, Wisconsin

DIMITRI D. MARKOV, MD, Assistant Professor, Department of Psychiatry, Thomas Jefferson University, Philadelphia, Pennsylvania

BARBARA E. McDERMOTT, PhD, Associate Professor of Clinical Psychiatry, University of California, Davis School of Medicine, Department of Psychiatry and Behavioral Sciences, Division of Psychiatry and the Law, Sacramento; and Research Director, Clinical Demonstration/Research Unit, Napa State Hospital, Napa, California

LORENZO NORRIS, MD, Clinical Instructor of Psychiatry, Department of Psychiatry, Medical Faculty Associates of George Washington University Hospital; and Director, Medical Wellness Clinic, George Washington University Hospital, Washington, District of Columbia

FRED OVSIEW, MD, Professor of Psychiatry, Department of Psychiatry, University of Chicago Medical Center, Chicago, Illinois

OLU OYESANMI, MD, Research Analyst, ECRI Institute, Plymouth Meeting, Pennsylvania

MARYLAND PAO, MD, Office of the Clinical Director, National Institute of Mental Health, National Institutes of Health, Bethesda, Maryland

RONALD SCHOUTEN, MD, JD, Associate Professor of Psychiatry, Harvard Medical School; and Director, Massachusetts General Hospital Law and Psychiatry Service, Boston, Massachusetts

GANESH SHANMUGAM, MD, Division of Allergy and Immunology, Department of Internal Medicine, University of Texas Southwestern Medical Center, Dallas, Texas

CHRISTOPHER L. SOLA, DO, Senior Associate Consultant, Department of Psychiatry and Psychology, Mayo Clinic; and Instructor in Psychiatry, Mayo Clinic College of Medicine, Rochester, Minnesota

JADE E. TIU, BA, Department of Psychiatry, Robert Wood Johnson Medical School-UMDNJ; and Department of Psychology, Rutgers University, Piscataway, New Jersey

SUSAN TURKEL, MD, Chief of Psychiatry-Neuropsychiatry, Childrens Hospital Los Angeles; and Associate Professor, Psychiatry, Pathology, and Pediatrics, University of Southern California Keck School of Medicine, Los Angeles, California

ROBERT L. WOOLFOLK, PhD, Department of Psychology, Rutgers University, Piscataway; and Department of Psychology, Princeton University, Princeton, New Jersey

PSYCHIATRIC CLINICS
OF NORTH AMERICA

Psychosomatic Medicine

CONTENTS VOLUME 30 • NUMBER 4 • DECEMBER 2007

Several classification issues regarding somatoform disorders are being debated as the process for revising the Diagnostic and Statistical Manual of Mental Disorders, Fifth Edition (DSM-V) unfolds over the next 5 years. Eight key questions center around the appropriate stakeholders for DSM-V, changes in terminology, movement of certain disorders within or outside of Axis I, the validity of symptom explanation as a core criterion, the status of functional somatic syndromes, the reliance on symptom counts, the reliability of lifetime symptom recall, and the value of symptom grouping. Somatic symptom measures are reviewed, and a brief self-rated scale is described in detail.

In this article the authors present their model of treatment for somatization disorder and related syndromes. It begins with a brief history of somatization followed by a discussion of theory and research on medically unexplained symptoms. Finally, it describes in some detail the authors' psychosocial treatment for medically unexplained symptoms, which uses methods from both cognitive behavioral therapy and experiential emotion-focused therapy.

Malingering of mental illness has been studied extensively; however, malingered medical illness has been examined much less avidly. While in theory any ailment can be fabricated or self-induced, pain–including lower back pain, cervical pain, and fibromyalgia-and cognitive deficits associated with mild head trauma or toxic exposure are feigned most frequently, especially in situations where there are financial incentives to malinger. Structured assessments have been developed to help detect both types of malingering; however, in daily practice, the physician should generally suspect malingering when there are tangible incentives and when reported symptoms do not match the physical examination or no organic basis for the physical complaints is found.

Legal Concerns in Psychosomatic Medicine

Rebecca W. Brendel and Ronald Schouten

In the practice of psychosomatic medicine, psychiatrists frequently encounter issues of legal concern. This article provides an overview of legal topics frequently encountered by the psychiatric consultant. One such area, discussed first in this article, is confidentiality and the management of private patient information. A second common interface between law and psychiatry is in the area of medical decision making. The psychiatric consultant is often asked to evaluate a patient's ability to accept or refuse treatment, and then make a determination of capacity. When the patient cannot give informed consent, an alternate decision maker must be found. Finally, malpractice liability is often a concern for the psychiatric consultant. Overall, psychiatrists should approach the care of patients foremost from a clinical perspective, while understanding the applicable laws and regulations of the jurisdictions in which they practice. In addition, clinicians should be aware of the legal and risk management resources available to them should a complex situation arise.

An Updated Review of Implantable Cardioverter/ Defibrillators, Induced Anxiety, and Quality of Life

J. Michael Bostwick and Christopher L. Sola

Despite overall favorable acceptance of implantable cardioverter-defibrillators (ICDs), patients may experience discharges as frightening and painful. The authors reviewed ICD-induced psychopathology in 2005. During the past 2 years the number of studies examining psychopathology and quality of life after ICD implantation has increased dramatically, warranting this update of that review. Variables assessed have included recipient age, gender, social support network, perception of control and predictability of shocks, and personality style. Now the picture of what is known is, if anything, cloudier than it was 2 years ago, with little definitive and much contradictory data emerging in most of these categories.

Psychiatric Aspects of Infertility and Infertility Treatments

Linda Hammer Burns

Infertility counseling, whether provided by a psychiatrist or another health care professional, involves the treatment and care of patients, not simply when they are undergoing fertility treatment but also with their long-term emotional well-being, and that of their children and the reproductive helpers who may assist them in achieving biologic or reproductive parenthood. They can educate patients about the side effects of infertility treatment medications and the impact of hormone shifts on psychologic well-being. They are also helpful with differential diagnoses among grief, depressions, and stress; in assessing psychologic preparedness; and in determining the acceptability and suitability of gamete donation, a gestational carrier, or surrogacy as a family-building alternative for individuals, couples, and reproductive collaborators.

Obesity is a systemic illness that affects virtually every organ system in the body. A presurgical psychiatric evaluation has been advocated as part of a multidisciplinary approach to bariatric surgery. This evaluation seeks to determine the patient's capacity to understand the risk and benefits of surgery and to appreciate the consequences of surgery. Given the comorbidity of psychiatric illness in the obese, the evaluation also screens for psychopathology, with particular attention paid to disorders of eating behavior. In the presurgical psychiatric evaluation a robust knowledge base concerning the various aspects of weight-loss surgery is essential.

The consultation psychiatrist is frequently called on to assess patients in medical settings with primary or secondary hematologic disorders. This article addresses psychiatric issues that are specific to patients who have selected hematologic disorders, including B_{12} and folate deficiency, sickle cell disease, and hemophilia, discussing the diseases, their unique psychiatric manifestations, and approaches to management. A review of hematologic side effects of psychotropic medications is also included.

Lung disease is a prominent cause of morbidity and mortality worldwide. When a patient has a common lung disease, such as asthma, or a less prevalent one, such as idiopathic pulmonary fibrosis, psychiatric issues should be considered as an integral part of the care plan for each patient. There have been many studies of psychologic factors and psychiatric syndromes in various lung diseases and their treatment. In this article, the authors focus on an evidence-based approach to reviewing this clinical literature.

Patients who have epilepsy frequently have comorbid psychiatric disorders. Research into the relationship between seizures and psychiatric disorders has begun to reveal a complex relationship between neurobiology and behavior. This article reviews the diagnosis and treatment of mood disorders, psychotic disorders, and aggression in epilepsy. The psychopharmacology of anti-epileptic drugs and other psychotropics in epilepsy, including relevant information about drug–drug interactions, is summarized to assist with treatment decisions. Finally, a discussion of psychogenic seizures and epilepsy surgery reviews recent treatment recommendations.

Multiple sclerosis (MS) is the most common chronic disabling disease of the central nervous system in young adults. Early onset and long duration of disease result in tremendous individual, family, and societal costs as well as reductions in quality of life and work productivity. Persons who have MS have a higher prevalence of a number of psychiatric symptoms and disorders. This article seeks to summarize the existing literature on the epidemiology, impact, and treatment of psychiatric disorders among persons who have MS and to identify the areas in which further research is needed.

With the advent of new treatments for pediatric disorders, more chronically ill children and adolescents are surviving into adulthood than ever before. This article is aimed at helping psychiatric consultants understand how medical, developmental, and psychosocial needs are altered in adults who have grown up chronically ill as children. Congenital heart disease, cystic fibrosis, and rheumatologic disorders are discussed in detail as models to illustrate the impact of congenital malformations, genetic disorders, and typically adult disorders occurring in the pediatric age group.

Military, occupational, and environmental events can cause toxic injuries that require psychiatric diagnosis and treatment. This article reviews the psychiatric effects of neurotoxins, including nerve gases, ionizing radiation, insecticides, heavy metals, solvents, and other toxic agents. Diagnostic considerations and clinical tests for further evaluation of the numerous psychiatric conditions and symptoms caused by toxic exposures are discussed.

PSYCHIATRIC CLINICS
OF NORTH AMERICA

THE CLINICS ARE NOW AVAILABLE ONLINE!

Access your subscription at:
http://www.theclinics.com

PSYCHIATRIC CLINICS
OF NORTH AMERICA

Preface

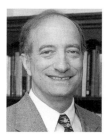 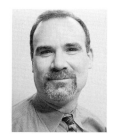 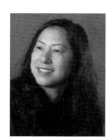

James L. Levenson, MD
David F. Gitlin, MD
Cathy Crone, MD

Guest Editors

The roots of Psychosomatic Medicine date back to the early twentieth century, at which time substantial work was focused on the relationship between "mind" and "soma." Walter Cannon's [1] seminal research on the physiology of emotions focused on the earliest biologic changes in World War I veterans who had "traumatic shock," resulting in the publication of *Bodily Changes in Pain, Hunger, Fear, and Rage* in 1915. This work led to his description of the "fight/flight response." Wolf and Wolff's [2] 1943 studies relating various emotional states to changes in gastric secretion helped to further this understanding of the interconnectedness of the brain and body. The term "psychosomatic medicine" was coined by Felix Deutch in 1922, and many of the leading psychiatrists during the 1930s to 1950s, including Deutch, Frances Dunbar, and Franz Alexander, focused on the development of theories explaining the causal relationship between emotions and physical illness.

These pioneering psychosomatic psychiatrists were followed by George Engel and Zbigniew Lipowski, who focused on the psychiatric phenomenology of medical illness. Ultimately, Consultation-Liaison Psychiatry evolved as a specialized area of psychiatric practice. Since the 1960s, all psychiatric residents have been expected to develop competency in this area of psychiatry [3]. Not surprisingly, this confluence of improved training and increased knowledge resulted in the development of numerous fellowship programs in Consultation-Liaison Psychiatry. By 1991, more than 50 fellowship programs existed nationwide. In 2001, The Academy of Psychosomatic Medicine applied to the American Board of Psychiatry and Neurology for the recognition of "Psychosomatic Medicine" as a subspecialty of psychiatry, choosing

0193-953X/07/$ – see front matter
doi:10.1016/j.psc.2007.08.003

© 2007 Elsevier Inc. All rights reserved.

to return to the name for the field imbedded in its history, its journals, and its national organizations. The Accreditation Council of Graduate Medical Education approved Psychosomatic Medicine as a psychiatric subspecialty in 2003 [4].

Today, Psychosomatic Medicine encompasses Consultation-Liaison Psychiatry and other aspects of the interface between medical and psychiatric illness. Previous issues of the *Psychiatric Clinics of North America* have reviewed advances in this interface under the name of Consultation-Liaison Psychiatry [5] and Psychiatry in the Medically Ill [6]. This issue uses the new name for the field and provides in-depth, up-to-date reviews of several medical illnesses and conditions in which psychiatric and emotional issues play a large role.

A key problem for all health care providers—and of particular interest to practitioners of psychosomatic medicine—is the patient with unexplained medical symptoms, many of whom have been considered to have somatoform disorders. As the process of developing the *Diagnostic and Statistical Manual of Mental Disorders, Fifth Edition* unfolds, there has been significant controversy regarding all of the Somatoform Disorders, as well as the category itself, in the *Diagnostic and Statistical Manual of Mental Disorders, Fourth Edition*. Kroenke provides insight into these diagnostic controversies and makes suggestions for the future. Woolfolk and colleagues begin with a brief history of somatization and a review of theory and research on medically unexplained symptoms; then, they focus in detail on describing a psychosocial treatment that they developed for somatization, which uses methods from cognitive behavioral therapy and experiential emotion-focused therapy. McDermott and Feldman tackle the challenging area of malingering. They explore the roots of malingering, describe a variety of tools to identify these individuals more effectively, and discuss a variety of potential interventions for medical providers in its management.

Physicians frequently face complex medical-legal issues, and this is particularly important in psychosomatic medicine. Brendel and Schouten, trained as psychiatrists and attorneys, provide expert review of the common issues of legal concern that are encountered in the practice of psychosomatic medicine, including confidentiality, competency and capacity determination, informed consent, substitute decision-making, and malpractice.

With the rapid advances occurring in medicine and surgery, psychosomatic medicine psychiatrists have had to develop expertise in several unique medical domains. Bostwick and Sola review psychiatric and psychosocial aspects of implantable cardiac defibrillators. They also discuss new assessment tools and treatment of associated psychopathology through psychoeducation, psychotherapy, and psychotropic medication. Burns provides an analysis of several psychiatric issues in the area of infertility, including the psychologic distress of infertility itself, the psychosocial stresses of infertility treatment, and potential secondary psychiatric symptomatology. Norris reviews current medical and psychiatric issues relevant to bariatric surgery, an increasingly popular intervention for the growing population of patients who have severe obesity and related medical complications.

Many medical and neurologic illnesses have been associated closely with psychiatric comorbidity. Becker and colleagues review common hematologic problems in Psychosomatic Medicine, including vitamin B_{12} and folate deficiency, sickle cell disease, and hemophilia, as well as hematologic side effects and relevant drug interactions of psychiatric medications. Shanmugam and colleagues discuss psychiatric issues in important lung diseases, including asthma, chronic obstructive pulmonary disease, cystic fibrosis, acute respiratory failure, idiopathic pulmonary fibrosis, and sarcoidosis and psychiatric syndromes that mimic respiratory diseases. Marcangelo and Ovsiew review the psychiatric issues that are associated with epileptic disorders. They note that there often is confusion about what constitutes psychiatric symptomatology secondary to seizures and what often is concurrent with seizures/epilepsy. Chwastiak and Ehde provide a comprehensive review of multiple sclerosis, with particular focus on the psychiatric features of this neurologic illness. Turkel and Pao provide an overview of the psychiatric issues facing children who develop chronic and severe medical illnesses. They examine several specific conditions, including cystic fibrosis, juvenile rheumatoid arthritis, and congenital heart disease, with special attention to the changes in psychiatric issues as these children progress into adulthood. Brown reviews the psychiatric effects of neurotoxins that may result from military, occupational, or environmental exposures, including nerve gases, ionizing radiation, insecticides, heavy metals, solvents, and other toxic agents, focusing on diagnostic considerations and clinical testing.

James L. Levenson, MD

E-mail address: jlevenson@mcvh-vcu.edu

David F. Gitlin, MD

E-mail address: dgitlin@partners.org

Cathy Crone, MD

E-mail address: cathy.crone@inova.com

References

[1] Cannon WB. Bodily changes in pain, hunger, fear, and rage. New York: D. Appleton & Company; 1915.
[2] Wolf S, Wolff HG. Human gastric secretion. New York: Oxford Press; 1943.
[3] Gitlin DF, Schindler BA, Stern TA, et al. Recommended guidelines for consultation-liaison psychiatric training in psychiatry residency programs. A report from the Academy of Psychosomatic Medicine Task Force on Psychiatric Resident Training in Consultation-Liaison Psychiatry. Psychosomatics 1996;37(1):3–11.
[4] Gitlin DF, Levenson JL, Lyketsos CG. Psychosomatic medicine: a new psychiatric subspecialty. Acad Psychiatry 2004;28(1):4–11.
[5] Levenson JL, editor. Consultation-liaison psychiatry. Psychiatric Clin North Am 1996; 19:413–637.
[6] Levenson JL, Trzepacz PT, Lyketsos CG, editors. Psychiatry in the medically ill. Psychiatric Clin North Am 2002;25:1–251.

Psychiatr Clin N Am 30 (2007) 593–619

PSYCHIATRIC CLINICS
OF NORTH AMERICA

ELSEVIER
SAUNDERS

Somatoform Disorders and Recent Diagnostic Controversies

Kurt Kroenke, MD[a,b,*]

[a]Indiana University School of Medicine, Indianapolis, IN, USA
[b]Regenstrief Institute, RG-6, 1050 Wishard Boulevard, Indianapolis, IN 46202, USA

S omatic symptoms account for more than half of all ambulatory visits or nearly 400 million clinic visits in the United States alone each year [1]. Moreover, counting only those who volunteer a somatic complaint may underestimate the true prevalence. Surveys using checklists of 15 to 20 common symptoms find that medical outpatients typically endorse a median of four symptoms as bothersome [2–4]. A survey asking 3000 primary care patients whether or not they had been bothered in the past 4 weeks by one or more of 15 common somatic symptoms revealed prevalences ranging from 23% to 63% for 12 of the symptoms [5]. Fig. 1 shows prevalences of the 10 most common symptoms and illustrates that that approximately one fourth of patients rate their symptoms as severe (ie, they have been "bothered a lot" by a particular symptom). For example, 33% report having been bothered by stomach pain, and 8% noted their pain was severe, whereas 53% reported headache, and 14% considered it severe.

Because of this high prevalence of somatic symptoms, somatoform disorders are one of the most common categories of mental disorders in general medical patients, with a prevalence similar to that of depressive or anxiety disorders [6,7]. Somatoform disorders also have an independent effect on disability and on impairment in multiple domains of health-related quality of life comparable to the effects of depression and anxiety [8]. There are two additional negative consequences germane to somatoform disorders. One is the excess health care costs resulting from high numbers of health care visits and repeated diagnostic testing, including invasive procedures, costly treatments, and hospitalization [9]. The second consequence is the adverse impact on the clinician-patient relationship. Somatoform disorders are rated by practitioners as among the most difficult of all conditions, far more challenging than other medical or mental disorders [10]. Some of this difficulty may be attributable to the perceived lack of effective treatments for somatoform

*Regenstrief Institute, RG-6, 1050 Wishard Boulevard, Indianapolis, IN 46202. *E-mail address*: kkroenke@regenstrief.org

0193-953X/07/$ – see front matter © 2007 Elsevier Inc. All rights reserved.
doi:10.1016/j.psc.2007.08.002

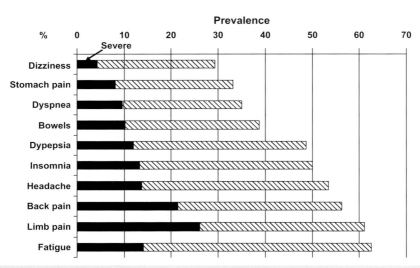

Fig. 1. Ten most prevalent symptoms in a survey of 3000 primary care patients. Symptoms for which the patient had been "bothered a lot" are indicated by the black part of the bar and defined as severe. Two other symptoms had a prevalence rate greater than 20% (ie, palpitations [29%] and chest pain [23%]). (*Data from* Kroenke K, Spitzer RL, Williams JBW. The PHQ-15: validity of a new measure for evaluating the severity of somatic symptoms. Psychosom Med 2002;64:258–66.)

disorders. Other reasons may be a clinician's inability to proffer a satisfactory explanation for the many and perplexing symptoms, a patient's negative experiences with previous health care providers, and complicating personality and interpersonal factors.

There have been recent advances in understanding the epidemiology, evaluation, and treatment of somatoform disorders that facilitate a more positive approach to patient management. In particular, considerable deliberations have occurred among experts regarding the optimal classification of somatoform disorders, including key questions and potential recommendations for revisions to the *Diagnostic and Statistical Manual of Mental Disorders, Fifth Edition* (*DSM-V*) and the *International Statistical Classification of Diseases, 11th Revision* (*ICD-11*). Integral to classification and treatment of any mental disorder is the development of a validated means of measuring the severity of a disorder and its response to treatment. The principal aim of this article is to summarize recent thinking regarding the classification of somatoform disorders, and a secondary aim is to highlight a practical means of measuring somatic symptom severity. Treatment of somatoform disorders and related conditions manifested by poorly explained somatic symptoms is covered elsewhere in this issue (see the article by Woolfolk, Allen, and Tiu) and in several recent comprehensive reviews [11–16].

DEFINING SOMATIC SYMPTOMS, PHYSICAL/MEDICAL COMORBIDITY, AND SOMATIZATION

Somatoform disorders cannot be discussed without briefly defining several key but sometimes misconstrued terms. Symptoms commonly are labeled "somatic" in psychiatry and other mental health disciplines, in part to distinguish bodily symptoms from cognitive, emotional, or other types of non-somatic symptoms. In contrast, general medical, surgical, and other non–mental health disciplines more often refer to bodily symptoms as "physical" symptoms. The distinction is not solely semantic. Labeling a symptom as somatic conjures up the terms, "somatization" and "somatoform," and, thereby, a poorly understood bodily symptom inadvertently may assume a psychologic cause. Somatic symptoms commonly are an admixture of physical and psychologic factors rather than purely the result of one or the other—an alloy rather than a single metal.

The term, "physical," also may have different nuances in psychiatry and medicine. In psychiatry, general medical disorders also are referred to as "physical" disorders. When using the term, "physical comorbidity," psychiatrists may be referring to patients who have mental disorders who also have (1) well-defined general medical disorders (eg, diabetes, coronary artery disease, or asthma) or (2) somatic symptoms only (eg, headache, low back pain, or fatigue). The first type of comorbidity more commonly is referred to in the general medical setting as "medical" (rather than physical) comorbidity. Again, being clear on what is meant when using the terms, physical or medical comorbidity, is important, because although mental disorders frequently overlap with medical disorders and somatic symptoms, the nature, implications, and impact of this overlap may differ.

Somatization likewise may have several definitions. Most agree with the core elements initially described by Lipowski: (1) one or more somatic symptoms that (2) lack an adequate medical explanation, (3) cause patient distress, and (4) prompt health care seeking behavior [17]. Some may disagree with the fourth behavioral component as a necessary criterion. After all, seeking health care is not required as core to the definition of most other mental or medical disorders. Cancer, hypertension, schizophrenia, and major depression exist in the general population whether or not individuals seek care for these conditions. Alternatively, the ubiquitous nature of somatic symptoms mandates setting some thresholds to separate most "persons" who suffer from common symptoms from the smaller subset of "patients" who are seeking or require care [18]. In 1961, Kerr White [19] reported that 80% of individuals in the general population experience one or more symptoms, of which only one fourth seek care. This finding was confirmed by Green and colleagues [20] 40 years later. Other epidemiologic studies similarly have shown that only a minority of individuals experiencing symptoms ultimately seek health care [21,22].

The real divide in defining somatization, however, centers on the role of psychologic factors. One view is that psychologic factors are essential to the definition, either as causal or contributory to the development and maintenance of somatization. A second view is more atheoretic, arguing that somatization consists of the four core features, whether or not there are apparent or latent psychologic components. Advantages of the latter include the fact that many somatizing patients deny or resist psychologic explanations; that later editions of *DSM* progressively have become less psychodynamic or etiologic in their definitions of mental disorders; that assigning putative mechanisms, either physical or psychologic, to poorly understood somatic symptom disorders is speculative; and that "medically unexplained" should not be synonymous with "psychiatrically explained" [23]. In this article, the term, somatization, is used in accordance with the four core criteria of Lipowski and does not presume that the presentation of distressing somatic symptoms is presumptive evidence of a psychiatric disorder.

CLASSIFYING SOMATOFORM DISORDERS
Background
A vigorous debate has occurred over the past several years regarding the current classification of somatoform disorders, with opinions ranging from the radical abolishment of the entire category to more subtle refinements. The more extreme view is articulated by Mayou and colleagues in a position paper [24], whereas a more diverse range of positions is represented in a recent series of eight articles in a 2006 issue of the *Journal of Psychosomatic Research* [25–32]. A 2007 consensus paper emanating from a series of workshops spearheaded by the Conceptual Issues in Somatoform and Similar Disorders (CISSD) work group and involving more than 20 experts from the United States and Europe recently was published in *Psychosomatics* [33]. Finally, the American Psychiatric Association (APA) convened a research conference as a prelude to revising *DSM-V*, entitled "Somatic Presentations of Mental Disorders," the proceedings of which will be published in a forthcoming issue of *Psychosomatic Medicine*.

Key Questions
The CISSD work group identified eight key questions, summarized in Table 1, along with brief comments regarding each question. The first three questions are not addressed further in this article but are elaborated in greater detail elsewhere [33]. Questions 4 and 5 are discussed , followed by comments on questions 6, 7, and 8.

Should "explanation" remain a core construct in diagnosing somatoform disorders?
This question remains the most contentious issue in classifying somatoform disorders. There is one major argument and several secondary arguments against including explanation (or the lack thereof) as a criterion in defining somatoform disorders. One secondary argument is that inter-rater reliability on the exact cause of somatic symptoms may be modest at best [34,35]. Another secondary argument is that more recent revisions of *DSM* have moved away from mechanistic or explanatory criteria for disorders toward a largely atheoretic, phenomenologic approach.

The major argument, however, is that diseases and symptoms often defy simple one-to-one mapping. Increasingly, research shows that dichotomizing somatic symptoms as "medically explained" versus "medically unexplained" is at the least overly simplistic and may be even misleading and counter-therapeutic. Instead, symptoms fall along a spectrum of medical-psychiatric causation, as illustrated in Fig. 2. At the middle is a large group of "symptom-only" diagnoses, flanked on either side by several types of disorders on the boundary between medical and psychiatric explanation. Although the divided line may seem to separate medical from psychiatric etiologies, this discussion of each of the five categories highlights the artificial nature of this dualistic conceptualization.

Symptom-only conditions. Multiple studies have shown that at least a third to half of all somatic symptoms are medically unexplained in general practice and population-based studies [36]. In the most rigorous of these studies [37], two physician raters independently reviewed all medical chart information and found that a high proportion of symptoms (with the exception of upper respiratory complaints, such as cough, sore throat, and rhinorrhea) were medically unexplained (Fig. 3). Although the figure lumps idiopathic and psychiatric causes into the same group, chart review revealed a documented psychiatric cause in only a minority of the cases. In short, common symptoms most often were idiopathic, with neither a medical nor psychiatric explanation proffered by a clinician. Similar findings recently were reported for somatic symptoms evaluated in medical and surgical specialty clinics where, again, a substantial proportion of symptoms remained unexplained [38].

Functional somatic syndromes. These syndromes consist of a cluster of somatic symptoms for which the cause is understood poorly and includes disorders such as irritable bowel syndrome, fibromyalgia, chronic fatigue syndrome, temporomandibular disorder, interstitial cystitis, and others. Experts question whether or not these are separate disorders or, instead, part of a group of poorly explained somatic conditions sharing common features [39,40]. First, literature syntheses have revealed that these disorders frequently overlap, at the level of specific syndromes (half to two thirds of patients who have one syndrome also suffer from one or more additional syndromes) [41] and in terms of individual symptoms [42]. Second, they are similar in terms of psychiatric comorbidity. Henningsen and colleagues [43] reviewed 244 studies of irritable bowel syndrome, nonulcer dyspepsia, fibromyalgia, and chronic fatigue syndrome in which the co-occurrence of depression and anxiety was assessed. The association of the four functional somatic syndromes with depression and anxiety was highly significant when compared with healthy persons and controls who had medical disorders of known organic pathology. The effect sizes were of only moderate magnitude, however, suggesting that at least a portion of the somatic symptomatology was independent of depression and anxiety. Third, functional somatic syndromes respond similarly to certain therapies traditionally considered "psychologic" treatments, such as antidepressants and cognitive-behavioral therapy [11,12,15]. For all of these reasons, the CISSD

Table 1
Key questions to consider in revising the classification of somatoform disorders

Key question	Comments
1. Who should be the stakeholders for *DSM-V*?	Besides the traditional stakeholders of mental health professionals, educators, and payers: • The acceptability and usefulness of any classification should be vetted with primary care and other nonpsychiatric clinicians who provide most of the care for patients who have somatoform disorders. • Efforts to engage patients are important to reduce the degree to which clinicians use different labels when talking with one another versus with patients.
2. Should some terms and concepts, such as somatization and somatoform, be abolished?	Some stigma has attached to these labels, partly because of negative clinician and societal attitudes. There are cultural differences in the acceptability of these terms, however, as with other terms, such as functional, medically unexplained, and psychosomatic. It also was argued that until positive attitudes develop toward caring for these disorders, stigma may attach quickly to any new labels.
3. Should the conditions currently diagnosed as somatoform disorders remain a psychiatric disorder on Axis I?	When the main feature is that of somatic symptoms (albeit "medically unexplained"), some believed the default should be to code the disorder on Axis III along with other general medical conditions. Others argued that some payment systems require an Axis I diagnosis to reimburse mental health care. Short of abolishing the category of somatoform disorders, one proposal is to require psychologic criteria in addition to unexplained somatic symptoms as part of the case definition.
4. Should "explanation" remain a core construct in diagnosing somatoform disorders?	Arbitrating the "cause" of a somatic symptom in the midst of potential physical and psychologic factors is complicated in many patients and subject to substantial inter-rater variability. Increasingly, a spectrum of medical-to-psychologic causation (see Fig. 1) is recognized.

(continued on next page)

Key question	Comments
Table 1 *(continued)*	
5. How should functional somatic syndromes be classified?	These common yet poorly understood somatic syndromes (eg, irritable bowel syndrome, fibromyalgia, and chronic fatigue syndrome) are classified on Axis III as general medical conditions. They frequently overlap with one another, however, and share some features in common with somatoform disorders. At the same time, the grouping into discrete "medical" disorders has seemed to have some heuristic value in terms of patient acceptability, research, and clinical care.
6. Should symptom counts be used to define somatoform diagnoses?	There is a continuous relationship between somatic symptom count and adverse consequences of somatization. Nonetheless, symptom thresholds are used for major depression, panic disorder, and other mental disorders. Many do agree that in addition to simple symptom counts, other psychologic criteria should be required for a somatoform diagnosis.
7. Is inquiry about lifetime recall of symptoms necessary?	There is accumulating evidence that lifetime recall of specific symptoms is unreliable. At the same time, somatoform diagnoses that are based on multiple unexplained symptoms are more stable. A consensus is emerging that inquiry should focus on current rather than lifetime symptoms.
8. Is symptom grouping useful?	SD originally depended on a lengthy checklist of somatic symptoms, both rare and common. *DSM-IV* purportedly simplified the diagnosis by requiring only eight symptoms out of four organ groups. The list of symptoms mandating inquiry, however, was not specified and presumably still could be very lengthy. The number and types of symptoms that need to be asked about and the added value of symptom grouping remain inconclusive.

Data from Kroenke K, Sharpe M, Sykes R. Revising the classification of somatoform disorders: key questions and preliminary recommendations. Psychosomatics 2007;48(4):277–85.

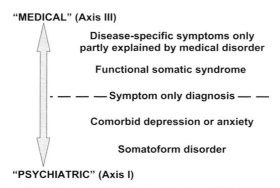

"MEDICAL" (Axis III)

Disease-specific symptoms only
partly explained by medical disorder

Functional somatic syndrome

— — — — Symptom only diagnosis — —

Comorbid depression or anxiety

Somatoform disorder

"PSYCHIATRIC" (Axis I)

Fig. 2. The spectrum of medical-psychiatric causes of somatic symptoms.

proposed a separate key question (see number 5 in Table 1) regarding how functional somatic disorders should be classified.

Disease-specific symptoms only partly explained by a medical disorder. One of the most surprising findings emerging from recent research is the frequency with which symptoms presumed to be the result of a specific medical disorder may be the result, at least in part, of nonspecific or psychiatric factors. Two studies in particular warrant comment. The first is a recent symptom survey of nearly 3500 patients 60 years and older attending primary care clinics [44]. The presence of 10 chronic medical disorders was noted, including coronary artery disease, congestive heart failure, obstructive lung disease, diabetes, hypertension, arthritis, chronic liver disease, stroke, chronic renal disease, and cancer. Chest pain was only moderately more prevalent in patients who had coronary artery

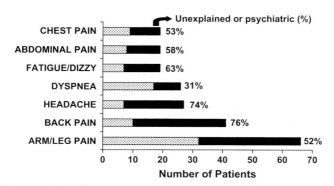

Fig. 3. Frequency of common somatic symptoms in a random sample of 289 primary care patients and the proportion of symptoms that are medically unexplained or psychiatric in presumed cause. (*Data from* Khan AA, Khan A, Harezlak J, et al. Somatic symptoms in primary care: etiology and outcome. Psychosomatics 2003;44(6):471–8.)

disease (31%) and congestive heart failure (27%) than in patients who had the eight noncardiac conditions (median = 20%; range, 14%–28%). Likewise, dyspnea was reported by 70%, 57%, and 53% of patients who had obstructive pulmonary disease, congestive heart failure, and coronary artery disease, respectively, compared with a median of 40% (range, 33%–45%) in patients who had the seven noncardiac, nonpulmonary conditions. Pain in the arms or legs was reported by 78% of patients who had arthritis compared with a median of 65% (range, 33% to 68%) in patients who had the nine other conditions. Other symptoms that are not unique to a particular organ system had a similar prevalence (ie, narrow range) across all 10 conditions, such as fatigue (median = 60%; range, 49%–64%), bowel complaints (median = 36%; range, 33%–39%), headache (median = 30%; range, 23%–38%), and dizziness (median = 29%; range, 25%–34%).

A second study was a literature synthesis that examined the association of comorbid depression or anxiety with medical symptom burden in patients who had arthritis (rheumatoid and osteoarthritis), diabetes, heart disease (coronary artery disease and congestive heart failure), and pulmonary disease (asthma and chronic obstructive pulmonary disease) [45]. A total of 31 studies involving 16,922 patients was reviewed, including seven studies (n = 5943) of diabetes, nine studies (n = 2593) of pulmonary disease, nine studies (n = 5900) of cardiac disease, and six studies (n = 2486) of arthritis. Patients who had chronic medical illness and comorbid depression or anxiety compared with those who had chronic medical illness alone reported significantly higher numbers of medical symptoms when controlling for severity of medical disorder. Across the four categories of common medical disorders, disease-specific somatic symptoms (eg, chest pain in patients who had coronary artery disease, dyspnea in patients who had pulmonary disease, or joint pain in patients who had arthritis) were associated at least as strongly with depression and anxiety as they were with objective physiologic measures of the medical disorder.

Comorbid depression and anxiety. As discussed previously, depression and anxiety frequently are comorbid with functional somatic syndromes and common medical disorders and increase the burden of somatic symptoms specific to these conditions. There also are many studies that demonstrate a powerful relationship between nonspecific somatic symptom reporting and the presence and severity of depression and anxiety.

Although the specific type of symptom is not particularly important in terms of predicting depression or anxiety, the number of symptoms is. Two primary care studies totaling 1500 patients demonstrate a strong relationship between the number of somatic symptoms endorsed by patients as currently bothersome and the likelihood of a coexisting depressive or anxiety disorder [3,46]. As the number of somatic symptoms endorsed as currently bothersome on a 15-symptom questionnaire increased from 0–1 to 2–3 to 4–5 to 6–8 to ≥ 9 symptoms in these two studies, the likelihood of a depressive or anxiety disorder increased from 4–7% to 18–22% to 31–35% to 52–61% to 78–81%, respectively. Like the erythrocyte sedimentation rate (ESR) for physical inflammatory disorders, the somatic symptom count is an ESR equivalent for potential "psychopathologic inflammation."

Among patients referred to three specialty clinics (gastroenterology, rheumatology, and neurology), depression was present in one fourth to one third of patients in each clinic, and depressed patients were only approximately one fourth as likely to have a physical diagnosis established as an explanation for their symptoms triggering the referral [47]. There are several comprehensive reviews of the comorbidity between somatic symptoms, depression, and anxiety [36,47–50].

Somatoform disorders. Somatoform disorders typically are the residuum of somatic symptoms "not better accounted for" or "not fully explained" by another medical or psychiatric disorder. The four common categories of somatic symptoms (summarized previously), however, emphasize the challenges in relying on explanation (or lack thereof) as a core criterion in defining somatoform disorders. It may be more important to consider other positive psychologic criteria characteristic of somatizing patients (eg, excessive illness worry or health anxiety, inordinate health care use, or catastrophizing) rather than over-reliance on a tenuous negative criterion (ie, lack of an explanation).

Should symptom counts be used to define somatoform diagnoses?
The diagnosis of somatization disorder (SD) and its more prevalent lower threshold variants typically requires a certain number of somatic symptoms. Many studies indicate that there is a continuous relationship between increasing somatic symptom counts and functional impairment, childhood and family risk factors, psychiatric comorbidity, health care use, and other measures of construct validity [3,51–55]. There does not seem to be a clear-cut symptom count threshold that justifies a specific cutpoint. At the same time, operational cutpoints are established for other continuous psychiatric (eg, depression and anxiety) and medical (eg, hypertension, diabetes, and hyperlipidemia) disorders. One alternative is to require "positive" psychologic/behavioral criteria in addition to medically unexplained symptoms for a somatoform diagnosis. Another is to use somatic symptom count and severity as a dimensional rather than categorical criterion, which is consistent with what also is considered for other disorders in *DSM-V.*

Is inquiry about lifetime recall of symptoms necessary?
In a large World Health Organization study (WHO), Simon and Gureje [56] found that only 39% of "lifetime" symptoms reported at baseline were recalled at 1-year follow-up. At the disorder level, a similar number of patients met criteria for SD at baseline and 1-year follow-up (74 and 70 patients, respectively), although only 21 patients met criteria at both time points. The same investigators examined the stability of abridged SD (defined as six lifetime medically unexplained symptoms in women or four in men) and found that half the cases of this subthreshold form of SD at baseline persisted at 1-year follow-up [57].

Leiknes and colleagues [58] found that recall of medically explained symptoms also was unreliable with the passage of time. Rief and Rojas [59] recently reviewed nine studies that examined the stability of syndromes characterized by multiple somatic complaints. Collectively, these studies confirmed that lifetime recall of individual symptoms is unreliable but that the reporting of multiple unexplained somatic symptoms is a more stable phenomenon over time. Counting only current symptoms but requiring a lower symptom threshold (eg, three or more unexplained symptoms) has been shown to capture most patients who have full or abridged SD [54]. Finally, focusing on current symptoms not only is more efficient in a busy practice setting but also is more relevant to patients seeking treatment.

Is symptom grouping useful?
The original criteria for Briquet's syndrome, from which *DSM-III* criteria for SD were derived, required at least one symptom in 9 of 10 possible groups. *DSM-III* dropped requirements about the number of groups, because the total number of somatization symptoms correlated highly with the number of somatization groups. *DSM-IV* resurrected a requirement for number of groups: at least four pain symptoms, two gastrointestinal symptoms, one conversion symptom, and one sexual symptom. In essence, a trade-off occurred by lowering the symptom count but making it necessary to "fill" four symptom groups for the diagnosis. Although proponents of this change believed it would make diagnosing SD less cumbersome, the clinical usefulness [60] of this revision has not been tested. The abbreviated criteria for SD in the *ICD-10* require symptoms to be distributed over at least two of four groups (cardiopulmonary, gastrointestinal, genitourinary, and skin and pain symptoms), although the conversion symptom category required in *DSM-IV* is excluded altogether.

Studies using factor analysis in different patient populations have tended to show a cardiopulmonary cluster (sometimes with autonomic symptoms), a gastrointestinal cluster, and a musculoskeletal/pain cluster [54,61,62]. Although initial work suggested the presence of a neurologic (conversion) symptom cluster [63], later empiric studies have failed to confirm this [61,64], even when enriched with neurologic patients [62]. Pseudoneurologic symptoms seem to have a strong association with psychopathology in general (rather than somatoform disorders uniquely) [65] and are the least likely somatic symptoms to persist [57]. Even when studies have identified symptom clusters, they have tended to reveal a single predominant somatization factor [33]. Finally, studies have not shown any substantial difference between the low base rates of SD defined according to *DSM-IV* versus *DSM-III* criteria, suggesting both may be unduly restrictive in identifying clinically relevant somatoform disorders [66].

Potential Recommendations for Revising the *Diagnostic and Statistical Manual of Mental Disorders, Fifth Edition*
Table 2 summarizes the current somatoform disorders as defined by *DSM-IV* and potential revisions suggested by the CISSD work group. There are several caveats. Although the CISSD is an ad hoc group that includes many

Table 2
Diagnostic and Statistical Manual of Mental Disorders, Fourth Edition somatoform disorders and potential recommendations for revising Diagnostic and Statistical Manual of Mental Disorders, Fifth Edition as outlined by the Conceptual Issues in Somatoform and Similar Disorders work group

Disorder	DSM-IV definition (abbreviated)	Potential recommendations for DSM-V
Somatization disorder (SD)	Polysymptomatic disorder that begins before age 30 years, extends over a period of years, and is characterized by a combination of pain. gastrointestinal, sexual, and pseudoneurologic symptoms	1) Make this a more inclusive (less restrictive) diagnosis, because DSM-IV SD identifies only a small proportion of the patients who have clinically relevant persistent somatic symptoms seen in clinical practice. This can be done by broadening the definition of SD to include lesser numbers of symptoms or by adding an abridged version of SD as a new category (see recommendations for undifferentiated somatoform disorder) 2) Focus on current symptoms only (rather than lifetime recall). 3) Consensus was not achieved on whether or not to retain explanation as a core construct or the role of symptom groups and checklists.
Undifferentiated somatoform disorder	One or more unexplained physical complaints, lasting at least 6 months, that are below the threshold for a diagnosis of SD.	1) Delete this overly inclusive category with uncertain clinical usefulness. 2) Consider instead an abridged version of SD with a lower symptom threshold but including positive psychologic and behavioral criteria typical of somatizing patients. See Table 4.
Conversion disorder	Unexplained symptoms or deficits affecting voluntary motor or sensory function that suggest a neurologic condition. Psychologic factors are judged causative or contributory.	1) Either keep in somatoform disorders or move to dissociative disorders 2) There was not strong consensus on revisions to this disorder.

(continued on next page)

	Table 2 (continued)	
Disorder	DSM-IV definition (abbreviated)	Potential recommendations for DSM-V
Hypochondriasis	Preoccupation with the fear of having, or the idea that one has, a serious disease based on the person's misinterpretation of bodily symptoms or bodily functions.	1) Change the name to "health anxiety disorder" 2) Refine the criteria based on recent empiric research [77,78]. 3) Either keep in somatoform disorders or move to anxiety disorders.
Pain disorder	Pain is the predominant focus of clinical attention. In addition, psychologic factors are judged to have an important role in its onset, severity, exacerbation, or maintenance.	1) Delete this category from Axis I. 2) Instead, code the specific type of pain conditions on Axis III (eg, low back pain, headache, fibromyalgia, and noncardiac chest pain) 3) If psychologic factors also are present, code these as a dual diagnosis on Axis I, as a discrete disorder (eg, major depression or panic disorder) or as psychologic factors affecting a general medical condition. 4) As in DSM-IV, pain symptoms still count toward the diagnosis of full or abridged SD if other criteria are met.
Body dysmorphic disorder	Preoccupation with an imagined or exaggerated defect in physical appearance	1) Keep in somatoform disorders or move to obsessive-compulsive disorder. 2) This category was not discussed in detail by the CISSD.
Somatoform disorder not otherwise specified (NOS)	Disorders with somatoform symptoms that do not meet the criteria for any of the specific somatoform disorders.	1) This category was not discussed by the CISSD 2) If DSM-V retains an NOS option for other categories of mental disorders, it likely will need to do so for somatoform disorders also.

Adapted from Kroenke K, Sharpe M, Sykes R. Revising the classification of somatoform disorders: key questions and preliminary recommendations. Psychosomatics 2007;48(4):277–85.

international experts on somatoform disorders, it was neither appointed nor sanctioned by the APA or WHO, the organizations authorized to approve revisions of *DSM* and *ICD*, respectively. As such, the CISSD recommendations should be considered advisory rather than official. Also, there were some suggestions for which the CISSD achieved near consensus but other issues where opinions diverged considerably.

The recommendations outlined in Table 2 are discussed in detail elsewhere [33]. A brief discussion of major issues and residual controversies is provided here. Most patients who have somatoform disorders are cared for outside the mental health setting, in primary care and in medical and surgical specialty clinics. In these settings, full or abridged versions of SD, undifferentiated somatoform disorder, and pain disorder are the categories applicable to the majority of patients [26]. As such, these categories occupied much of the time spent by the CISSD in its proceedings. Although hypochondriacal beliefs and attitudes are prevalent among somatizing patients, it seems that a formal diagnosis of hypochondriasis is not applied commonly to patients by mental health specialists or other types of clinicians. Conversion disorder (CD) and body dysmorphic disorder are less frequent conditions and received only a modest or minimal amount of attention by the CISSD, respectively.

Somatization disorder, lower threshold variants, and undifferentiated somatoform disorder

A major topic and area of general consensus was that the criteria for the diagnosis of SD were too restrictive. At the same time, undifferentiated somatoform disorder was believed overly inclusive, with unproved clinical usefulness. SD as currently defined represents a small subgroup of patients who have severe somatization and fails to capture many individuals who have more moderate yet clinically significant somatization. For example, SD is present in less than 0.5% of the general population and only 1% to 4% of patients presenting in general practice [67]. In contrast, abridged SD is present in up to 4% of the general population and up to 20% of general practice patients.

As shown in Table 3, different methods of defining lower-threshold somatization reveal a 10% to 22% prevalence in various outpatient samples [5,68–70].

Table 3
Prevalence of somatization in the outpatient practice setting

Author	Setting	N	Definition*	Prevalence
Gureje [68]	General practice	5438	Abridged SD	20%
Escobar [69]	General practice	1456	Abridged SD	22%
Kroenke [70]	General practice	1000	MSD (8%) or somatoform disorder NOS (4%)	12%
Kroenke [5]	General practice	3000	PHQ-15 score ≥15	10%
Kroenke [5]	Obstetrics-gynecology	3000	PHQ-15 score ≥15	10%

*Abridged somatization disorder (SD) defined as 6 lifetime medically unexplained symptoms in women (4 in men) derived from a possible list of 37 somatic symptoms. Multisomatoform disorder (MSD) defined as 3 current medically unexplained symptoms derived from a possible list of 15 somatic symptoms with at least a 2-year history of unexplained symptoms, whereas somatoform disorder NOS has the same 3-symptom threshold as MSD but not the chronicity criterion. PHQ-15 is the Patient Health Questionnaire 15-item somatic symptom scale, which ranges from a score of 0 to 30.

Gureje and colleagues [68] analyzed data from a WHO study of mental disorders in general practice conducted in 14 countries, in which they found a much higher prevalence of abridged than full SD (19.7% versus 2.8%). Although there was moderate geographic variation (eg, highest rates in South America), abridged SD was common across all cultures. Although most outpatient studies have been conducted in general practice/primary care settings, Kroenke and colleagues [5] found similar rates of somatization in obstetrics-gynecology practices. Also, the types of lower-threshold somatization (summarized in Table 3) all are associated with substantial functional impairment, excess health care use, and high rates of psychiatric comorbidity, in particular depression and anxiety. As shown in Fig. 4, patients who have lower threshold types of somatization have impairment on multiple domains of health-related quality of life closer to full SD than to patients who do not have somatization [54]. Fig. 4 shows four of the eight 36-Item Short-Form Health Survey (SF-36) scales; results on the four scales not shown were similar.

Although most agree that a lower threshold category is warranted, there are a variety of options for constituting such a category. Several conditions have empiric data supporting their validity, such as abridged SD [69], multisomatoform disorder (MSD) [70], bodily distress disorder [62], and medically unexplained symptom (MUS) spectrum disorder [71]. There also are other published proposals [26,66,72,73]. Finally, example criteria were discussed by CISSD participants and outlined in Table 4 to stimulate ongoing discussion and refinement [33]. There was general agreement that besides mere somatic symptom counts, psychologic and behavioral criteria characteristic of somatizing patients should be included in revised definitions of SD or its lower threshold variants.

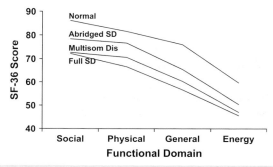

Fig. 4. Health-related quality of life scores on four SF-36 scales in a weighted sample of primary care patients classified as full (n = 139) and abridged (n = 84) SD, MSD (n = 85), and normal (n = 89) (ie, neither of the three disorders). (*Data from* Kroenke K, Spitzer RL, deGruy FV, et al. A symptom checklist to screen for somatoform disorders in primary care. Psychosomatics 1998;39(3):263–72.)

Table 4
Example criteria for a more inclusive definition of somatization disorder[a,b]

A. Physical symptoms that currently are bothersome and not explained better by another medical or psychiatric disorder. Somatic symptoms that are core criteria for depressive or anxiety disorders are not counted toward diagnosis of somatic symptom disorder.
B. Symptoms cause significant occupational or social impairment.
C. One or more of the symptoms has been present most of the time for at least 6 months.
D. Two or more of the following:
   1. Multiple physical symptoms: symptoms that cluster in a single somatic syndrome, such as irritable bowel syndrome or fibromyalgia, count as one rather than multiple symptoms.
   2. Attributional component: continues to attribute the symptoms to an undiagnosed general medical disorder despite an adequate or repeated medical work-up
   3. Affective component: health anxiety, manifested by fear of having a serious disease (but not intense or persistent enough to fulfill the criteria for health anxiety disorder)
   4. Cognitive component, such as rumination about bodily symptoms, selective attention to or frequent checking of symptoms, or catastrophizing (ie, fearing progression or bad outcomes despite reassurance)
   5. Behavioral component, such as high number of health care visits, requests for repeated testing, seeking care from multiple providers for the same symptoms.

[a]There was not unanimous agreement on these criteria; these were initial suggestions from CISSD workshop participants. Also, various names were proposed (eg, somatic symptom disorder, physical symptom disorder, MSD, polysomatoform disorder, and bodily distress disorder) but no consensus was achieved.
[b]Additional specifiers might be duration (eg, chronic defined as greater than 2 years) and severity (eg, defined by scores on a somatic symptom rating scale).
   From Kroenke K, Sharpe M, Sykes R. Revising the classification of somatoform disorders: key questions and preliminary recommendations. Psychosomatics 2007;48(4):277–85.

Pain disorder

There was widespread agreement about deleting pain disorder from the category of somatoform disorders. Although *DSM-IV* was intended to be largely atheoretic and free of unsupported mechanisms as diagnostic criteria, pain disorder and CD violate this principle. Criterion C for pain disorder specifies, "psychological factors are judged to have an important role in the onset, severity, exacerbation, or maintenance of the pain." Although pain frequently is comorbid with depression, the triangular relationship between pain, depression, and somatoform disorders and its directionality is complex [50,74]. Pain disorder is researched infrequently as a somatoform diagnosis, and even pain experts argue against an Axis I diagnosis [75,76]. Assigning an Axis I diagnosis to a small subset of chronic pain patients not only is arbitrary and stigmatizing to them but also inadvertently may underestimate the role of psychologic factors in the much larger group of patients who have chronic pain. Thus, the recommendation when pain is the predominant complaint is to code the pain symptoms on Axis III with concomitant psychiatric comorbidity coded on Axis I. When pain coexists with poorly explained nonpain complaints, however, and patients manifest other characteristics of somatization (see Table 4), a somatoform diagnosis also is still possible.

Hypochondriasis

There have been several evidence-based reviews on the criteria for hypochondriasis that should be considered when revising *DSM-V* [77,78]. For example, the ineffectiveness of medical reassurance is shown to be an unreliable criterion for hypochondriasis [77,79]. One consensus CISSD recommendation is that the term itself has become so pejorative that the name should be changed, possibly to health anxiety disorder. There is disagreement as to whether or not the condition should remain in the somatoform disorder category or moved to the anxiety disorder category. Opinions also differ as to whether or not hypochondriasis/health anxiety should remain a discrete disorder or be rolled into SD and its lower threshold variants as one of the criteria or domains.

Conversion disorder

There are several debates regarding CD. First, some experts believe it should be moved from somatoform disorders to dissociative disorders. Second, if CD is moved out of the somatoform disorder category, would individual pseudoneurologic symptoms not meeting full criteria for CD still count toward a diagnosis of SD? Third, some wonder why neurologic symptoms warrant a separate disorder distinct from other medically unexplained symptoms. Fourth, CD is the one condition besides pain disorder that formally implicates psychologic mechanisms, a criterion that is hard to verify, not required for other somatoform disorders, and divergent from the largely atheoretic, phenomenologic nature of *DSM-IV.* Fifth (as discussed previously) analysis of somatic symptom groups in clinical and population samples often fail to reveal a neurologic symptom cluster. Sixth, pseudoneurologic symptoms are the least likely to persist at follow-up [57].

Miscellaneous issues

There are four other topics emanating from the CISSD that deserve commentary:

1. One radical proposal is to largely abolish the category of somatoform disorders and move all conditions manifested principally by MUS to Axis III. Although several experts in somatoform disorders endorse this position [24,27], many others disagree [25,28].
2. Some believe that the terms, "somatization" and "somatoform," no longer should be used because, like hypochondriasis, they have acquired negative connotations. Moreover, many clinicians, even if they use these terms in the medical records, use different terminology when communicating with patients, which makes terms, such as somatoform, a code between clinicians, often for disorders they find frustrating to manage. Alternatives proposed for SD include, "physical symptom disorder," "somatic symptom disorder," "bodily distress disorder," and "MSD." Others note that somatoform is a useful term in some cultures (eg, Germany), and that any new diagnostic label ultimately will become tainted unless attitudes and skills of clinicians toward managing these disorders improve.

3. All agree that language potentially pejorative to patients should be avoided. Examples found in the *DSM-IV* chapter on somatoform disorders include terms, such as, "doctor-shopping," "pseudo-neurological," "inconsistent historians," "misinterpretation of bodily symptoms," and the use by patients of "colorful, exaggerated terms" to describe their symptoms.
4. The APA and WHO should work together to make *DSM-V* and *ICD-11* compatible with respect to the categories, disorders, and criteria for mental disorders. For example, decisions should be made about conditions that appear in one system (eg, neurasthenia and somatoform autonomic dysfunction in *ICD-10*) but not in another (in this case, *DSM-IV*).

MEASURING SOMATIC SYMPTOMS

The assessment and outcome monitoring of many medical disorders rely on measurement (eg, blood pressure readings in hypertension, serum glucose in diabetes, peak flow in asthma, and noninvasive assessment of coronary perfusion in cardiovascular disease). Validated measures traditionally have been used in psychiatric research but not routinely in clinical practice. Several brief self-rated measures have been evaluated, however, for use in depression [80], and the recent Sequenced Treatment Alternatives to Relieve Depression trial has proved that depression measures are useful in monitoring and tailoring treatment [81].

Measures can have a variety of uses, including screening, diagnosis, assessment of severity, and gauging treatment decisions. The latter use is relevant particularly to patients and clinicians to monitor and adjust therapy to optimize outcomes. Therefore, measures that have served as the primary outcome in treatment trials are potential candidates for use in clinical practice. A literature synthesis of 34 randomized controlled trials for treatment of somatoform disorders recently was completed [16]. The primary outcome measures used in these trials are summarized in Table 5. In addition to the length of the measure, scoring range, and number of trials in which each measure was used, additional pragmatic information is provided. Although clinical trials require outcome measures with robust psychometric characteristics, such as validity and sensitivity to change, uptake into clinical practice also depends on practical considerations, such as availability (eg, Has the actual scale been published in one or more articles and, thus, is easily accessible to clinicians?), brevity and ease of scoring, mode of administration (self-rated versus interviewer), and cost of the measure (ie, proprietary versus public domain).

The Symptom Checklist (SCL)-12 is the 12-item somatization scale of the SCL-90 [82,83] and has been used in the largest number of trials. It is a brief self-rated scale that is scored easily. The only potential drawback is that the SCL-90 is proprietary. There is an older version of the measure, which was published in the medical literature and sometimes is used in research [84]. The revised version recommended by the developers, however, is proprietary and needs to be purchased for use. In addition to its somatization scale, the SCL-90 includes scales that assess depression, anxiety, and several other domains.

Table 5

Measures used in randomized clinical trials of somatoform disorders to assess treatment outcomes

Scale	Description	Items	Response set[a]	Score range	Self-rated	No. of trials	Diagnostic[b]	Availability[c]
SCL-12 [82–84]	SCL-90 somatization scale	12	5	0–48	Yes	10	No	Wide use but proprietary (costs to use)
PHQ-15 [5]	PHQ somatic symptom severity scale	15	3	0–30	Yes	2	No	Free to use, published
SOMS [87,88]	Screening for Somatoform Symptoms scale	53	5	0–206	Yes	4	Yes	Must be ordered from authors
HAM-A SOM [85,86]	Hamilton Anxiety Rating Scale–somatic anxiety subscale	7	5	0–28	No	3	No	Free to use, variably published
CGI-SD [89]	Clinical global impression of somatic symptom improvement	33	7	33–231	No	2	Yes	Uncertain
Whiteley Index [90,91]	Hypochondriacal attitudes and illness worries	14	2	0–14	Yes	4	No	Free to use, published.

[a]Number of response options per item.

[b]These measures also are designed to make *DSM-IV* and *ICD-10* somatoform diagnoses.

[c]SCL-90 is proprietary though earlier version (Hopkins Symptom Checklist) was published and often used. PHQ-15 and Whiteley Index are published fully in one or more journals and free to use. The HAM-A did not have an exactly worded scale provided in the original publication and extensive training is required; a structured interview guide has since been published, although how its operating characteristics compare with the original version are not well established. The SOMS and CGI-SD are referenced but not published in the original articles. Their authors need to be contacted to see about their availability.

All other measures in Table 5 have been used in a smaller number of trials (ie, two to four). The two other brief somatic symptom scales are the somatic anxiety subscale of the Hamilton Anxiety Rating Scale (HAM-A) and the Patient Health Questionnaire somatic symptom severity scale (PHQ)-15. The HAM-A is an anxiety outcome measure used commonly in clinical trials, and its somatic subscale is intended to measure seven somatic symptom clusters most likely associated with anxiety (muscular, sensory, cardiovascular, respiratory, gastrointestinal, genitourinary, and autonomic). The HAM-A is interviewer-administered rather than self-rated, a potential limitation in busy practice settings. A more important drawback is that in its original form, the scale had no instructions for administration or for scoring, and there are no scripted questions [85]. Thus, the method of administering each item and assigning the level of symptom severity can be arbitrary, which is why in clinical trials (its principal use), extensive training is required for reliable administration. A structured interview guide has been developed to improve reliability [86], although published comparisons with the original version are limited.

The PHQ-15, displayed in Fig. 5, is discussed in greater detail because the author and colleagues developed it, it is freely available for use in research and clinical practice, and it exemplifies a brief, easily scored, and valid measure of somatic symptom severity [5]. It includes 15 symptoms that account for more than 90% of symptoms seen in primary care (exclusive of self-limited upper respiratory symptoms, such as cough, nasal symptoms, sore throat, ear ache, and so forth). The PHQ-15 asks patients to rate how much they have been bothered by each symptom during the past month on a 0 ("not at all") to 2 ("bothered a lot") scale. Thus, the total score ranges from 0 to 30, with cutpoints of 5, 10, and 15, representing thresholds for mild, moderate, and severe somatic symptom severity, respectively. Therefore, the PHQ-15 can be used as a continuous or categorical measure of somatic symptom severity.

There are several factors arguing for the PHQ-15 as an excellent somatization measure. First, approximately 10% of outpatients have a score of 15 or greater, a prevalence consistent with other studies of clinically significant somatization. Second, increasing scores on the PHQ-15 are associated strongly with functional impairment, disability, and health care use. Third, items on the PHQ-15 overlap better with other validated somatization screeners than any other two screeners do with one another [26]. Fourth, it is an excellent measure for identifying high-utilizing somatizing patients in health care systems [9,87]. Fifth, total self-reported PHQ somatic symptom counts are shown to be highly associated with clinician-rated somatoform disorder symptom counts [88,89]. Sixth, there is emerging evidence that supports the PHQ-15's sensitivity to change in clinical trials as a primary [90] and secondary [91] outcome measure.

Additionally, the PHQ-15 can be used to make a diagnosis of MSD, which is defined as three or more medically unexplained PHQ-15 symptoms scored as 2 (ie, "bothered a lot") plus a several-year history of unexplained symptoms [70].

Physical Symptoms (PHQ-15)

During the <u>past 4 weeks</u>, how much have you been
bothered by any of the following problems?

	Not bothered at all [0]	Bothered a little [1]	Bothered a lot [2]
a. Stomach pain	☐	☐	☐
b. Back pain	☐	☐	☐
c. Pain in your arms, legs, or joints (knees, hips, etc.)	☐	☐	☐
d. Menstrual cramps or other problems with your periods [**Women only**]	☐	☐	☐
e. Headaches	☐	☐	☐
f. Chest pain	☐	☐	☐
g. Dizziness	☐	☐	☐
h. Fainting spells	☐	☐	☐
i. Feeling your heart pound or race	☐	☐	☐
j. Shortness of breath	☐	☐	☐
k. Pain or problems during sexual intercourse	☐	☐	☐
l. Constipation, loose bowels, or diarrhea	☐	☐	☐
m. Nausea, gas, or indigestion	☐	☐	☐
n. Feeling tired or having low energy	☐	☐	☐
o. Trouble sleeping	☐	☐	☐

Fig. 5. The PHQ-15.

MSD is believed a useful construct for capturing clinically significant somatization for several reasons. First, it has a primary care prevalence (8%–10%) consistent with other epidemiologic studies of clinically significant somatization. Second, it is associated with substantial functional impairment, disability, and health care use, even after controlling for comorbid depressive and anxiety disorders and comparable to other studies of somatization and somatoform disorders. Third, the majority (88%) of patients who have MSD also meet criteria for abridged or full SD [54]. Fourth, MSD is intermediate between abridged and full SD in terms of functional impairment, psychiatric comorbidity, family dysfunction, and health care use and costs. Fifth, the usefulness of MSD was acknowledged by *DSM-IV, Primary Care Version*, in which MSD was listed as a moderately severe form of undifferentiated somatoform disorder [92]. Sixth, it was used as an operational definition of somatization in an international study of mental disorders in primary care [93].

The Screening for Somatoform Symptoms (SOMS) is a self-rated questionnaire that includes all 33 physical complaints of the *DSM-IV* SD symptom list, the symptoms of *ICD-10* SD, and the *ICD-10* somatoform autonomic dysfunction symptom list [94]. Thus, in addition to assessing somatic symptom severity in general, it can serve as a diagnostic measure for two somatoform disorders. Originally published in German, an English-language version can be ordered from its authors [95]. Its length could be an advantage (ie, more comprehensive coverage of somatic symptoms) and a drawback (for clinicians seeking a brief measure in busy practice settings).

The Clinical Global Impression for Somatization Disorder (CGI-SD) scale yields a composite symptom severity rating made by a trained rater after questioning patients about the current frequency of, intensity of, and impairment caused by the 33 somatic symptoms that are assessed in assigning a *DSM-IV* diagnosis of SD [96]. The scale itself has not been published and the requirement for administration by a trained rate is a potential drawback. Finally, the Whiteley Index is not a somatization measure but a widely used self-rated measure of hypochondriacal attitudes and behaviors [97]. A seven-item version also is available [98].

Examples of other somatic symptom measures not used in the 34 trials of somatoform disorders but commonly used in psychosomatic research include the 17-item Psychosomatic Symptom Checklist [99,100], the 13-item Somatic Symptom Inventory [101], and the five-item Somatosensory Amplication Scale [102].

SUMMARY

Classification is not a trivial matter. In *Burmese Days*, George Orwell writes, "It is devilish to suffer from a pain that is all but nameless. Blessed are they who are stricken only with classifiable diseases! Blessed are the poor, the sick, the crossed in love, for at least other people know what is the matter with them and will listen to their belly-achings with sympathy." Patients who have somatoform disorders are particularly susceptible to this Orwellian lamentation. They are afflicted by symptoms that defy simple explanations. As detailed in this article, there is a spectrum of medical and psychiatric factors that can cause or contribute to somatic symptom burden.Research is continuing to reveal the central mechanisms that may provide a common pathway for physical and psychologic symptoms. The dualism that places some somatic symptom disorders on Axis I and others on Axis III gradually may fade in the coming decades as what the unifying causes are among common symptoms and the multicausal nature of many symptoms are discovered. Meanwhile, the classification systems should continue to operate on pragmatic principles where mechanistic explanations are lacking [103]. This will allow grouping patients into categories that inform research, scientific and patient communication, prognostication, and clinical management. Coupling a heuristic classification system with evidence-based measures for assessing severity and monitoring treatment outcomes are important steps in the optimal care of symptomatic patients.

References

[1] Schappert SM. National Ambulatory Medical Care Survey: 1991 summary. Adv Data 1993;230:1–16.

[2] Kroenke K, Arrington ME, Mangelsdorff AD. The prevalence of symptoms in medical outpatients and the adequacy of therapy. Arch Intern Med 1990;150:1685–9.

[3] Kroenke K, Spitzer RL, Williams JBW, et al. Physical symptoms in primary care: predictors of psychiatric disorders and functional impairment. Arch Fam Med 1994;3:774–9.

[4] Marple RL, Kroenke K, Lucey CR, et al. Concerns and expectations in patients presenting with physical complaints: frequency, physician perceptions and actions, and 2-week outcome. Arch Intern Med 1997;157:1482–8.

[5] Kroenke K, Spitzer RL, Williams JBW. The PHQ-15: validity of a new measure for evaluating the severity of somatic symptoms. Psychosom Med 2002;64:258–66.

[6] Spitzer RL, Williams JB, Kroenke K, et al. Utility of a new procedure for diagnosing mental disorders in primary care. The PRIME-MD 1000 study. JAMA 1994;272: 1749–56.

[7] Ormel J, Vonkorff M, Ustun TB, et al. Common mental disorders and disability across cultures. Results from the WHO Collaborative Study on psychological problems in general health care. JAMA 1994;272:1741–8.

[8] Spitzer RL, Kroenke K, Linzer M, et al. Health-related quality of life in primary care patients with mental disorders: results from the PRIME-MD 1000 study. JAMA 1995;274: 1511–7.

[9] Barsky AJ, Orav EJ, Bates DW. Somatization increases medical utilization and costs independent of psychiatric and medical comorbidity. Arch Gen Psychiatry 2005;62:903–10.

[10] Hahn SR. Physical symptoms and physician-experienced difficulty in the physician-patient relationship. Ann Intern Med 2001;134:897–904.

[11] O'Malley PG, Jackson JL, Santoro J, et al. Antidepressant therapy for unexplained symptoms and symptom syndromes. J Fam Pract 1999;48:980–90.

[12] Kroenke K, Swindle R. Cognitive-behavioral therapy for somatization and symptom syndromes: a critical review of controlled clinical trials. Psychother Psychosom 2000;69: 205–15.

[13] Allen LA, Escobar JI, Lehrer PM, et al. Psychosocial treatments for multiple unexplained physical symptoms: a review of the literature. Psychosom Med 2002;64:939–50.

[14] Raine R, Haines A, Sensky T, et al. Systematic review of mental health interventions for patients with common somatic symptoms: can research evidence from secondary care be extrapolated to primary care? BMJ 2002;325:1082.

[15] Jackson JL, O'Malley PG, Kroenke K. Antidepressants and cognitive-behavioral therapy for symptom syndromes. CNS Spectr 2006;11:212–22.

[16] Kroenke K. Efficacy of treatment for somatoform disorders: a review of randomized controlled trials. Psychosom Med, in press.

[17] Lipowski ZJ. Somatization: the concept and its clinical application. Am J Psychiatry 1988;145:1358–68.

[18] Eisenberg L. What makes persons "patients" and patients "well"? Am J Med 1980;69: 277–86.

[19] White KL. The ecology of medical care. N Engl J Med 1961;265:885–92.

[20] Green LA, Fryer GE, Yawn BP, et al. The ecology of medical care revisited. N Engl J Med 2001;344:2021–5.

[21] Banks MH, Beresford SA, Morrell DC, et al. Factors influencing demand for primary medical care in women aged 20–44 years: a preliminary report. Int J Epidemiol 1975;4: 189–95.

[22] Verbrugge LM, Ascione FJ. Exploring the iceberg: common symptoms and how people care for them. Med Care 1987;25:539–69.

[23] Jackson JL, Kroenke K. Managing somatization: medically unexplained should not mean medically ignored. J Gen Intern Med 2006;21:797–9.

[24] Mayou R, Kirmayer LJ, Simon G, et al. Somatoform disorders: time for a new approach in DSM-V. Am J Psychiatry 2005;162:847–55.

[25] Levenson JL. A rose by any other name is still a rose. J Psychosom Res 2006;60:325–6.

[26] Kroenke K. Physical symptom disorder: a simpler diagnostic category for somatization-spectrum conditions. J Psychosom Res 2006;60:335–9.

[27] Sykes R. Somatoform disorders in DSM-IV: mental or physical disorders? J Psychosom Res 2006;60:341–4.

[28] Hiller W. Don't change a winning horse. J Psychosom Res 2006;60:345–7.

[29] Sharpe M, Mayou R, Walker J. Bodily symptoms: new approaches to classification. J Psychosom Res 2006;60:353–6.

[30] Bradfield JW. A pathologist's perspective of the somatoform disorders. J Psychosom Res 2006;60:327–30.

[31] Creed F. Can DSM-V facilitate productive research into the somatoform disorders? J Psychosom Res 2006;60:331–4.

[32] De Gucht V, Maes S. Explaining medically unexplained symptoms: toward a multidimensional, theory-based approach to somatization. J Psychosom Res 2006;60: 349–52.

[33] Kroenke K, Sharpe M, Sykes R. Revising the classification of somatoform disorders: key questions and preliminary recommendations. Psychosomatics 2007;48:277–85.

[34] Kroenke K, Lucas CA, Rosenberg ML, et al. Causes of persistent dizziness: a prospective study of 100 patients in ambulatory care. Ann Intern Med 1992;117:898–904.

[35] Kroenke K. Studying symptoms: sampling and measurement issues. Ann Intern Med 2001;134:844–55.

[36] Kroenke K. Patients presenting with somatic complaints: epidemiology, psychiatric comorbidity and management. Int J Methods Psychiatr Res 2003;12:34–43.

[37] Khan AA, Khan A, Harezlak J, et al. Somatic symptoms in primary care: etiology and outcome. Psychosomatics 2003;44:471–8.

[38] Reid S, Wessely S, Crayford T, et al. Medically unexplained symptoms in frequent attenders of secondary health care: retrospective cohort study. Br Med J 2001;322:1–4.

[39] Wessely S, Nimnuan C, Sharpe M. Functional somatic syndromes: one or many? Lancet 1999;354:936–9.

[40] Barsky AJ, Borus JF. Functional somatic syndromes. Ann Intern Med 1999;130:910–21.

[41] Aaron LA, Buchwald D. A review of the evidence for overlap among unexplained clinical conditions. Ann Intern Med 2001;134:868–81.

[42] Gardner JW, Gibbons RV, Hooper TI, et al. Identifying new diseases and their causes: the dilemma of illnesses in Gulf War veterans. Mil Med 2003;168:186–93.

[43] Henningsen P, Zimmermann T, Sattel H. Medically unexplained physical symptoms, anxiety, and depression: a meta-analytic review. Psychosom Med 2003;65:528–33.

[44] Sha MC, Callahan CM, Counsell SR, et al. Physical symptoms as a predictor of health care use and mortality among older adults. Am J Med 2005;118:301–6.

[45] Katon W, Lin EH, Kroenke K. The association of depression and anxiety with medical symptom burden in patients with chronic medical illness. Gen Hosp Psychiatry 2007;29: 147–55.

[46] Kroenke K, Jackson JL, Chamberlin J. Depressive and anxiety disorders in patients presenting with physical complaints: clinical predictors and outcome. Am J Med 1997;103: 339–47.

[47] Kroenke K. The interface between physical and psychological symptoms. Primary Care Companion J Clin Psychiatry 2003;5(Suppl 7):11–8.

[48] Katon W, Sullivan M, Walker E. Medical symptoms without identified pathology: relationship to psychiatric disorders, childhood and adult trauma, and personality traits. Ann Intern Med 2001;134:917–25.

[49] Kroenke K, Rosmalen JG. Symptoms, syndromes, and the value of psychiatric diagnostics in patients who have functional somatic disorders. Med Clin North Am 2006;90: 603–26.

[50] Henningsen P, Lowe B. Depression, pain, and somatoform disorders. Curr Opin Psychiatry 2006;19:19–24.

[51] Kisely S, Goldberg D, Simon G. A comparison between somatic symptoms with and without clear organic cause: results of an international study. Psychol Med 1997;27:1011–9.

[52] Katon W, Lin E, Von KM, et al. Somatization: a spectrum of severity. Am J Psychiatry 1991;148:34–40.

[53] Simon GE, Von Korff M. Somatization and psychiatric disorder in the NIMH Epidemiologic Catchment Area study. Am J Psychiatry 1991;148:1494–500.

[54] Kroenke K, Spitzer RL, deGruy FV, et al. A symptom checklist to screen for somatoform disorders in primary care. Psychosomatics 1998;39:263–72.

[55] Jackson J, Fiddler M, Kapur N, et al. Number of bodily symptoms predicts outcome more accurately than health anxiety in patients attending neurology, cardiology, and gastroenterology clinics. J Psychosom Res 2006;60:357–63.

[56] Simon GE, Gureje O. Stability of somatization disorder and somatization symptoms among primary care patients. Arch Gen Psychiatry 1999;56:90–5.

[57] Gureje O, Simon GE. The natural history of somatization in primary care. Psychol Med 1999;29:669–76.

[58] Leiknes KA, Finset A, Moum T, et al. Methodological issues concerning lifetime medically unexplained and medically explained symptoms of the Composite International Diagnostic Interview: a prospective 11-year follow-up study. J Psychosom Res 2006;61:169–79.

[59] Rief W, Rojas G. Stability of somatoform symptoms: implications for classification. Psychosom Med, in press.

[60] First MB, Pincus HA, Levine JB, et al. Clinical utility as a criterion for revising psychiatric diagnoses. Am J Psychiatry 2004;161:946–54.

[61] Simon G, Gater R, Kisely S, et al. Somatic symptoms of distress: an international primary care study. Psychosom Med 1996;58:481–8.

[62] Fink P, Toft T, Hansen MS, et al. Symptoms and syndromes of bodily distress: an exploratory study of 978 internal medical, neurological, and primary care patients. Psychosom Med 2007;69:30–9.

[63] Liu G, Clark MR, Eaton WW. Structural factor analyses for medically unexplained somatic symptoms of somatization disorder in the Epidemiologic Catchment Area study. J Psychosom Res 1997;42:245–52.

[64] Gara MA, Silver RC, Escobar JI, et al. A hierarchical classes analysis (HICLAS) of primary care patients with medically unexplained somatic symptoms. Psychiatry Res 1998;81: 77–86.

[65] Interian A, Gara MA, az-Martinez AM, et al. The value of pseudoneurological symptoms for assessing psychopathology in primary care. Psychosom Med 2004;66:141–6.

[66] Rief W, Heuser J, Mayrhuber E, et al. The classification of multiple somatoform symptoms. J Nerv Ment Dis 1996;184:680–7.

[67] Escobar JI, Burnam MA, Karno M, et al. Somatization in the community. Arch Gen Psychiatry 1987;44:713–8.

[68] Gureje O, Simon GE, Ustun TB, et al. Somatization in cross-cultural perspective: a World Health Organization study in primary care. Am J Psychiatry 1997;154:989–95.

[69] Escobar JI, Gara M, Silver RC, et al. Somatisation disorder in primary care. Br J Psychiatry 1998;173:262–6.

[70] Kroenke K, Spitzer RL, deGruy FV III, et al. Multisomatoform disorder. An alternative to undifferentiated somatoform disorder for the somatizing patient in primary care. Arch Gen Psychiatry 1997;54:352–8.

[71] Smith RC, Gardiner JC, Lyles JS, et al. Exploration of DSM-IV criteria in primary care patients with medically unexplained symptoms. Psychosom Med 2005;67:123–9.

[72] Fava GA, Freyberger HJ, Bech P, et al. Diagnostic criteria for use in psychosomatic research. Psychother Psychosom 1995;63:1–8.

[73] Rief W, Hiller W. Toward empirically based criteria for somatoform disorders. J Psychosom Res 1999;46:507–18.

[74] Bair MJ, Robinson RL, Katon W, et al. Depression and pain comorbidity: a literature review. Arch Intern Med 2003;163:2433–45.

[75] Sullivan M. Pain disorder: a case against the diagnosis. Int Rev Psychiatry 2000;12:91–8.

[76] Birket-Smith M, Mortensen EL. Pain in somatoform disorders: is somatoform pain disorder a valid diagnosis? Acta Psychiatr Scand 2002;106:103–8.

[77] Fink P, Ornbol E, Toft T, et al. A new, empirically established hypochondriasis diagnosis. Am J Psychiatry 2004;161:1680–91.

[78] Creed F, Barsky A. A systematic review of the epidemiology of somatisation disorder and hypochondriasis. J Psychosom Res 2004;56:391–408.

[79] Martin A, Jacobi F. Features of hypochondriasis and illness worry in the general population in Germany. Psychosom Med 2006;68:770–7.

[80] Williams JW Jr, Pignone M, Ramirez G, et al. Identifying depression in primary care: a literature synthesis of case-finding instruments. Gen Hosp Psychiatry 2002;24:225–37.

[81] Rush AJ, Trivedi MH, Wisniewski SR, et al. Acute and longer-term outcomes in depressed outpatients requiring one or several treatment steps: a STAR*D report. Am J Psychiatry 2006;163:1905–17.

[82] Derogatis L, Cleary P. Confirmation of the dimensional structure of the SCL-90: a study in construct validation. J Clin Psychol 1977;33:981–9.

[83] Derogatis L. SCL-90-R administration, scoring, and procedures manual. Towson (MD): Clinical Psychometrics Research; 1977.

[84] Derogatis LR, Lipman RS, Rickels K, et al. The Hopkins symptom checklist (HSCL): a self-report symptom inventory. Behav Sci 1974;19:1–15.

[85] Hamilton M. The assessment of anxiety states by rating. Br J Med Psychol 1959;32:50–5.

[86] Shear MK, Vander BJ, Rucci P, et al. Reliability and validity of a structured interview guide for the Hamilton Anxiety Rating Scale (SIGH-A). Depress Anxiety 2001;13:166–78.

[87] Barsky AJ, Orav EJ, Bates DW. Distinctive patterns of medical care utilization in patients who somatize. Med Care 2006;44:803–11.

[88] Rost KM, Dickinson WP, Dickinson LM, et al. Multisomatoform disorder: agreement between patient and physician report of criterion symptom explanation. CNS Spectr 2006;11:383–8.

[89] Interian A, Allen LA, Gara MA, et al. Somatic complaints in primary care: further examining the validity of the Patient Health Questionnaire (PHQ-15). Psychosomatics 2006;47:392–8.

[90] Kroenke K, Messina N III, Benattia I, et al. Venlafaxine extended release in the short-term treatment of depressed and anxious primary care patients with multisomatoform disorder. J Clin Psychiatry 2006;67:72–80.

[91] Kroenke K, West SL, Swindle R, et al. Similar effectiveness of paroxetine, fluoxetine, and sertraline in primary care: a randomized trial. JAMA 2001;286:2947–55.

[92] American Psychiatric Association. Diagnostic and statistical manual of mental disorders, 4th edition: primary care version (DSM-IV-PC). Washington, DC: American Psychiatric Association; 1995.

[93] Simon GE, Von Korff M, Piccinelli M, et al. An international study of the relation between somatic symptoms and depression. N Engl J Med 1999;341:1329–35.

[94] Rief W, Hiller W, Heuser J. SOMS—Das Screening fur Somatoforme Störungen. Manual zum Fragebogen (SOMS—the screening for somatoform symptoms). Bern: Huber; 1997.

[95] Rief W, Nanke A. Somatoform disorders in primary care and inpatient settings. Adv Psychosom Med 2004;26:144–58.

[96] Allen LA, Woolfolk RL, Escobar JI, et al. Cognitive-behavioral therapy for somatization disorder: a randomized controlled trial. Arch Intern Med 2006;166:1512–8.

[97] Pilowsky I. Dimensions of hypochondriasis. Br J Psychiatry 1967;113:89–93.

[98] Conradt M, Cavanagh M, Franklin J, et al. Dimensionality of the Whiteley Index: assessment of hypochondriasis in an Australian sample of primary care patients. J Psychosom Res 2006;60:137–43.

[99] Chibnall JT, Tait RC. The psychosomatic symptom checklist revisited: reliability and validity in a chronic pain population. J Behav Med 1989;12:297–307.

[100] Attanasio V, Andrasik F, Blanchard EB, et al. Psychometric properties of the SUNYA revision of the psychosomatic symptom checklist. J Behav Med 1984;7:247–58.

[101] Barsky AJ, Wyshak G, Klerman GL. Hypochondriasis: an evaluation of the DSM-III criteria in medical outpatients. Arch Gen Psychiatry 1986;43:493–500.

[102] Barsky AJ, Wyshak G, Klerman GL. The somatosensory amplification scale and its relationship to hypochondriasis. J Psychiatr Res 1990;24:323–34.

[103] Engel CC. Explanatory and pragmatic perspectives regarding idiopathic physical symptoms and related syndromes. CNS Spectr 2006;11:225–32.

Psychiatr Clin N Am 30 (2007) 621–644

PSYCHIATRIC CLINICS
OF NORTH AMERICA

ELSEVIER
SAUNDERS

New Directions in the Treatment of Somatization

Robert L. Woolfolk, PhD[a,b,*], Lesley A. Allen, PhD[c],
Jade E. Tiu, BA[a,c]

[a]Department of Psychology, Rutgers University, 152 Frelinghuysen Road, Piscataway,
NJ 08854, USA
[b]Department of Psychology, Princeton University, Green Hall, 18 Turner Court,
Princeton, NJ 08544, USA
[c]Department of Psychiatry, Robert Wood Johnson Medical School-UMDNJ,
671 Hoes Lane, Piscataway, NJ 08854, USA

In this article the authors present their model of treatment for somatization disorder (SD) and related syndromes. It begins with a brief history of somatization followed by a discussion of theory and research on medically unexplained symptoms. Finally, it describes in some detail the authors' psychosocial treatment for medically unexplained symptoms [1], which uses methods from both cognitive behavioral therapy and experiential emotion-focused therapy.

Somatization is among the most puzzling phenomena that health care workers encounter. In somatization physical symptoms occur in the absence of any identifiable bodily mechanism. The causes of somatization that health care workers are able to implicate are neither proximate nor somatic, seeming instead to be indirect and to be characterized most aptly as psychologic or cultural. Somatization seems to be universal, found in all present societies and in all past societies for which there are relevant records.

At the dawn of the psychoanalytic era, Breuer and Freud [2] developed the concept of "conversion," a process whereby intrapsychic activity putatively brings about somatic symptoms. Although Freud later broke with Breuer and created the substantial edifice of psychoanalysis, his work on hysteria provided a blueprint for and harbinger of later theoretical explanations of somatization. Here the ideas of early emotional trauma or intrapsychic conflict as the cause of physical symptoms began to take shape. This work also introduced the notion of a physical symptom as an unconscious form of communication, as a device for securing secondary gain, or a means for avoiding emotional pain. The notion of the transduction of psychologic conflict into bodily symptoms was disseminated widely as psychoanalysis began to dominate psychiatry.

*Corresponding author. E-mail address: woolfolk@princeton.edu (R.L. Woolfolk).

0193-953X/07/$ – see front matter
doi:10.1016/j.psc.2007.07.001
© 2007 Elsevier Inc. All rights reserved.
psych.theclinics.com

Stekel [3] coined the term "somatization" (*somatisieren*) during the early 1920s and defined it as "the conversion of emotional states into physical symptoms."

A landmark in the descriptive psychopathology of somatization was the seminal monograph of Paul Briquet [4], *Triaté Clinique et Thérapeutique de L'hystérie.* The current conception of SD derives directly from this paper. Briquet's meticulous and exhaustive listing of the symptomatology of hysteria remains unsurpassed. Briquet, in fact, described three related syndromes: conversion phenomena, hysterical personality, and multiple chronic unexplained somatic symptoms [5,6]. These three syndromes overlapped somewhat in symptomatology, and they often were observed to co-occur. Briquet's perspicuous work was revived by Purtell, Robins, and Cohen [7] and was developed further by members of the illustrious Washington University department of psychiatry. Perley and Guze [8] published a list of 57 symptoms, commonly reported by women diagnosed as having hysteria, that were clustered in 10 different areas. These investigators were the first to suggest specific criteria for the diagnosis of hysteria: the presence of 25 symptoms from at least 9 of the 10 symptom areas [9]. Later, this list of 57 symptoms was expanded to include 59 symptoms, and the term "Briquet's syndrome" was adopted [10]. The criteria for Briquet's syndrome subsequently were incorporated into the Feighner criteria [11], the precursor to the symptom set that appeared in the third edition of the *Diagnostic and Statistical Manual of Mental Disorders* (DSM-III) [12]. In that volume the theoretically neutral term "somatization" was preferred to the more traditional terminology. Although some of the traditional language remains in the fourth edition of the DSM (DSM-IV) (eg, "conversion disorder"), the word "hysteria" no longer appears [13]. The ninth edition of the World Health Organization's (WHO) *International Classification of Diseases* (ICD-9) [14], a more cosmopolitan nosology of somatic and mental disorders published a year earlier than DSM-III, retains much of the earlier terminology, including "neurasthenia" as well as "hysteria." The ICD-10 [15] has shifted in the direction of the DSM, although without banishing all the classical vocabulary.

SD is diagnosed, according to the DSM-IV [13], when a patient has at least four unexplained pain complaints (eg, in the back, chest, joints), two unexplained gastrointestinal complaints (eg, nausea, bloating), one unexplained sexual symptom (eg, sexual dysfunction, irregular menstruation), and one pseudoneurologic symptom (eg, seizures, paralysis, numbness). For a symptom to be counted toward the diagnosis of SD, it must be medically unexplained or substantially in excess of the associated medical pathology. Also, each symptom must prompt the seeking of medical care or interfere with the patient's functioning.

The differences in the diagnostic criteria of DSM-III, DSM-III-R, DSM-IV, and ICD-10, although subtle in some instances, may be responsible for some of the inconsistencies in the epidemiologic findings. Some epidemiologic research has suggested that SD is relatively rare. In the Epidemiological Catchment Area (ECA) study [16], the largest survey of SD (performed in a community sample of 20,000 people across five sites in the United States), the lifetime prevalence of DSM-III SD was 0.13%. Prior research had resulted in higher estimates, ranging from 0.4% to 2% of the population, for Perley-Guze's hysteria [17,18]. Not surprisingly, SD seems to be more common in primary care settings than in community populations. In the WHO Cross-National Study of Mental Disorders in Primary Care [19], which assessed 5438 primary care patients at 15 centers in 14 countries, the prevalence of SD was 0.9% and 2.8%, as defined by DSM-III-R and ICD-10, respectively. Smaller studies conducted in primary care settings have estimated the prevalence of DSM-III-R SD to range from 1.0% in a sample of 685 patients [20] to 5.0% in a sample of 222 patients [21].

For a number of reasons, several authorities suggest the actual prevalence of SD may be substantially higher than the literature suggests. First, autobiographic memory of past psychiatric symptoms, including somatization symptoms, is unreliable [22,23]. Individuals seem to forget (or at least fail to report) previously reported symptoms that are no longer troublesome [22,23]. Given that the diagnosis of SD requires patients to describe both current and remitted symptoms, and the latter often are not recalled, these studies probably underestimate the true occurrence of SD. Second, the diagnosis of SD requires that a physical examination and diagnostic tests be performed or that medical records be reviewed to determine the nature of each symptom. Such extensive investigations of physical symptoms are too costly to incorporate into large epidemiologic studies. The third argument for the underestimation of prevalence rates has to do with the conjecture that physicians are more likely to make the somatization diagnosis than are nonphysician diagnosticians [24,25]. Presumably, physicians are better able to distinguish between a medically sound explanation for a symptom and the patient's "medical sounding" explanation for that symptom. Because nonphysicians conducted assessments without access to medical records in the ECA and WHO studies cited previously, SD may have been underdiagnosed in those studies. At the one site in the ECA study where physicians evaluated symptom reports to determine whether symptoms were medically explained, the prevalence of SD was higher than at the other sites [26].

Patients diagnosed as having the most severe form of somatization, SD, have been shown to incur health care expenses that are nine times the United States average, and they consume disproportionate amounts of the time and energy of health care providers [27]. In addition to the extensive direct costs, SD creates enormous indirect costs to the economy in the form of lost work productivity. Individuals diagnosed as having SD report being bedridden for 2 to 7 days per month [27,28]. SD is not only costly but also is difficult to treat successfully. In a longitudinal study following patients who had SD who were receiving standard medical care, only 31% recovered after 15 years [29]. Typically, patients who have SD are dissatisfied with the medical services they receive and repeatedly change physicians [30]. These "treatment-resistant" patients frustrate health care providers with their frequent complaints and dissatisfaction with treatment [30]. Not one controlled medication trial for SD has been published, to the authors' knowledge. Anecdotal evidence suggests many patients diagnosed as having SD refuse to take medication, and those who do so frequently report adverse medication side effects [31]. The story is much the same with other polysymptomatic somatoform disorders [32]. As of this writing, pharmacologic treatment has had minimal success in somatization.

SUBTHRESHOLD SOMATIZATION

Some investigators have encouraged broadening the somatization construct to include the many patients affected by unexplained symptoms not numerous enough to meet criteria for full SD. Both the ICD-10 and the DSM-IV include residual diagnostic categories for subthreshold somatization cases. In the DSM-IV, undifferentiated SD is a diagnosis characterized by one or more medically unexplained physical symptom(s) lasting for at least 6 months [13]. The ICD-10's criteria for undifferentiated SD differ from the DSM-IV's in that ICD-10 requires multiple unexplained symptoms lasting for at least 6 months [15]. The ICD-10 provides an additional category for subthreshold SD, somatoform autonomic dysfunction, for cases of three or more unexplained symptoms of autonomic arousal [15]. The authors are aware of no published data that establish the validity of any of these three diagnostic categories.

Two research teams have suggested categories for subthreshold somatization other than those described in the DSM-IV and the ICD-10. Escobar and colleagues [33] proposed the label "abridged somatization" be applied to men experiencing four or more unexplained physical symptoms or to women experiencing six or more unexplained physical symptoms. Kroenke and colleagues [34] suggested the category of "multisomatoform disorder" to describe men or women currently experiencing at least three unexplained physical symptoms and reporting a 2-year history of somatization. Both these subthreshold somatization categories seem to be significantly more prevalent than full SD, described earlier. Abridged somatization has been observed in 4.4% of community samples [33] and in 16.6% to 22.0% of primary care samples [19,20,35]. The occurrence of multisomatoform disorder has been estimated at 8.2% of primary care patients [34].

The demographic characteristic most often associated with somatization is gender. In the ECA study, women were 10 times more likely than men to meet criteria for SD [36]. Gender differences, although not as extreme, also have been found in most studies employing subthreshold somatization categories, such as Escobar's abridged somatization or Kroenke's multisomatoform disorder [34,37]. A more complex picture of the association between gender and somatization was suggested by the WHO's Cross-National study [19] in which female primary care patients were more likely than their male counterparts to meet the ICD-10 criteria for full SD but were no more likely to meet Escobar's abridged somatization criteria. At least on the severe end of the continuum, SD is uncommon in men. Gender differences are less obvious in the various subthreshold syndromes.

Current thinking is that the low prevalence of SD in men may be explained, in part, by stereotypic male traits, such as a disinclination to admit discomfort and an unwillingness to seek medical treatment [38]. Also, physicians may be less likely to consider somatization as a possible explanation for a man's symptoms than for a woman's symptoms [39]. Gender biases may cause physicians to communicate with and treat male patients differently from the ways in which they communicate with and treat female patients. At this juncture, there are only conjectural explanations for the different rates of somatization in men and women.

Ethnicity, race, and education have been associated with SD and subthreshold somatization. Epidemiologic research has shown somatization patients were more likely to be female, nonwhite, and less educated than nonsomatizers [16,19]. Findings on ethnicity have been less consistent across studies. In the ECA study [16], Hispanics were no more likely than non-Hispanics to meet criteria for SD. The WHO study [19], conducted in 14 different countries, revealed a higher incidence of somatization, as defined by either ICD-10 or Escobar's abridged criteria, in Latin American countries than in the United States.

Findings on the relationship between age and somatization have been somewhat consistent. Most studies indicate that SD and abridged somatization are more common in middle-aged and older patients (over 45 years of age) than in younger patients [19,25]. Some research [16], however, has detected no association between SD and age. Children and adolescents, of course, are extremely unlikely to meet criteria for SD (and cannot, if one uses the DSM-IV criteria), perhaps because they have not lived long enough to acquire enough clinically significant somatization symptoms, especially sexual and menstrual symptoms.

CONCEPTUALIZATION OF SOMATIZATION

A biopsychosocial conceptualization of somatization leads to specific psychosocial treatment strategies that include cognitive, experiential, interpersonal, and behavioral interventions. This model of somatization emphasizes the interaction of physiology, cognition, emotion, behavior, and environment (Fig. 1). Patients presenting with somatization have higher levels of physiologic arousal and are less likely to habituate to a stressful task than control subjects [40]. This physiologic arousal is compounded by a tendency to amplify somatosensory information; that is, these patients are hypersensitive to bodily sensations that are experienced as intense, noxious, and disturbing [41]. Further, somatization patients form negative cognitive appraisals of their physical sensations [42]. For example, they may believe that pain, fatigue, and/or discomfort of any kind are signs of disease. In addition to misinterpreting somatic sensations, some patients think catastrophically to the extent that they imagine persistent physical sensations to be a sign of some potentially fatal disease, such as cancer or AIDS.

Dysfunctional cognitions may elicit negative emotions or be elicited by negative emotions [43]. This cognition–emotion cycle may interact in a complex fashion with maladaptive behaviors. For example, thoughts of possible illness

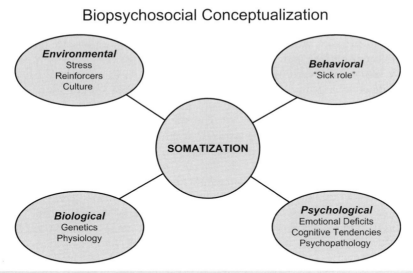

Fig. 1. Biopsychosocial conceptualization.

give rise to feelings of anxiety, dysphoria, and frustration, which are likely to generate and maintain physiologic arousal and physical symptomatology. Intending to prevent injury or exacerbation of symptoms, somatoform patients typically withdraw from their normal activities [27,28,44]. Such time away from activities provides opportunities for additional attention to be focused on physical health. Furthermore, patients suffering from these physical symptoms, distorted cognitions, and negative affect may seek repeated contact with physicians and request medical tests. Physicians, in turn, attempting to conduct thorough evaluations and avoid malpractice suits, may encourage somatizing behavior by ordering unnecessary diagnostic procedures. Chronic medical testing may ingrain patients in the "sick role" and reinforce somatizers' maladaptive belief that any physical symptom indicates organic pathology. Also, unnecessary medical procedures, if implemented, may result in iatrogenic illness.

Dysfunctional emotional processing also has been associated with somatization. These patients tend to score higher than medical patients and/or nonpatient controls on scales of neuroticism and negative affect [45–48]. Alexithymia, literally meaning "having no words for emotions or feelings," has been implicated in somatization by various theorists. The Toronto Alexithymia Scale, in particular the subscale assessing difficulties identifying feelings and distinguishing emotions from bodily sensations, has been shown to be associated positively with somatization [49]. Other authorities have discussed the "hysterical" emotional styles of these patients [50,51]. The authors' impression is that, although some somatizers manifest attenuated emotional processing and obliviousness to affect, others seem to have exaggerated emotional reactions. Some patients display each style, at different times. Contemporary theory in cognitive neuroscience suggests that emotional processing provides an important source of information about one's reactions to one's environment [52,53]. Incomplete or distorted emotional processing, in a sense, deprives individuals of data that are important to effective problem solving. Poor understanding of the emotional domain also may result in unresolved negative affective states and a prolongation of the physiologic arousal that accompanies negative affect. Clinicians often report that the affect of somatizers seems incongruent with eliciting circumstances, being either disproportionately flat or exaggerated. Both clinical impressions and the research literature suggest that somatizers fail to integrate and/or express fully their cognitive and affective responses to their environment. Using standard cognitive-behavioral therapy to challenge cognitions that are disconnected from affective experiences seems misguided and unproductive. Thus, the authors have aimed to design a treatment that helps patients access, process, and accept their implicit cognitive and affective responses.

ASSESSMENT

When patients present for psychiatric treatment, the first priority is to clarify the presenting problem(s) and related medical pathology and psychopathology. The authors recommend a thorough review of medical and psychiatric history as well as a discussion of current occupational, social, and physical functioning. Whenever possible such information is requested from patients' physician and family members as well as from the patients themselves.

A diagnosis of DSM-IV SD (or of moderate levels of somatization) requires clinicians to review a patients' lifetime history of 33 different physical symptoms and to determine the status of those symptoms, a time-consuming and complex task. Because most clinicians make diagnostic decisions based on unstructured patient interviews, many symptoms experienced by somatizers may never be discussed. Histories of somatization symptoms and abnormal illness behavior may be obscured by patients' narratives of their lives.

More accurate diagnoses may be achieved using a structured interview schedule, such as the Structured Clinical Interview for DSM-IV Disorders (SCID) [54] and a medical history review. The SCID provides questions to guide the clinician through the diagnostic criteria for the somatoform disorders (SD, hypochondriasis, undifferentiated somatoform disorder, pain disorder, and body dysmorphic disorder) as well as the other major psychiatric disorders. The SD section of the SCID requires the clinician ask in detail about the patient's lifetime experience with each physical symptom. The impact of each symptom experienced on the patient's behavior is explored. Also, patients are asked for medical diagnoses and medical recommendations for each symptom. Because patients' responses to questions about the organic basis of symptoms are not necessarily reliable, patients' physicians are consulted. Only medically unexplained symptoms are counted toward the somatization diagnosis.

Although the somatization section of the SCID may seem tedious to the clinician, the authors have found very few somatization patients respond negatively to its administration. In fact, most seem to appreciate the interviewer's careful attention to their somatic symptomatology. The authors have come to view the SD section of the SCID as a means of enhancing the patient–clinician bond. For many somatization patients, this interview is the first time a health care practitioner has evaluated each of the patient's symptoms extensively.

In addition to enhancing the patient–clinician relationship, the SCID, medical history review, and physician consultation can facilitate differential diagnosis. General medical conditions, such as rheumatoid arthritis or inflammatory bowel disease, may be excluded. The interviewer can distinguish between hypochondriasis and somatization by clarifying whether the distress is caused more by the patient's interpretations of symptoms (for example, that the reoccurrence of the symptoms suggests a fatal illness) or by the symptoms themselves. Also, because the SCID requires the clinician to inquire into the patient's lifetime experience with other psychiatric disorders (affective, anxiety disorders, psychotic, and substance dependence disorders), psychiatric explanations for symptoms can be excluded. Of course, the presentation of a general medical condition or a nonsomatoform psychiatric illness does not exclude the possibility of comorbid SD. In fact, these comorbid conditions present some of the most complex cases.

TREATMENT

When the authors began their work on SD, neither pharmacologic nor psychosocial treatment of SD had been shown to yield substantial clinical benefit. The most efficacious intervention for SD at that time was the psychiatric consultation intervention developed by Smith's group [55,56]. The consultation intervention consists of a letter sent to primary care physicians describing SD and providing recommendations to guide primary care. The recommendations, as shown in Box 1, were simple. Patients whose primary physicians had received the consultation letter exhibited better health outcomes (ie, better physical functioning and lower cost of medical care) than those whose physicians had not received the letter [55,56].

The authors' research group recently has published a controlled trial in which patients diagnosed as having SD treated with individual affective cognitive-behavioral therapy (ACBT) in conjunction with standard medical care augmented by Smith's psychiatric consultation letter experienced significantly greater reductions in physical discomfort and disability than those receiving only augmented standard medical treatment [57]. ACBT also was associated with higher levels of clinically significant improvement (ie, "much" or "very much" improvement as judged by a clinician blind to the patient's treatment condition) and lower health care costs than seen in the control condition. The benefits of ACBT were maintained 1 year after treatment had ended

Box 1: Recommendations in the psychiatric consultation letter sent to treating physicians

- Schedule appointments with patients on a regular basis instead of "as needed" appointments.
- Perform brief physical examinations focusing on the area of discomfort at each visit.
- Avoid unnecessary diagnostic procedures, invasive treatments, and hospitalizations.
- Avoid explaining symptoms with statements such as "Your symptoms are all in your head."

[57]. The efficacy of this treatment, applied to subthreshold somatization, also was demonstrated in a primary care setting [58].

Components of the Therapy

The components of ACBT are relaxation training, behavioral management, cognitive restructuring, emotion identification, emotion regulation, and interpersonal skills training. Given that somatization patients typically seek relief from their physical ailments, not from emotional distress, they begin treatment more willing to learn behavioral skills than to explore emotional issues. The first sessions are skill focused (ie, training patients in relaxation and behavioral management). These initial sessions are designed to reduce discomfort, to introduce patients to the potential benefits of psychotherapy, and to establish a therapeutic alliance in a fashion that is consistent with patients' tastes, proclivities, and expectations. The second phase of treatment is a cognitive-emotional elicitation/regulation module intended to enhance patients' understanding of their thoughts and feelings so they can interact more effectively with their environments. The third phase of treatment aims to enhance interpersonal functioning and to confront and alter the "sick role."

The individual treatment begins with training in relaxation [59,60]. Emphasis is placed on incorporating relaxation into daily life, before and during stressful situations, and in response to feelings of physical discomfort. Relaxation serves a number of functions in the treatment of somatization. It may interrupt the muscle tension–pain cycle found in patients who have chronic pain [61]. It may reduce generalized physiologic arousal or physiologic reactivity [62]. Finally, cognitive benefits may result from patients' observations that they are not completely helpless victims of their symptoms but instead have some control over them [62].

Once patients begin using one form of relaxation, training in behavioral management begins. This module of treatment aims to increase gradually patients' vocational, social, and self-care activities and to improve patients' mood and physical robustness. Also, sleep hygiene and stimulus control techniques are taught, as needed. The acquisition of these skills also may contribute to each patient's sense of self-efficacy in various areas and reduce feelings of powerlessness.

The cognitive-emotional elicitation/regulation module aims to help patients differentiate and understand their thoughts and feelings so that they can interact more effectively with their environments. The atmosphere of these sessions is more psychotherapeutic and less psychoeducational than that of the earlier sessions. Cognitive and emotion-focused strategies [63,64] in this module are integrated and individualized using case-based formulations [65].

Patients begin by monitoring their thoughts and emotions associated with changes in their physical symptoms. Experiential techniques, such as focusing [66] and techniques from Gestalt therapy [67], are used to assist patients in attending to, identifying, labeling, accepting, and expressing their thoughts and emotions. In the authors' experience, somatization patients typically are disinclined to focus intensively on their emotional experiences. These patients, however, are willing to explore emotions co-occurring with their physical symptoms and to try to make sense of those emotions by examining associated thoughts and behaviors. Once a patient's unique patterns of cognitive and emotional tendencies are identified, a semi-standardized, case-based formulation is used to guide the treatment. Emotional elicitation may be emphasized to help assimilate previously disowned or disavowed cognitive and/or emotional experiences. For example, if it is agreed that the patient inhibits feelings of anger, portions of treatment sessions and homework may be devoted to facilitating the introspection, identification, labeling, and, perhaps, the expression of anger. Alternatively, emotional regulation strategies, including relaxation, distraction, and cognitive restructuring, may be implemented for dysfunctional, destructive, exaggerated, or uncontrollable emotions. Determining which emotions, for a given individual in a given situation, need to be sought or amplified and which need to be examined through the lens of associated cognition or attenuated is a task that is central to the integration of cognitive and emotion-focused methods.

Cognitive interventions are based on cognitive treatment programs for stress management [68] and pain management [69]. Cognitive errors characteristic of this population, such as thinking catastrophically about somatic symptoms, are addressed with cognitive restructuring techniques. Distraction is taught to reduce excessive attention paid to their physical sensations. Also, patients explore the function that the "sick role" plays in their social world. Specifically, they examine whether they derive secondary gains from their physical symptoms and disability. Treatment helps patients develop alternative strategies for attaining those gains derived from the sick role.

Therapeutic Techniques

The therapeutic posture the authors assume with patients and the rationale for treatment that they present to patients are among the most important elements of their therapy. Their attitude toward patients is empathic and interested. They begin by asking patients about their physical symptoms and about the impact those symptoms have on their lives. The questions about the particular nature of the symptoms, such as the types of pain (eg, stabbing, pounding, burning, aching), and the situations in which symptoms typically occur provide therapists with important information while concurrently validating patients' discomfort. Patients' beliefs about their physical symptoms and past coping techniques are explored also. Throughout this discussion and throughout the entire treatment, the therapist strives to acknowledge the physical symptoms and the distress associated with them. The therapist's efforts to validate the patient's discomfort and distress are critical to the development of therapeutic rapport. Because patients presenting with somatization symptoms are so accustomed to being discounted or dismissed by their health care providers, patients often become more willing to engage in treatment after they feel understood by the therapist.

After communicating a considered appreciation of the patient's difficulties, the therapist describes the treatment's rationale. A biopsychosocial model of physical symptoms is proposed. Here, the therapist's stance is empathic and nonconfrontational. For patients who attribute their symptoms to an unknown biologic mechanism or to toxic aspects of the physical environment, the therapist suggests that even if symptoms are caused by some organic pathology or by environmental agents, stress is likely to exacerbate them. In this way, the therapist aims to expand and to create variations in patients' explanations of their symptoms but is careful not to contradict patients' beliefs directly. Faulty beliefs about symptoms are challenged more effectively in future sessions after some trust and credibility have been established.

The treatment is described as "stress management." The rationale presented is that because stress is likely to aggravate physical symptoms, the reduction of stress is likely to alleviate physical discomfort. Many patients are open to this idea, and, indeed, some already believe that stress might have a physical impact upon their bodily sensations or may have played a role in their underlying but unknown pathology. Most somatizing patients, however, would not accept the notion that their physical symptoms are entirely a direct product of stress. Therefore, it is important that therapists clarify that stress is only one factor contributing to patients' physical discomfort. The avowed aim of this treatment is, by limiting the adverse influence of stress, to give patients control over the aspects of their illness that can be controlled.

Almost all patients diagnosed as having somatization syndromes have had extensive, unsatisfying, and futile encounters with the health care system. Typically, the authors' intervention is the latest in a long line of treatments, all of which have been failures. Given that their expectations are low, patients must be motivated to come to therapy, despite minimal initial hope of success. The author's patients report that what keeps them coming back is the opportunity to be treated by someone who cares about them and who makes a respectful effort to understand what their lives are like.

In treatment the authors place a great emphasis on psychotherapy as a caring encounter. They emphasize this quality to a greater degree than do many expositions of cognitive-behavioral therapy, a treatment that usually is associated with a didactic therapist–patient relationship, without the emotional intensity of older more traditional forms of psychotherapy, such as psychoanalysis or client-centered therapy. Although it is true that in ACBT the therapist functions as a teacher and a trainer, the therapist also is a confidant and a helper who must earn the patient's trust through being truthful, caring, and empathic. The kind of caring encounter that is based on genuine and sincerely felt compassion is essential to the effective treatment of these patients. These patients, in many cases, have not been treated with kindness or courtesy. In offering civility and sympathy, the authors' therapy often proves to be a corrective emotional experience. Caring and empathy are not, in themselves, sufficient to produce change in these patients, but they can be important elements in restoring confidence in the health care system and the patients' resolve to attempt to cope with what can be great discomfort and disability.

Relaxation

The authors typically teach diaphragmatic breathing for the first month of treatment and an abbreviated progressive muscle relaxation for the second month of treatment. Diaphragmatic breathing can be used in concert with progressive muscle relaxation. The authors believe that relaxation training is most effective when it enables the trainee to learn how to relax on any given occasion and throughout the day, as opposed to extended sessions occurring once or twice per day to achieve an especially deep state of lowered arousal at scheduled times.

The therapist introduces diaphragmatic breathing and explains that the long-term goal is for the patient to breathe abdominally as much as possible. Regular abdominal breathing takes time to establish if it is a departure from the patient's typical practice. Over the course of treatment, the patient is asked to practice breathing abdominally between sessions and to report back on her progress. Eventually, breathing abdominally may coincide with reductions in tension and discomfort, although patients should be warned not to be disappointed if they initially experience little significant relief.

The crucial challenge in relaxation training is helping patients use the techniques on a regular basis. The considerable amount of therapy time used to describe, practice, and effectively implement relaxation techniques indicates the importance the authors place on using them. Even though training in relaxation often is completed by the eighth week of treatment, the authors continue to inquire into patients' use of relaxation throughout their work with them. Some patients learn to use both abbreviated progressive muscle relaxation and abdominal breathing, either in combination or separately. Others have a strong preference for one method or the other. The authors attempt to train patients in the two forms of relaxation and to allow the patient to decide ultimately which to employ. At this point the research literature cannot demonstrate that any form of systematic relaxation will be superior to others for a given individual [62]. What is clear, however, is that relaxation is beneficial only if it is used.

Behavioral management

Behavioral methods are based largely on the principles of classical and operant conditioning. Existing pathogenic contingencies of reinforcement are replaced with salutary ones. For example, patients learn to connect with friends and family by engaging with them in pleasurable activities instead of interacting with them through activities focused on the patients' physical discomfort. Exercise assignments are designed to be pleasurable and commensurate with patients' physical capacities, so that exercise eventually may be reinforced by inherent natural contingencies. Overall, the acquisition of a broader repertory of activities also may enhance a patient's self-efficacy in multiple areas and reduce feelings of infirmity and powerlessness.

Activity pacing is an important topic to address when discussing the initiation of a new activity. The authors' clinical experience and some research suggest that some, if not many, somatization patients have perfectionistic tendencies driving them to overachieve [70,71]. The authors believe that many of these patients may have difficulty moderating their activity levels; they overfunction at times and underfunction at other times. Of course, by the time they reach a psychotherapist's office, they are underfunctioning in important areas of their lives. Nevertheless, once they have been convinced to undertake an activity, they may be inclined to "overdo" it. Because somatization patients may overfunction or strive for perfection in therapy, the therapist emphasizes the importance of making small changes in a specific behavior at first and subsequently instituting gradual increases in that activity over the course of therapy. Other ways in which activity pacing is incorporated into therapy is by persuading patients to take frequent breaks in the midst of their daily routines.

Many patients who have somatization syndromes report significant sleep disturbance [72]. Failure to receive adequate restorative sleep is a contributory factor exacerbating many psychiatric disorders. In somatizers sleep loss is correlated almost invariably with a worsening of symptoms. The authors now believe that treating insomnia early and aggressively is a key to successful treatment of somatization.

Many of the authors' patients, especially those not working outside their homes, engage in sleep practices that may increase the likelihood of insomnia, such as taking naps during the day, keeping erratic sleep schedules, and watching television in bed. To combat poor sleep habits, the authors provide patients with brief psychoeducational training in sleep hygiene and stimulus control techniques [73].

To increase the likelihood that behavioral changes become a permanent part of patients' lives, they are discussed throughout treatment. The therapist monitors all changed behaviors every week of treatment.

Identifying thoughts and feelings

The cognitive-emotional elicitation/regulation components of treatment aim to help patients differentiate and understand their thoughts and feelings so that they can interact more effectively with their environments. The atmosphere of sessions devoted to this enterprise is more psychotherapeutic and less psychoeducational than that of the earlier sessions that are focused on relaxation training and making behavioral changes.

Patients begin this phase of treatment by monitoring the thoughts and emotions that are associated with changes in their physical symptoms. Experiential techniques, such as focusing [66] and techniques from Gestalt therapy [67], are used to assist patients in attending to, identifying, labeling, accepting, and expressing their thoughts and emotions. In the authors' experience, somatization patients are disinclined to focus intensively on their emotional experiences. These patients, however, often are willing to explore emotions co-occurring with their physical symptoms and to try to make sense of those emotions by examining the associated thoughts and behaviors.

Symptom-monitoring forms are introduced to help patients focus their attention on thoughts and feelings between sessions (Fig. 2). These forms are analogous to dysfunctional thought records used with depressed patients [74]. The authors' symptom-monitoring forms require patients to describe two specific moments each day: (1) when their physical symptoms are relatively severe and (2) when their physical symptoms are relatively less severe and they are experiencing greater relative comfort. Because the goal is to increase patients' awareness rather than to assess symptom severity, it is not critical that the patient write about "the most uncomfortable" or "the least uncomfortable" period of the day. The authors aim for a record of representative "physically uncomfortable" and "physically less uncomfortable" episodes. Ideally, these entries are made as proximate as possible to the occurrence of the episodes. On days without significant variation in physical discomfort, patients are instructed to choose, retrospectively, episodes of relative comfort and discomfort. At the moment of recording, patients note the time of day, the physical symptoms experienced, the environmental circumstances, and thoughts and emotions concurrent with the physical symptoms. The monitoring forms can be used to detect patterns in symptoms and in the relationships among symptoms, thoughts, and emotions.

Although patients complete symptom-monitoring forms in response to changes in symptomatology, the exercise is intended to increase patients' awareness of the situations, thoughts, and feelings that coincide with these symptomatic fluctuations. Of course, given this population's tendency to attend to their physical sensations excessively, the authors' aim is not to encourage additional "body scanning." Increased awareness of physical changes and of the psychosocial context in which these sensations occur, however, is helpful in ascertaining connections between symptoms and stress.

An initial task is to teach patients to distinguish between physical sensations and emotions and to differentiate thoughts from emotions. For example, if

Symptom Monitoring Forms (used in treatment)

Date/Time	Physical Symptoms *Rate the intensity (0-5)*	Situation *What were you doing at that moment?*	Emotion *What did you feel? Rate the intensity (0-100)*	Thought *What were you thinking about at that moment? What was going through your mind at that moment?*

Rating Scale for Physical Symptoms

0 = no physical discomfort
1 = slight physical discomfort, discomfort can be ignored
2 = mild physical discomfort, discomfort can't be ignored but doesn't interfere at all
3 = moderate physical discomfort, discomfort interferes with concentration
4 = severe physical discomfort, discomfort interferes with many activities
5 = very severe physical discomfort, discomfort requires bed-rest

Rating Scale for Emotions

0 = no experience of the specified emotion
1 = the slightest degree possible of the specified emotion
.
.
.
100 = the most intense experience of the specified emotion

Fig. 2. Symptom-monitoring form.

a patient says that her physical sensations included anxiety, the therapist might reply, "I would consider anxiety an emotion, not a physical sensation. So, let's put that in the emotion column. But, sometimes people have physical sensations that accompany anxiety. Did you feel anything in your body, any physical sensation, at that time that coincided with the anxiety?" Similarly, if a patient says that she felt stupid, the therapist should (1) label this experience as that of the evaluative cognition that "I am stupid," (2) distinguish cognition and emotion, and (3) question the patient about the emotion that coincided with that cognition. Also, emphasis is placed on learning to differentiate among emotions: patients are asked to use specific emotion terms such as "sad," "worried," or "annoyed," instead of more nebulous emotion terms such as "stressed," "bad," or "upset."

Many patients presenting with somatization struggle with the self-awareness activities because of difficulties in identifying and differentiating among their thoughts and feelings. Whatever the cause of this difficulty (eg, alexithymia, repressive coping), the authors' efforts focus on enhancing awareness and acceptance of thoughts and feelings. Many patients find that recognizing and expressing thoughts and/or feelings may be the most difficult component of treatment. Nevertheless, these initial skills must be mastered before cognitive restructuring techniques can be taught. Disputing cognitions is futile unless one can identify one's thoughts and feelings. The heightening of patients' self-awareness is facilitated by therapists' refraining from disputing cognitions until a thorough investigation of emotions and their companion cognitions has been conducted. The authors want patients to be able to experience and communicate emotions during a session. This work in session is extended to the patient's life outside of therapy by means of homework assignments that call on the patient to identify and record emotions, as well as associated physical symptoms and thoughts.

Cognitive restructuring

An important component of treatment is to help patients examine their cognitive tendencies. After reviewing a few weeks of a patient's symptom-monitoring forms, the therapist will have a sense of the patient's typical dysfunctional thinking patterns. Typical cognitive errors that the authors have observed include perfectionistic thoughts, catastrophic thoughts (about physical symptoms as well as other life events), overestimating the possibility of negative outcomes, "should" statements, and dichotomous thinking. The authors' sense is that at the core of these errors is a global negative perception of self as being inadequate or unlovable. Although many patients may not acknowledge seeing themselves as inadequate or unlovable, especially in a brief episode of treatment, thoughts about being weak, vulnerable, undesirable, unattractive, or helpless may not be far from the surface when the "meaning" of a thought is explored. Once such dysfunctional beliefs are identified, the authors use cognitive restructuring techniques [68].

Addressing illness behavior

In hopes of interrupting the dysfunctional pattern of physical symptoms prompting physician visits that fail to alleviate or even exacerbate those symptoms, the therapist helps the patient learn to reconsider the thoughts fueling illness behavior. Their patients often make comments like, "There must be something wrong with me that my doctor hasn't found." If such a belief is sound, the rational response is to seek additional diagnostic procedures. Such beliefs may be assailable, however. Patients are encouraged to look at the evidence supporting or undermining that belief. Questions like, "What makes you think there is something medically wrong with you?" or "What evidence is there that the doctor has missed something?" are followed by "What evidence is there that you may not have a serious medical problem?" Also, patients are questioned about the advantages and disadvantages of having another diagnostic procedure. They are asked what would convince them that they are not suffering from the illness they fear. The grounds for the falsification of beliefs are explored extensively to demonstrate that one can never be 100% certain of perfect health. In addition to challenging patients' beliefs associated with illness behavior, the therapist constructs behavioral experiments in which patients test the consequences of avoiding (or, at least, delaying) physician visits. Symptom-monitoring forms are used to assess the impact of modifying this aspect of illness behavior. If patients can delay a physician visit long enough, the somatization symptom that initially prompted the intent to seek medical treatment may subside.

The goal of the sick role discussion is to provide patients with some insight into any secondary gain they might derive while experiencing pain or discomfort and to examine the possibility that illness behavior has become habitual. Having identified the secondary gain, the therapist and patient collaborate to find alternative methods for attaining the sick role's benefits. For example, if the patient's spouse is especially nurturing when the patient is in pain, the authors help the patient ask directly for more attention and affection.

Examining the sick role's benefits is a sensitive issue because family, friends, and physicians may have accused the patient of faking, imagining, or exaggerating symptoms. Thus, the therapist is careful not to imply that the patient is choosing to experience his or her symptoms. The discussion will be fruitless if the patient becomes defensive. Because of the sensitivity of this topic, the authors typically defer its discussion until the third month of treatment.

To avoid raising the patient's defenses initially, the discussion begins by focusing on the patient's perceptions of other people who have been ill, other people whom the patient knows or has known well. The therapist asks who, in the patient's family and social circle, had health problems during the patient's childhood (or during the patient's adulthood, if no one had health problems during the patient's childhood). In the authors' clinical experience, as in research by Craig and colleagues [75], many patients meeting criteria for a somatoform disorder report having observed illness during childhood in either a family member or a close friend. The patient is asked to describe the individual who was ill and to talk about the ways in which that person's life was affected by illness or physical discomfort. Specifically, the therapist asks about the sick person's missed opportunities and missed experiences and how others responded to the person. Next, the therapist inquires into the "silver lining" that being unhealthy may have had for the sick person: "Were there any benefits of being unhealthy for that individual?" If the patient believes there were no benefits, the therapist may ask specifically about each of the following possible benefits: receiving special attention or nurture, avoiding undesirable activities, avoiding arguments, gaining a special role in the family, or diminishing one's own expectations for oneself. Usually the patient acknowledges that the ill individual experienced some benefits from his or her illness.

Having discussed another person's experiences with illness, the therapist shifts the discussion to the impact of illness on the patient's life. The therapist begins with inquiries into the patient's experience of illness as a child: "How did others respond to you when you were sick or in pain as a child?" "Were you taken to the doctor or did you miss school when you were sick?" "Did you receive special attention or treatment when you were sick?" Afterwards, questions focus on the impact of illness during the patient's adult life: "In previous sessions we discussed the many disadvantages of your health problems these days. Are there any advantages to being sick?"

Although almost all of the authors' patients have acknowledged that some benefits accrue from "being sick," therapists often feel anxious during this discussion. It may seem likely that explicit discussion with the patient about the sick role will undermine the therapeutic relationship. In the authors' experience, however, no patient has withdrawn prematurely from treatment after discussing the sick role. Although the topic is sensitive, it can be examined productively.

Often the discussion of the sick role begins to provide a rationale for assertiveness training because it may reveal deficits in the patient's assertiveness. If the patient is deriving substantial attention or nurture through being sick, he or she also may be deficient in the ability to ask directly for attention and nurture. Patients who avoid undesirable activities by being sick may have difficulty setting limits on others. One advantage of the sick role is that people can be rewarded without having to ask directly for what they want. The sick role tends to undermine assertiveness and to provide few opportunities to hone skills of self-assertion, except perhaps in interactions with health care providers.

If the patient acknowledges that the sick role has become "second nature," the authors may borrow a technique of fixed-role therapy [76] and have the patient attempt to play the part of a "healthy person" in one or more activities. One method is to ask the patient to find a role model who is not impaired and to imitate that person's behavior. Another is to have the patient ask the question, "What would a healthy person do in this situation?" and then act out the answer. Occasionally, as much psychologic research has shown, changes in attitudes and emotions follow changes in behavior rather than preceding them. Expanding the range of the patient's behavior before the patient feels "healthy enough" can be effective, if the approach is used judiciously. How much to push somatizers to extend themselves is a matter of clinical judgment. Good therapeutic decisions in this area tend to optimize treatment outcomes.

Assertiveness

At this point in treatment, the therapist will have assessed for deficits in the patient's assertiveness. Some patients assert themselves effectively and have their needs met in some, but not all, situations. Some patients can assert themselves only in regard to certain kinds of needs. Other patients can assert their needs when they are aware of them but may not always be aware of what those needs might be. Other patients have pervasive, traitlike deficits in assertiveness across virtually all areas of their lives. In the authors' experience, all somatization patients have difficulty expressing their thoughts and feelings assertively in, at least, some situations.

The therapist begins by defining assertiveness and explaining the rationale for helping the patient act more assertively in some situations. The authors define assertiveness as an open and honest expression of one's thoughts and feelings that avoids blaming or attacking others. Much of ACBT treatment, up to this point, has provided the groundwork for becoming assertive. For example, the self-awareness exercises and symptom-monitoring forms direct the patient to pay attention to his or her thoughts and feelings. The first stage of acting assertively involves identifying thoughts and feelings. The second stage, valuing one's thoughts and feelings, is implicit in and fostered by some of the behavioral techniques. By taking time to relax and to engage in pleasurable activities, patients, in effect, are affirming the value and legitimacy of taking care of themselves.

Before being introduced to the third stage of assertiveness, patients may need additional work on the first and second stages. Specifically, patients might be asked to track their thoughts and feelings when interacting with others between therapy sessions. (At this point in treatment, unassertive individuals often can identify their thoughts and feelings when they are alone, but they may have difficulty being self-aware while interacting with others, especially others who are accustomed to or expect them to be unassertive.) A homework assignment might be to ask, "What do I think and feel?" during various interactions with others. For patients who continue to have trouble valuing their thoughts and feelings, the therapist should use the technique from fixed-role therapy [76]. Patients are directed to role-play in the outside world, to behave as they would if they really did think their own feelings and needs were important. Through this device, assertive behavior, with a tone of conviction, can be practiced, and the patient can witness its often-successful results. Occasionally patients adopt and assimilate features of this more assertive persona.

The third stage of assertiveness involves communicating one's thoughts, feelings, desires, and needs with "I statements." The therapist suggests the patient use the following statement as a model, "I feel _____, when you _____." An example of content in this form is, "I felt worried when you didn't call to tell me you'd be late coming home from work last night."

By making such a statement, this individual is taking responsibility for her feelings as opposed to blaming others (eg, "You're so selfish not to have called"). Also, the statement is indisputable, because it is an expression of the patient's emotional reaction. The result is that the person being spoken to is somewhat less likely to react defensively than if attacked or explicitly criticized; the person addressed also may be less likely to attempt to refute the assertion itself.

Sessions with spouse or significant other
The goals of including the significant other (domestic partner/spouse) in treatment are to obtain additional information about the patient, to gain the significant other's support for the treatment, and to alter behaviors of the significant other that may reinforce the patient's symptoms or illness behavior. The authors consider this aspect of the treatment to be so valuable that, even when working within their 10-session treatment format, they ask the patient's significant other to attend 1 to 3 of the 10 sessions.

The authors typically invite the significant other to participate in a conjoint session within the first month of treatment. The rationale for meeting together with the patient and significant other is to encourage an open dialogue. In the authors' experience, the therapeutic relationship is not always strong enough to tolerate a therapist's meeting separately with a significant other, because some patients readily become suspicious that "behind my back" others are minimizing their degree of discomfort. Although the authors would like to begin deriving the benefits of including the significant other in treatment as soon as possible, for logistical reasons they typically delay the first conjoint session until they have had some time to develop rapport with the patient. They find the third or forth session works well as an initial conjoint session.

The focus of the conjoint session(s) includes discussions about the rationale for a "stress management" treatment and about how such a treatment could be maximally helpful to the patient. The therapist asks the significant other to comment on the impact of stress on the patient's physical symptoms. Also, the impact of the patient's physical symptoms on the patient's and significant other's lives is examined. Here the authors aim to elicit information and to suggest that the significant other's involvement in treatment may benefit both parties. Reducing the likelihood that the significant other will undermine the treatment is critical.

After clarifying the treatment's rationale, the therapist attempts to determine whether the significant relationship has been impaired by the patient's illness. Somatizers' tendencies to withdraw from activities may diminish pleasure in their significant others' lives as well as in their own. When a patient foregoes couple's activities, such as eating at restaurants, going to movie theaters, dancing, or hiking, the domestic partner and the relationship may suffer. The patient and significant other are asked to think about activities they once and might, yet again, enjoy together. Afterwards, the couple and therapist collaborate to develop a plan for increasing pleasurable conjoint activities. Reengaging in these activities may increase satisfaction with the relationship as well as reduce the patient's focus on his or her symptoms.

A subsidiary aim of the conjoint sessions is to address the couple's communication about the patient's physical symptoms. Initially the therapist asks the couple to describe a few recent discussions about the patient's physical symptoms. Both members of the couple are asked to describe what each said about the symptoms and what each thought and felt at that time. Afterwards, the therapist summarizes and reflects on the couple's communication about the patient's symptoms. Suggestions for alternative modes of interacting, which are less likely to reinforce illness behavior, are provided.

SUMMARY

Patients who have multiple medically unexplained symptoms have baffled and perplexed health care professionals for many years. Given the substantial costs of somatization to both patients and the health care system, there is a pressing need for effective treatments. This article describes a recently developed, evidence-based psychosocial treatment for medically unexplained symptoms and the therapeutic rationale that underlies it. The authors' work provides efficacious treatment options for this refractory and debilitating set of disorders.

References

[1] Woolfolk RL, Allen LA. Treating somatization: a cognitive-behavioral approach. New York: Guilford Press; 2007.

[2] Breuer J, Freud S. Studies on hysteria. Harmondsworth (UK): Penguin; 1974 [Strachey J, Strachey A, Trans.] [original work published 1895].

[3] Stekel W. In: Peculiarities of behaviour, vols. 1–2. London: Williams and Norgate; 1924.

[4] Briquet P. Traité clinique et thérapeutique de l'hystérie. Paris: Bailliére & Fils; 1859.

[5] Dongier M. Briquet and Briquet's syndrome viewed from France. Can J Psychiatry 1983;6: 422–7.

[6] Mai FM, Merskey H. Briquet's treatise on hysteria. A synopsis and commentary. Arch Gen Psychiatry 1980;37:1401–5.

[7] Purtell JJ, Robins E, Cohen ME. Observations on clinical aspects of hysteria: a quantitative study of 50 hysteria patients and 156 control subjects. JAMA 1951;146:902–9.

[8] Perley MJ, Guze SB. Hysteria—the stability and usefulness of clinical criteria. N Engl J Med 1962;266:421–6.

[9] Guze SB. The diagnosis of hysteria: what are we trying to do? Am J Psychiatry 1967;124: 491–8.

[10] Guze SB, Woodruff RA, Clayton PJ. Sex, age, and the diagnosis of hysteria (Briquet's syndrome). Am J Psychiatry 1972;129:745–8.

[11] Feighner JP, Robins E, Guze SB, et al. Diagnostic criteria for use in psychiatric research. Arch Gen Psychiatry 1972;26:57–63.

[12] American Psychiatric Association. Diagnostic and statistical manual of mental disorders. 3rd edition. Washington, DC: American Psychiatric Association; 1980.

[13] American Psychiatric Association. Diagnostic and statistical manual of mental disorders. 4th edition. Washington, DC: American Psychiatric Association; 1994.

[14] World Health Organization. The ICD-9 classification of mental and behavioral disorders: diagnostic criteria for research. Geneva (Switzerland): World Health Organization; 1979.

[15] World Health Organization. The ICD-10 classification of mental and behavioral disorders: diagnostic criteria for research. Geneva (Switzerland): World Health Organization; 1993.

[16] Robins LN, Reiger D. Psychiatric disorders in America: the Epidemiological Catchment Area study. New York: Free Press; 1991.

[17] Weissman MM, Myers JK, Harding PS. Psychiatric disorders in a U.S. urban community: 1975-1976. Am J Psychiatry 1978;135:459–62.

[18] Woodruff RA Jr, Clayton PJ, Guze SB. Hysteria: studies of diagnosis, outcome, and prevalence. JAMA 1971;215:425–8.

[19] Gureje O, Simon GE, Ustun T, et al. Somatization in cross-cultural perspective: a World Health Organization study in primary care. Am J Psychiatry 1997;154:989–95.

[20] Kirmayer LJ, Robbins JM. Three forms of somatization in primary care: prevalence, co-occurrence, and sociodemographic characteristics. J Nerv Ment Dis 1991;179:647–55.

[21] Peveler R, Kilkenny L, Kinmonth AL. Medically unexplained physical symptoms in primary care: a comparison of self-report screening questionnaires and clinical opinion. J Psychosom Res 1997;42:245–52.

[22] Simon GE, Gureje O. Stability of somatization disorder and somatization symptoms among primary care patients. Arch Gen Psychiatry 1999;56:90–5.

[23] Simon GE, Von Korff M. Recall of psychiatric history in cross-sectional surveys: implications for epidemiologic research. Epidemiol Rev 1995;17:221–7.

[24] Martin R. Somatoform disorders in the general hospital setting. In: Judd FK, Burrows GD, Lipsitt DR, editors. Handbook of studies on general hospital psychiatry. New York: Elsevier; 1991. p. 251–65.

[25] Swartz M, Blazer D, George L, et al. Somatization disorder in a community population. Am J Psychiatry 1986;143:1403–8.

[26] Swartz M, Hughes D, George L, et al. Developing a screening index for community studies of somatization disorder. J Psychiatr Res 1986;20:335–43.

[27] Smith GR, Monson RA, Ray DC. Patients with multiple unexplained symptoms: their characteristics, functional health, and health care utilization. Arch Intern Med 1986;146:69–72.

[28] Katon W, Lin E, Von Korff M, et al. Somatization: a spectrum of severity. Am J Psychiatry 1991;148:34–40.

[29] Coryell W, Norten SG. Briquet's syndrome (somatization disorder) and primary depression: comparison of background and outcome. Compr Psychiatry 1981;22:249–56.

[30] Lin EH, Katon W, Von Korff M, et al. Frustrating patients: physician and patient perspectives among distressed high users of medical services. J Gen Intern Med 1991;6:241–6.

[31] Murphy GE. The clinical management of hysteria. JAMA 1982;247:2559–64.

[32] Fallon BA. Pharmacotherapy of somatoform disorders. J Psychosom Res 2004;56: 455–60.

[33] Escobar JI, Burnam MA, Karno M, et al. Somatization in the community. Arch Gen Psychiatry 1987;44:713–8.

[34] Kroenke K, Spitzer RL, de Gruy FV, et al. Multisomatoform disorder: an alternative to undifferentiated somatoform disorder for the somatizing patient in primary care. Arch Gen Psychiatry 1997;54:352–8.

[35] Escobar JI, Waitzkin H, Silver RC, et al. Abridged somatization: a study in primary care. Psychosom Med 1998;60:466–72.

[36] Swartz M, Landermann R, George L, et al. Somatization. In: Robins LN, Reiger D, editors. Psychiatric disorders in America. New York: Free Press; 1991. p. 220–57.

[37] Escobar JI, Rubio-Stipec M, Canino G, et al. Somatic Symptom Index (SSI): a new and abridged somatization construct. J Nerv Ment Dis 1989;177:140–6.

[38] Wool CA, Barsky AJ. Do women somatize more than men? Gender differences in somatization. Psychosomatics 1994;35:445–52.

[39] Golding JM, Smith GR, Kashner M. Does somatization disorder occur in men? Clinical characteristics of women and men with multiple unexplained physical symptoms. Arch Gen Psychiatry 1991;48:231–5.

[40] Rief W, Shaw R, Fichter MM. Elevated levels of psychophysiological arousal and cortisol in patients with somatization syndrome. Psychosom Med 1998;60:198–203.

[41] Barsky AJ. Amplification, somatization, and the somatoform disorders. Psychosomatics 1992;33:28–34.

[42] Rief W, Hiller W, Margraf J. Cognitive aspects of hypochondriasis and the somatization syndrome. J Abnorm Psychol 1998;107:587–95.

[43] Teasdale JD. Negative thinking in depression: cause, effect or reciprocal relationship? Adv Behav Res Ther 1983;5:3–25.

[44] Allen LA, Escobar JI, Lehrer PM, et al. Psychosocial treatments for multiple unexplained physical symptoms: a review of the literature. Psychosom Med 2002;64:939–50.

[45] Blakely AA, Howard RC, Sosich RM, et al. Psychiatric symptoms, personality, and ways of coping in chronic fatigue syndrome. Psychol Med 1991;21:347–62.

[46] Epstein SA, Kay G, Clauw D, et al. Psychiatric disorders in patients with fibromyalgia. A multicenter investigation. Psychosomatics 1999;40:57–63.

[47] Noyes R, Langbehn DR, Happel RL, et al. Personality dysfunction among somatizing patients. Psychosomatics 2001;42:320–9.

[48] Talley NJ, Boyce PM, Jones M. Is the association between irritable bowel syndrome and abuse explained by neuroticism? A population-based study. Gut 1998;42:47–53.

[49] De Gucht V, Heiser W. Alexithymia and somatisation: quantitative review of the literature. J Psychosom Res 2003;54:425–34.

[50] Kirmayer LJ, Robbins JM, Paris J. Somatoform disorders: personality and the social matrix of somatic distress. J Abnorm Psychol 1994;103:125–36.

[51] Kaminsky MJ, Slavney PR. Hysterical and obsessional features in patients with Briquet's syndrome (somatization disorder). Psychol Med 1983;13:111–20.

[52] Izard CE. Four systems for emotion activation cognitive and noncognitive processes. Psych Rev 1993;100:68–90.

[53] LeDoux JE. Emotion: clues from the brain. Ann Rev Psychol 1995;46:209–35.

[54] First MB, Spitzer RL, Gibbon M, et al. Structured clinical interview for DSM-IV axis I disorders (SCID-I). Washington, DC: American Psychiatric Press; 1997.

[55] Smith GR, Monson RA, Ray DC. Psychiatric consultation letter in somatization disorder. N Engl J Med 1986;314:1407–13.

[56] Smith GR, Rost K, Kashner M. A trial of the effect of a standardized psychiatric consultation on health outcomes and costs in somatizing patients. Arch Gen Psychiatry 1995;52:238–43.

[57] Allen LA, Woolfolk RL, Escobar JI, et al. Cognitive-behavioral therapy for somatization disorder: a randomized controlled trial. Arch Intern Med 2006;166:1512–8.

[58] Escobar JI, Gara MA, Diaz-Martinez AM, et al. Effectiveness of a non-pharmacological intervention in primary care patients with medically unexplained symptoms. Ann Fam Med 2007;5:328–35.

[59] Fried R. The role of respiration in stress and stress control: toward a theory of stress as a hypoxic phenomenon. In: Lehrer PM, Woolfolk RL, editors. Principles and practice of stress management. 2nd edition. New York: Guilford; 1993. p. 301–31.

[60] Bernstein D, Carlson CR. Progressive relaxation: abbreviated methods. In: Lehrer PM, Woolfolk RL, editors. Principles and practice of stress management. 2nd edition. New York: Guilford; 1993. p. 53–87.

[61] Linton SJ. Chronic back pain: integrating psychological and physical therapy–an overview. Behav Med 1994;20:101–4.

[62] Lehrer PM, Woolfolk RL. Research on clinical issues in stress management. In: Lehrer PM, Woolfolk RL, editors. Principles and practice of stress management. 2nd edition. New York: Guilford; 1993. p. 521–38.

[63] Kennedy-Moore E, Watson JC. Expressing emotion. New York: Guilford; 1999.

[64] Greenberg LS. Emotion-focused therapy. Washington, DC: American Psychological Association; 2001.

[65] Persons JB. Cognitive therapy in practice: a case formulation approach. New York: W.W. Norton; 1989.

[66] Gendlin ET. Focusing. New York: Bantam; 1981.

[67] Perls F. The Gestalt approach and eyewitness to therapy. Palo Alto (CA): Science and Behavior Books; 1973.

[68] Beck AT. Cognitive approaches to stress. In: Lehrer PM, Woolfolk RL, editors. Principles and practice of stress management. 2nd edition. New York: Guilford; 1993. p. 333–72.

[69] Philips HC, Rachman S. The psychological management of chronic pain: a treatment manual. 2nd edition. New York: Springer Publishing Co; 1996.

[70] Surawy C, Hackmann A, Hawton K, et al. Chronic fatigue syndrome: a cognitive approach. Behav Res Therapy 1995;33:535–44.

[71] Ware NC. Society, mind and body in chronic fatigue syndrome: an anthropological view. In: Bock GR, Whelan G, editors. Chronic fatigue syndrome. Chichester (UK): Wiley; 1993. p. 62–82.

[72] Affleck G, Urrows S, Tennen H, et al. Sequential daily relations of sleep, pain intensity, and attention to pain among women with fibromyalgia. Pain 1996;68:363–8.

[73] Morin CM. Insomnia: psychological assessment and management. New York: Guilford Press; 1993.

[74] Beck AT, Rush AJ, Shaw BF, et al. Cognitive therapy of depression. New York: Guilford Press; 1979.

[75] Craig TKJ, Cox AD, Klein K. Intergenerational transmission of somatization behaviour: a study of chronic somatizers and their children. Psychol Med 2002;32:805–16.

[76] Kelly GA. The psychology of personal constructs. New York: Norton; 1955.

Malingering in the Medical Setting

Barbara E. McDermott, PhD[a,b,*], Marc D. Feldman, MD[c]

[a]University of California, Davis School of Medicine, Department of Psychiatry
and Behavioral Sciences, Division of Psychiatry and the Law, 2230 Stockton Blvd, 2nd Floor,
Sacramento, CA 95817, USA
[b]Clinical Demonstration/Research Unit, Napa State Hospital, 2100 Napa Vallejo Hwy, Napa,
CA 94558, USA
[c]The University of Alabama, Tuscaloosa, 2609 Crowne Ridge Court, Birmingham,
AL 35243–5351, USA

"**M**alingering" is defined as the conscious feigning, exaggeration, or self-induction of illness (either physical or psychological) for an identifiable secondary gain [1]. In the medical setting, that secondary gain can be diverse, including the receipt of monies (legal settlements or verdicts, worker's compensation, disability benefits); the procurement of abusable prescription medications, such as opioids or benzodiazepines; the avoidance of unpleasant work or military duty; or simply access to a warm, dry hospital bed. In other cases, the incentives can be more subtle, such as avoidance of onerous household responsibilities. Malingering is distinguished from factitious disorder by its motivation: in clear-cut cases, the malingerer consciously falsifies or induces illness or symptoms for a specific purpose that is identifiable, once details of the malingerer's life are known. In contrast, in factitious disorder, symptom production is conscious for a primary gain: the assumption of the "sick role" [2]. The reasons that the individual desires the sick role are presumably primarily unconscious [3]. In psychiatry, malingering of mental illness is often suspected in both criminal and civil cases, where the secondary gain can be substantial [4,5]. As noted, malingering in the medical setting has not been studied as extensively. This article discusses the various disorders most commonly malingered in the medical setting, the frequency of such malingering, methods for detection, and finally, recommendations for intervention.

CLASSIFICATION

Diagnostic confusion between malingering and mental disorders, particularly factitious disorder, can be traced to Asher's [6] original description of

*Corresponding author. University of California, Davis School of Medicine, Department of
Psychiatry and Behavioral Sciences, Division of Psychiatry and the Law, 2230 Stockton
Blvd, 2nd Floor, Sacramento, CA 95817. E-mail address: bemcdermott@ucdavis.edu
(B.E. McDermott).

0193-953X/07/$ – see front matter
doi:10.1016/j.psc.2007.07.007

© 2007 Elsevier Inc. All rights reserved.
psych.theclinics.com

Munchausen syndrome. Asher attributed several possible motives to Munchausen syndrome, including "a desire to escape from the police" and "a desire to get free board and lodgings for the night" (339), motives that would now clearly be classified as malingering. The tendency to include malingering within the factitious disorder spectrum was further reinforced by Spiro [7], who recommended that in individuals with Munchausen syndrome, "malingering should only be diagnosed in the absence of psychiatric illness and the presence of behavior appropriately adaptive to a clear-cut long-term goal" (569). Thus, according to Spiro, an individual with a psychiatric disorder of any type cannot be deemed a malingerer. There are, however, many examples of patients with factitious disorder who also malinger [8]. Eisendrath [9] described three such individuals, all of whom entered into civil litigation as a result of their feigned physical illnesses. In each case, it appeared that the feigned illness was intended to allow the individual to assume the sick role and only later was used to pursue financial incentives.

The term "malingering by proxy" has been suggested [10] for those cases in which illness is fabricated in a child for secondary gain—for example, for the purpose of obtaining social assistance benefits [11]. The literature contains several case reports of parents who report, or induce their children to report, disability for the purpose of litigation and ultimately remuneration [12,13].

Various types of malingerers have been identified. As described by Resnick [14], their behaviors can include pure malingering, partial malingering, and false imputation. In pure malingering, the individual is fabricating a condition that does not exist and has never existed. In partial malingering, the individual is exaggerating symptoms that actually exist. False imputation refers to an individual's ascribing symptoms to a cause that is actually unrelated. For example, in personal injury litigation, an individual might claim pain from a motor vehicle accident when in fact the pain is secondary to an unrelated fall. Most detection methods target either pure or partial malingering, as the presumption in false imputation is that the symptom is real; only the source of the symptom is in question.

The Diagnostic and Statistical Manual, 4th edition text revision (DSM-IV-TR) [15] classifies malingering with a "V" code, indicating, "Other conditions that may be the focus of clinical attention." In this nomenclature, malingering is not considered to be a mental disorder. Instead, by definition it is "the intentional production of false or grossly exaggerated physical or psychological symptoms motivated by external incentives" (739). The DSM provides four guidelines for when to suspect malingering, including (1) the evaluation occurs in a medico-legal context, (2) a discrepancy exists between the person's claims and objective findings, (3) the individual is uncooperative during the diagnostic evaluation and is noncompliant with the prescribed treatment regimen, and (4) antisocial personality disorder is present. However, many experts consider this definition overly broad and inclusive, leading to the risk of overidentification of patients as malingerers. For example, Rogers [16] noted that use of these guidelines as criteria for detecting malingering (ie, an individual who meets two of the four criteria) leads rather impressively to the correct classification of approximately two-thirds of true malingerers. However, he determined that this strategy led to the overclassification of true psychiatric patients as malingerers. Rogers concluded that persons meeting two of the four DSM-IV-TR criteria have only a one in five chance of being true malingerers. An 80% false positive rate is inordinately high and generally considered unacceptable.

Rogers [17] described three models to explain the underlying motivation of an individual who malingers: the pathogenic model, the criminological model, and the adaptational model. Although the pathogenic model no longer receives general support [18], it warrants an historical discussion. In this model, the malingerer's motivation is based on true pathology. The production of symptoms is postulated to be an effort to gain control over real symptoms. The eventual outcome is the replacement of feigned symptoms with real ones. However, research has not shown this prediction to hold true [19]. The criminological model presumes an underlying "badness" of the malingerer and is based on the DSM suggestions for when to be suspicious of malingering. As Rogers [20] noted, "a bad person in bad circumstances (legal difficulties) who is performing badly (uncooperative)" (7) is considered highly likely to malinger in the criminological model. Finally, the motivation can be understood within the adaptational model, wherein the malingerer evaluates the cost-benefit of his or her options. In this model, malingering may be more likely under three circumstances: (1) when the context is adversarial, (2) when the personal stakes are high, and (3) when there are no viable alternatives. An individual feigning mental illness when faced with a life sentence is an example of this model. It is important to note that these models only provide explanations for the behavior; they are not intended as prescriptions for the detection of malingering.

In a study evaluating the correlates of malingering, Sierles [21] asked 172 Veterans Administration patients and 160 medical students, a control group, to complete a questionnaire designed to assess the frequency and potential indicators of malingering in various types of patients. The sample included patients from acute medical, surgical, psychiatric, substance dependence, and alcohol detoxification services. The questionnaire contained a list of 59 problems; the individuals were asked if they had ever reported any of these as problems for which a physician could find no organic basis, and a malingering index score was calculated. An individual was considered to have a pattern of medically unexplained symptoms if 20 or more items from the list were endorsed. In addition, Sierles included items that were indicative of the respondent's being sociopathic. He found that being a sociopath and having a drug or alcohol diagnosis increased the likelihood of malingering. The study revealed that, of the individuals evaluated, medical and surgical patients were the least likely to admit ever to having malingered; they received a malingering index score even slightly lower than that of the medical students.

DIFFERENTIAL DIAGNOSIS

There are five conditions from which malingering must be differentiated: undetected physical pathology, three of the somatoform disorders, and factitious disorder.

Undetected or Underestimated Physical Illness

Malingering, like somatoform disorders and factitious disorder, is a diagnosis of exclusion. Patients who present with unexplained somatic complaints may actually have an illness that is not detected during an initial evaluation, or even with subsequent testing. Physicians may be inclined at that point to presume the patient is malingering. While it may be nearly impossible to rule out every conceivable occult physical pathology that is responsible for the presentation of a patient who might be malingering, physicians should reasonably consider whether the evaluation has been adequate. Further testing must be balanced with the possibility of a nonorganic etiology, as physicians can engender serious iatrogenic problems by overtesting and overtreating. A rule of thumb is to seriously consider and evaluate malingering before advancing to highly esoteric physical diagnoses.

Pain Disorder and Somatization Disorder

Cases of pain disorder involve persistent complaints of pain that are not accounted for by tissue damage. Somatization disorder cases involve chronic, unpleasant symptoms (often including pain) that appear to implicate multiple organ systems. In both, it is presumed that the patient actually experiences the pain he or she is reporting. The pain complaints may covary with psychological stressors. Unlike malingering, the pain reported in these disorders is not under conscious control, nor is it motivated by external incentives. However, there are no reliable methods for affirmatively establishing that pain and other complaints are unconscious and involuntarily produced [22].

Hypochondriasis

Hypochondriasis is diagnosed in patients who unconsciously interpret physical sensations as indicative of serious disease. The patient may present with minor pains that he or she fears indicate some unrecognized, potentially life-threatening illness. These patients are eager to undergo diagnostic evaluations of all kinds. In contrast, the malingerer is often uncooperative with the diagnostic process and, unlike those with hypochondriasis, is unlikely to show any relief or pleasure (albeit temporary) in response to negative test results. When hypochondriac patients do simulate or self-induce illness, the deceptions reflect a desperate need to convince physicians to perform further tests [22].

Factitious Disorder with Predominantly Physical Signs and Symptoms

As in malingering, factitious physical disorders involve the feigning, exaggeration, or self-induction of medical illness. However, the fraudulent complaints cannot be adequately explained by external incentives. Rather, the factitious disorder patient will welcome the chance to undergo medical and surgical procedures—including those that most people would seek to avoid—because they find the sick role intrinsically gratifying. Malingerers, conversely, seek to minimize medical contacts through which their deceptions might be uncovered.

EPIDEMIOLOGY

While almost any medical illness can be malingered, there is evidence that certain types of medical problems are more likely to be malingered than others. In a study of over 30,000 cases referred to 144 neuropsychologists, the most likely ailment to be malingered was mild head injury, followed by fibromyalgia or chronic fatigue syndrome, pain, neurotoxic disorders, electrical injury, seizure disorders, and moderate or severe head injury [23]. In another report, malingerers more commonly presented with cervical pain and repetitive strain injuries, accessing general practitioners, rheumatologists, neurologists, and orthopedic and hand surgeons [22]. These differences are likely reflective of the types of individuals surveyed: neuropsychologists are more likely to evaluate individuals referred for head trauma, while general practitioners are more likely to be contacted for pain complaints.

Just as the frequency of malingered mental illness varies depending on the context (ie, criminal, civil, or military evaluations), estimates of malingering in the medical setting vary considerably. For example, in a study surveying 105 board-certified orthopedic surgeons and neurosurgeons from six states, estimates of the percentages of their patients with low back pain who were malingering varied widely, from a low of 1% to a high of 75% [24]. However, the majority of the surgeons made low estimates, with 78% indicating that 10% or fewer of their patients malingered their pain. Factors that surgeons most strongly considered in making their estimates were not in fact related to secondary gain, but were more closely associated with inconsistencies in the medical examination. The two inconsistencies most frequently cited as suggestive of malingering were weakness in the exam not seen in other activities, and disablement disproportionate to the objective findings. Other studies suggest that the incidence of malingered pain is significantly higher. For example, estimates of malingering range from 25% to 30% for fibromyalgia cases [25], with similar results found for patients malingering chronic pain [26].

The literature also contains inconsistencies regarding the incidence of malingering in mild head trauma, with some authors suggesting that malingering is common [27–29] and others suggesting that it is rare [30]. Rogers [31] estimated that approximately half of the individuals evaluated for personal injury claims were feigning all or part of their cognitive deficits. In a meta-analysis of the effect of financial incentives on neuropsychological symptoms, Binder and colleagues [32] reaffirmed that compensation is critical. Their results indicated that more abnormalities and disabilities were reported in patients with financial incentives, even if injuries were less severe. The highest rates of malingering of medical illness appear related to personal injury litigation, worker's compensation, or disability claims [23]. For example, Greiffenstein and colleagues [33] found a 37% base rate of malingering in individuals with mild head injury who were seeking compensation of some sort. Along these lines, several studies have indicated that patients with milder injuries or fewer symptoms were more likely to seek compensation [34,35]. Symptoms appearing long after the alleged injury—which have been shown to be less likely to have an organic etiology [36]—occurred more frequently in patients pursuing financial compensation. Similarly, a shorter duration of amnesia was correlated with failure to return to work. Larrabee [37], in a review of 11 studies, found a prevalence rate of malingering of 40% in 1,363 patients who were seeking compensation for a mild head injury. Various signs were suggested as indicative of the possibility of malingering, including a severity of impairment that is inconsistent with mild trauma, discrepancies in the records, inconsistencies in self-report versus observed behavior, and implausible self-reported symptoms. In support of these detection strategies, Binder and colleagues [38] found that 95% of authentic mild head trauma cases evidence no impairment three months after the trauma.

In the aforementioned study of 144 neuropsychologists [23], estimates of malingering varied by referral type. When the referral was made secondary to a personal injury claim, estimates of malingering were 30%; for disability or worker's compensation cases, estimates were as high as 33%. Malingering was estimated in 23% of individuals facing criminal cases. In contrast, the estimate was only 8% for cases without any known external incentive. When patients were in litigation, the neuropsychologists estimated that 41% referred for mild head injury were malingering, as compared with 37% for fibromyalgia and 33% for pain. They also determined that when patients were referred by defense attorneys for civil cases, estimates for malingering were even higher. These results suggest that, in contrast to malingered mental illness, which more often occurs in the context of criminal charges to reduce or eliminate sentencing, the malingering of physical illness is substantially related to financial incentives.

DIAGNOSIS

In addition to the office or hospital, malingerers also often present to emergency departments or urgent care centers, generally "doctor-shopping" if their initial efforts to procure secondary gain (ie, abusable medications for their own use or for resale) are unmet by the physicians seen initially. When pursuing drugs, they may report an unusually large number of drug allergies to steer the physician toward prescribing their drug of choice, or simply insist on a specific product, such as meperidine (Demerol).

The malingerer who seeks to avoid an immediate predicament might feign an acute problem, while those seeking a permanent disability judgment will feign a subacute medical problem that is recognizable to the examiner when the malingerer's stressors are known [22].

Physicians are trained to assess and treat individuals who actually have medical or mental health symptoms. A health care provider's natural inclination—one reinforced by education and training—is to accept the person's reported symptoms at face value. Rosenhan [39] conducted a famous study that demonstrated clinicians' tendency to blindly accept reported mental health symptoms. In this study, eight nonmentally ill individuals presented to a psychiatric hospital alleging that they were hearing very atypical voices. Based on this one reported symptom, every person was admitted to the hospital and given a diagnosis of schizophrenia, even though each person ceased reporting any symptoms after admission.

Clinicians should be aware that malingering for compensation of various types may be unplanned. The patient may seize upon an incidental workplace or motor vehicle accident as a fortuitous opportunity for financial gain. It also appears, at least anecdotally, that there is an increased frequency of disability claims in families in which a family member has already been declared disabled.

Citing Hamilton and Feldman [22], "it is against [the malingerer's] interests to acknowledge any improvement in their condition or even any palliative effects of medicine, corrective surgery, or physical therapy. The one exception to this may be in cases of sophisticated patients who admit to partial or temporary relief of pain to enhance their credibility" (448).

Eisendrath, Rand, and Feldman [40] offered a list of potential correlates of illness deception (Box 1). However, their validity and reliability have not been formally researched.

DETECTION OF MALINGERED PAIN

The detection of malingered pain is often extremely difficult, in large part because the experience of pain is so subjective [41,42]. Additionally, as is so often cited for malingered mental illness, it is much easier to malinger that with which you have had experience.[1] It is relatively easy to malinger pain because everyone has had the experience of pain and therefore knows how it should appear to others. Hamilton and Feldman [22] note that the malingerer's pain complaint "will vary according to the medical sophistication of the patient; they may present with diffuse pain, or patterns of pain that are not consistent with known medical conditions or with the anatomy of the peripheral nervous system" (444-5). In particular, these cases may present as specific maladies, such as repetitive strain injury or variable limb pain (ie, in reflex sympathetic dystrophy, fibromyalgia, or chronic fatigue syndrome), though the bulk of the literature has focused on low back pain or pain related to the cervical and thoracic spine (especially whiplash injuries). The malingerer commonly knows the characteristics of the pain associated with the condition he or she is feigning. One unfortunate result of the wide availability of high quality medical information on the Internet is that malingerers now have abundant guidance on how to convincingly display pain and disability [22].

There are no objective laboratory tests that allow examiners to independently quantify pain without the use of patient self-report. Although initially thermography was considered to be promising as an independent method for evaluating pain, it has fallen out of use because it was shown to be

---

[1]Although technically, Resnick would describe this phenomenon as partial malingering.

Box 1: Potential indicators of malingering

1. The signs and symptoms do not improve with treatment. There is escalation of symptoms, relapse, or new complaints apparently in the service of keeping the caregivers engaged.

2. The magnitude of symptoms consistently exceeds what is usual for the disease or there is evident dishonesty about the presentation of symptoms.

3. Some findings are determined to have been self-induced, or at least worsened through self-manipulation.

4. There are remarkable numbers of tests, consultations, and treatment efforts, to no avail.

5. The individual disputes test results that do not support the presence of authentic disease.

6. The individual accurately predicts physical deteriorations.

7. The individual "doctor shops" and has sought treatment at an unusual number of facilities.

8. The individual emerges as an inconsistent, selective, or misleading source of information.

9. The individual refuses to allow the treatment team access to outside information sources.

10. There is a history of so many medical treatments for secondary problems that the impression is created that the individual must be astonishingly unlucky. (This "black cloud" phenomenon may strain credulity to the breaking point.)

11. Deception is explicitly considered by at least one health care professional, if evidenced merely by a brief chart entry.

12. The individual does not follow treatment recommendations and is intensely disruptive.

13. The individual focuses on his or her self-perceived "victimization" by medical personnel and others.

14. There is consistent evidence from laboratory or other tests that disproves information supplied by the individual.

15. The individual has had exposure to a model of the ailment they are falsifying (eg, a relative with a similar ailment).

16. Even while pursuing medical or surgical assessment, the individual vigorously opposes psychiatric assessment and treatment.

17. During interviews, the individual makes statements to strengthen his or her case that nevertheless contradict the records.

18. There is evidence for external incentives for illness or incapacity.

Adapted from Eisendrath SJ, Rand DC, Feldman MD. Factitious disorders and litigation. In Feldman MD, Eisendrath SJ editors. The spectrum of factitious disorders. Washington (DC): American Psychiatric Press, Inc., 1996. p. 65–82; with permission.

nonspecific [43]. While the self-report Minnesota Multi-Phasic Personality Inventory, 2nd edition (MMPI-2) [44] has been used with considerable success in identifying malingering of mental illness [45], it is less effectively used with malingered medical illnesses. However, in one study [46], MMPI-2 profiles were compared between pain patients who were and were not involved in litigation. The investigators found that pain patients in litigation endorsed more obvious and fewer subtle items. They found inconsistent support for using the "Conversion V" as an identifier of litigants. These results provide modest support for the use of the MMPI-2 in the detection of malingered pain. However, although many patients in litigation are also malingering, the two groups may not be identical in regards to psychological profiles.

The Symptom Checklist-90-Revised (SCL-90-R) [47], a self-report checklist containing 90 items targeting a wide range of psychological problems, also has been used to identify genuine pain patients. In a simulation study, Wallis and Bogduk [48] found that, consistent with research on the simulation of mental illness, patients who malinger pain frequently "overendorse" symptoms. Simulators scored significantly higher than true whiplash patients on all SCL-90-R subscales.

In a study designed to evaluate the effectiveness of three scales in identifying malingerers, Larrabee [49] found that one instrument, the Modified Somatic Perception Questionnaire; [50], distinguished malingerers from nonmalingerers with a sensitivity and specificity of 0.90. In a series of simulation studies, McGuire and colleagues [51] evaluated the effectiveness of using the Pain Patient Profile (P3); [52] in identifying malingerers. The P3 contains three clinical scales: depression, anxiety, and somatization, as well as a validity scale. They found that simulators were more likely to score above a t-score of 55 on all three scales, although the depression scale had the highest positive and negative predictive power. The investigators concluded that this instrument shows promise in the detection of malingered pain, though the inventory and its use require more study.

Several studies have been designed to evaluate whether facial expressions of pain are useful in identifying simulators. Various investigators have found that judges consistently ascribed higher levels of pain to simulators, even when given feedback or advance warning [53,54]. Thus, attempting to detect malingering by evaluating the degree of the patient's pained expression appears fruitless.

Regarding physical examinations, expected signs of injury or disease will be absent or inadequate to account for the patient's reported degree of pain. Because they are still commonly applied, "Waddell signs" will be mentioned. In the 1980s, Waddell indicated that certain signs were suggestive of nonorganic pain or "illness behavior" [55,56]. These signs were divided into five general categories, including tenderness, simulation, distraction, regional, and overreaction. Table 1 presents the complete list of signs. Since being published, these signs of illness behavior have often been viewed as suggestive of malingering. However, in a review of the literature on this point, Fishbain and colleagues [57] found inconsistent evidence. In one study, Waddell signs were

Table 1
Waddell signs

Category	Sign
Tenderness	Superficial skin tender to light touch
	Nonanatomic deep tenderness not localized to one area
Simulation	Axial loading on skull induces lower back pain
	Shoulder and pelvis rotated in same plane induces pain
Distraction	Difference in straight leg raising in supine versus sitting position
Regional	Many muscle groups evidence weakness
	Sensory loss in stocking or glove distribution
Overreaction	Disproportionate facial or verbal expressions

associated with poorer outcomes, but the signs did not discriminate organic from nonorganic pain [58].

In a review examining various physical tests of malingering [58], including Waddell signs, the investigators found support for using two (of the seven described) for detecting nonorganic symptoms. The two for which the investigators found consistent support were both for detecting nonorganic paralysis. The Hoover's test [59] and the abducter test [60], both of which involve manipulation of the legs, show promise in detecting malingered leg paresis. In an article written for family physicians, Kiester and Duke [61] offered additional suggestions for detecting malingered pain including, for example, checking shoes for uneven wear in patients limping into the office; manual laborers claiming inability to work but having callouses, dirt, or lacerations on their hands; and patients who do not injure themselves upon fainting or collapsing. The reader is also referred to the groundbreaking and colorful books on malingering by Gavin [62] and Collie [63], in which other clues to malingering, many still viable, are presented.

DETECTION OF MALINGERED HEAD TRAUMA

While pain is ubiquitous, fortunately head trauma and subsequent cognitive deficits are relatively uncommon. As a result, the associated patterns of test results expected from certain central nervous system injuries may be less well known to the casual observer. Thus, standard neuropsychological assessments can be useful in identifying individuals who exaggerate such deficits. Various instruments have been developed to detect this type of malingering.

The assessments of malingered head trauma and related cognitive deficits fall into six general types of detection strategies [31]: the floor effect, performance curve, magnitude of errors, symptom validity testing, atypical presentation, and psychological sequelae. The floor effect refers to the inability of individuals to perform extremely simple tasks. The Rey 15-item memory test [64] is an example of such an assessment. This test requires that individuals remember a set of 15 letters, numbers, and geometric shapes that are in fact quite simple. Individuals attempting to malinger memory deficits often miss more than truly impaired individuals do because of their efforts at deception. The performance curve strategy is based on the supposition that malingerers do not distinguish between easy and difficult items. Thus, their performance curve can be compared with those of individuals with true deficits and discrepancies noted. The Validity Indicator Profile [65] is an example of this strategy. The magnitude of errors method is derived from research indicating that malingerers give larger numbers of near misses and grossly wrong responses to standardized tests [66]. Symptom validity testing requires a forced choice assessment (ie, the patient must choose between two or more responses). Response rates below chance are indicative of malingering. The Victoria Symptom Validity Test [67] is an example of this type of assessment. Atypical presentation occurs when the response patterns exhibited are significantly different from those of true patients. The primary limitation of this method of detection is that nonmalingerers can sometimes exhibit this pattern. For example, in a simulation study using the Bender Gestalt [68], standard scoring did not identify malingerers from nonmalingerers. However, in this study, a forensic psychologist was able to identify simulators with 100% accuracy. The final method is psychological sequelae and is based on research that suggests that individuals malingering medical illnesses are likely to exaggerate psychological symptoms as well [69–71].

Recently, response time has been proposed as an additional strategy. Resnick [72] theorized that increased response latency may occur for two reasons: simulators may overestimate the response time in individuals with a true traumatic brain injury, and latency may be increased secondary to the time it takes a malingerer to decide on an appropriate (wrong) response. Several investigators have examined this strategy with inconsistent results. For example, Rees and his colleagues [73], on the Test of Malingered Memory (TOMM), found that simulators have longer reaction times on correct responses. Strauss and colleagues [74,75] found that reaction time was longer on a symptom validity task in simulators (as compared with controls) and that this difference was more pronounced with more difficult items. In contrast, Rose and colleagues [76] found that controls and simulators had the same reaction time to a digit recognition test. However, the combination of response latency and number of correct responses improved the discriminating ability of the test.

Several authors have provided guidelines for when to suspect malingering of cognitive deficits. Greiffenstein and colleagues [77] indicated that the examiner should suspect malingered memory deficits under the following circumstances: (1) poor performance on two or more standard neuropsychological assessments, (2) complete disability in a social role, (3) inconsistency between reported symptom history and other sources of information, and (4) remote memory loss. Pankratz and Binder [78] suggested seven behaviors that are indicative of malingering and require further exploration. The first and foremost is dishonesty: if patients misrepresent details of their lives, they may also be misrepresenting their symptoms. Additionally, the following six are suggestive of malingering: (1) inconsistency between reported and observed symptoms, (2) inconsistency between physical and neuropsychological findings, (3) resistance to or avoidance of standardized tests, (4) failure on measures designed to detect malingering, (5) functional findings on medical examination, and (6) delayed cognitive complaints following trauma.

Faust and Ackley [79] also suggest six behaviors that are indicative of feigned cognitive deficits: (1) poor effort, (2) exaggerated symptoms, (3) production of nonexistent symptoms, (4) distortion of history regarding symptoms, (5) distortion of premorbid functioning, and (6) denial of strengths. Slick and colleagues [80] have proposed a much more complicated schema for the detection of malingered cognitive deficits, which includes four criteria, designated as Criteria A through D. Criterion A is the presence of financial incentive. Criterion B includes evidence of exaggeration on neuropsychological tests. Criterion C includes evidence of false or exaggerated self-report, and Criterion D is that both criteria B and C cannot be accounted for by psychiatric, neurological, or developmental factors. An individual can be considered a "probable malingerer" when Criterion A is met and two or more items (of a list of six) are met from Criterion B or one from B and one from C (of a list of five). Possible malingering is defined as the presence of Criterion A plus two (or more) items from Criterion C. More simply put, these investigators believe that self-report evidence (other than an admission of malingering) is only suggestive of malingering; evidence of malingering on standard neuropsychological testing is necessary to be more definitive.

In a recent survey of neuropsychologists who consistently practice in the area of compensation claims [81], more than 45% indicated that they routinely use the TOMM [82], and more than 33% indicated that they use the Rey 15-item Test [64]. As suggested, both instruments were designed specifically for the detection of malingering. Other specialized tests were used with less frequency. An exhaustive list of instruments developed for the purpose of detecting malingered cognitive deficits is beyond the scope of this article. However, Table 2 provides a list of the more commonly used assessment tools and many more are discussed by Pope at http://www.kspope.com/assess/malinger.php. Most of these instruments require administration by a psychologist with specific training.

OTHER MALINGERED ILLNESSES

While pain (ie, lower back pain, cervical pain—primarily from whiplash injuries—and fibromyalgia) and mild head injury (including associated cognitive

Table 2
Selected memory and cognitive tests

Memory tests	Ease of administration	Brief description
Victoria Symptom Validity Test	Requires training	Computer administered, forced choice; 24 easy, 24 difficult items, response time also recorded
Rey 15-item	Simple	15 different items shown, told to reproduce as many as can
Test of Memory Malingering (TOMM)	Requires training	2 alternative forced choice, 50 target pictures, recognize from 50 presentations of 2 pictures
Portland Digit Recognition Test	Requires minimal training	72 items, 26 easy, 36 hard; verbal presentation of 5-digit number, 5, 10 & 30 sec. delay
Digit memory test	Requires minimal training	3 blocks of 24 5-digit numbers; forced choice with 5, 10 & 15 sec. delay
Reliable digit span	Requires training on Wechsler Adult Intelligence Scale (WAIS-III)	Based on WAIS-III digit span subtest; sum longest string of digits passed on both trials forward and backward
Word Completion Memory Test (WCMT)	Requires training	2 subtests: Inclusion (30 items), Exclusion (30 items); copies and rates words; is a priming task
Word Memory Test (WMT):	Requires minimal training	20 linked word lists; oral and computerized version
Other cognitive deficits	Ease of administration	Brief description
Validity Indicator Profile	Requires training	100 problems assessing nonverbal abstraction; 78 word definition problems; 2 alternative forced choice
Cognitive behavioral driver's inventory	Requires training	10 tasks in part adapted from other instruments; requires specialized equipment
Computerized assessment of response bias	Requires training	Computer administered; 25 trials of 5-digit string; response time also recorded

deficits and memory loss) are the most common medical illnesses feigned, the literature reveals various other illnesses that may be malingered. For example, both cognitive deficits and psychological sequelae are frequently attributed to toxic exposures, especially because the injuries related to such exposure may be ambiguous [83]. Psychogenic seizures are another ailment identified in some malingering investigations. In a study of psychogenic seizures, Abubakr and colleagues [84] found that almost 22% of the patients were malingering and all but one had financial incentives to do so. Similar results were found by Cragar and colleagues [85]. Huang [86] even reported a case of an individual malingering HIV illness to obtain housing.

While malingering can occur in any setting for multiple reasons, malingering in the medical setting is often associated with financial incentives. As indicated, the detection of malingering can be complex and may involve specialized testing. However, the hallmark of malingering is the inconsistency between reported symptoms and collateral reports, observed behaviors, and physical and psychological assessments.

TREATMENT

When a determination of malingering is made, the clinician is faced with the dilemma of how to "treat" a nondisorder. Depending on the situation, the clinician may elect to confront the individual with the assessment. Pankratz and Erickson [87] emphasize the importance of permitting the malingerer to save face. Kiester and Duke [61] recommend explaining to patients that they do not have a serious problem and that deterioration is not expected. They also recommend assisting in replacing the patient's illness behavior with other, more psychologically healthy behaviors. However, these interventions are predicated on a certain level of psychological health. When there are substantial secondary gains, such as large sums of money, such interventions may well be ineffective. In these cases, referral to a mental health professional also may be fruitless. In some cases, though, such a referral facilitates an exploration of some of the psychological or social deficits for which the patient compensates through his or her malingering.

Any attempted management of malingering must first be based on an understanding of the motivations for symptom production [88]. Blatant malingering may arise from the same types of enduring personality traits that are observed in antisocial personality disorder (ASPD), such as a tendency to manipulate others for personal gain. A number of other psychological problems—some viewed as treatable and others as refractory, such as ASPD—may contribute to the drive to malinger. These problems include anxiety, depression, and other personality disorders more amenable to intervention. Treatment of these underlying or coexisting mental disorders may reduce the patient's self-perceived need to malinger.

Overall, management of milder forms of malingering may benefit from the kinds of interventions advocated for factitious disorder [89]. They are beyond the scope of this article. It is important to note, however, that caregivers' aversion to malingering can translate into overly harsh confrontations and dismissals from further care. Consistent with the face-saving strategies noted, a nonconfrontational approach can allow the patient to relinquish the complaints without admitting that symptoms have been falsified.

References

[1] Fishbain DA. Secondary gain concept—definition problems and its abuse in medical-practice. J Pain 1994;3:264–73.

[2] Parsons T. The social system. Glencoe (IL): Free Press; 1951.

[3] Eisendrath SJ. Psychiatric aspects of—chronic pain. Neurology 1995;45:S26–34.

[4] Rogers R, Sewell KW, Goldstein AM. Explanatory models of malingering: A prototypical analysis. Law Hum Behav 1994;18:543–52.

[5] Rogers R. Conducting Insanity Evaluations. New York: Van Nostrand Reinhold; 1986.

[6] Asher R. Munchausen's syndrome. Lancet 1951;1:339–41.

[7] Spiro HR. Chronic factitious illness: Munchausen's syndrome. Arch Gen Psychiatry 1968;18:569–79.

[8] Feldman MD. Illness or illusion? Distinguishing malingering and factitious disorder. Prim Psychiatry 1995;2:39–41.

[9] Eisendrath SJ. When Munchausen becomes malingering: Factitious disorders that penetrate the legal system. Bull Am Acad Psychiatry Law 1996;24:471–81.

[10] Bools C. Factitious illness by proxy: Munchausen syndrome by proxy. Br J Psychiatry 1996;169:268–75.

[11] Cassar J, Hales E, Longhurst J, et al. Can disability benefits make children sicker. J Am Acad Child Adolesc Psychiatry 1996;35:700–1.

[12] Stutts JT, Hickey SE, Kasdan ML. Malingering by proxy: a form of pediatric condition falsi-fication. J Dev Behav Pediatr 2003;24:276–8.

[13] Lu PH, Boone KB. Suspect cognitive symptoms in a 9-year-old child: malingering by proxy? Clin Neuropsychol 2002;16:90–6.

[14] Resnick PJ. The detection of malingered mental illness. Behav Sci Law 1984;2:20–38.

[15] American Psychiatric Association: Diagnostic and statistical manual of mental disorders, 4th edition, text revision. Washington (DC): American Psychiatric Association; 2000.

[16] Rogers R. Development of a new classificatory model of malingering. Bull Am Acad Psychiatry Law 1990;18:323–33.

[17] Rogers R. Models of feigned mental illness. Prof Psychol Res Pr 1990;21:182–8.

[18] Vitacco JM, Rogers R. Assessment of malingering in correctional settings. In: Scott CL, Gerbasi JB, editors. Handbook of correctional mental health. Washington (DC): American Psychiatric Publishing; 2005. p. 133–53.

[19] Resnick PJ. Malingered psychosis. In: Rogers R, editor. Clinical assessment of malingering and deception. 2nd edition. New York: Guilford; 1997. p. 47–67.

[20] Rogers R. Introduction. In: Rogers R, editor. Clinical assessment of malingering and deception. 2nd edition. New York: Guilford Press; 1997. p. 1–9.

[21] Sierles FS. Correlates of malingering. Behav Sci Law 1984;2:113–8.

[22] Hamilton JC, Feldman MD. "Chest pain" in patients who are malingering. In: Hurst JW, Morris DC, editors. Chest pain. Armonk (NY): Futura Publishing Co., Inc.; 2001. p. 443–56.

[23] Mittenberg W, Patton C, Canyock EM, et al. Base rates of malingering and symptom exaggeration. J Clin Exp Neuropsychol 2002;24:1094–102.

[24] Leavitt F, Sweet JJ. Characteristics and frequency of malingering among patients with low back pain. Pain 1986;25:357–64.

[25] Gervais RO, Russell AS, Green P, et al. Effort testing in patients with fibromyalgia and disability incentives. J Rheumatol 2001;28:1892–9.

[26] Gervais RO, Green P, Allen LM, et al. Effects of coaching on symptom validity testing in chronic pain patients presenting for disability assessments. Journal of Forensic Neuropsychology 2001;2:1–19.

[27] Binder LM. Persisting symptoms after mild head injury: a review of the postconcussive syndrome. J Clin Exp Neuropsychol 1986;8:323–46.

[28] Binder LM. Assessment of malingering after mild head trauma with the Portland digit recognition test. J Clin Exp Neuropsychol 1993;15:170–82.

[29] Guilmette TJ, Whelihan W, Sparadeo FR, et al. Validity of neuropsychological test results in disability evaluations. Percept Mot Skills 1994;78:1179–86.

[30] Leininger BE, Gramling SE, Farrell AD, et al. Neuropsychological deficits in symptomatic minor head injury patients after concussion and mild concussion. Journal of Neurology, Neurosurgery & Psychiatry 1990;53:293–6.

[31] Rogers R, Harrell EH, Liff CD. Feigning neuropsychological impairment: a critical review of methodological and clinical considerations. Clin Psychol Rev 1993;13:255–74.

[32] Binder LM, Rohling ML. Money matters: meta-analytic review of the effects of financial incentives on recovery after closed-head injury. Am J Psychiatry 1996;153:7–10.

[33] Greiffenstein MF, Baker WJ. Miller was (mostly) right: head injury severity inversely related to simulation. Legal and Criminological Psychology 2006;11:131–45.

[34] Millis SR. The recognition memory test in the detection of malingered and exaggerated memory deficits. Clin Neuropsychol 1992;6:406–14.

[35] Alexander MP. Neuropsychiatric correlates of persistent post-concussive syndrome. J Head Trauma Rehabil 1992;7:60–9.

[36] Fenton G, McClelland R, Montgomery A, et al. The postconcussional syndrome: Social antecedents and psychological sequelae. Br J Psychiatry 1993;162:493–7.

[37] Larrabee GJ. Detection of malingering using atypical performance patterns on standard neuropsychological tests. Clin Neuropsychol 2003;17:410–25.

[38] Binder LM, Rohling ML, Larrabee GJ. A review of mild head trauma: I. meta-analytic review of neuropsychological studies. J Clin Exp Neuropsychol 1997;19:421–31.

[39] Rosenhan DL. On being sane in insane places. Science 1973;179:250–8.

[40] Eisendrath SJ, Rand DC, Feldman MD. Factitious disorders and litigation. In: Feldman MD, Eisendrath SJ, editors. The spectrum of factitious disorders. Washington (DC): American Psychiatric Press, Inc; 1996. p. 65–82.

[41] Cunnien AJ. Psychiatric and medical syndromes associated with deception. In: Rogers R, editor. Clinical assessment of malingering and deception. 2nd Edition. New York: Guilford; 1997. p. 23–46.

[42] Craig KD, Badali MA. Introduction to the special series on pain deception and malingering. Clin J Pain 2004;20:377–82.

[43] Mendelson G, Mendelson D. Malingering pain in the medicolegal context. Clin J Pain 2004;20:423–32.

[44] Butcher JN, Dahlstrom WG, Graham JR, et al. MMPI-2: manual for administration and Scoring. Minneapolis (MN): University of Minnesota Press; 1989.

[45] Rogers R, Sewell KW, Salekin RT. A meta-analysis of malingering on the MMPI-2. Assessment 1994;1:227–37.

[46] Dush DM, Simons LE, Platt M, et al. Psychological profiles distinguishing litigating and non-litigating pain patients: Subtle, and not so subtle. J Pers Assess 1994;62:299–313.

[47] Derogatis LR. Symptom Checklist-90-Revised (SCL-90-R): administration, scoring and procedures manual. Minneapolis (MN): National Computer Systems; 1994.

[48] Wallis BJ, Bogduk N. Faking a profile: can naive subjects simulate whiplash responses? Pain 1996;66:223–7.

[49] Larrabee GJ. Exaggerated pain report in litigants with malingered neurocognitive dysfunction. Clin Neuropsychol 2003;17:395–401.

[50] Main CJ. The modified somatic perception questionnaire (MSPQ). J Psychosom Res 1983;27:503–14.

[51] McGuire BE, Harvey AG, Shores EA. Simulated malingering in pain patients: A study with the pain patient profile. Br J Clin Psychol 2001;40:71–9.

[52] Tollison DC, Langley JC. Pain patient profile manual. Minneapolis (MN): National Computer Services; 1995.

[53] Craig KD, Prkachin KM, Grunau RV. The facial expression of pain. New York: Guilford Press; 1992.

[54] Poole GD, Craig KD. Judgments of genuine, suppressed, and faked facial expressions of pain. J Pers Soc Psychol 1992;63:797–805.

[55] Waddell G, McCulloch JA, Kummel E, et al. Non-organic physical signs in low-back pain. Spine 1980;5:117–25.

[56] Waddell G, Bircher M, Finlayson D, et al. Symptoms and signs: physical disease or illness behavior. Br Med J 1984;289:739–41.

[57] Fishbain DA, Cutler RB, Rosomoff HL, et al. Is there a relationship between nonorganic physical findings (Waddell signs) and secondary Gain/Malingering? Clin J Pain 2004;20: 399–408.

[58] Greer S, Chambliss L, Mackler L. What physical exam techniques are useful to detect malingering? J Fam Pract 2005;54:719–22.

[59] Hoover CF. A new sign for the detection of malingering and functional paresis of the lower extremities. J Am Med Assoc 1908;51:746–7.

[60] Sonoo M. Abductor sign: a reliable new sign to detect unilateral non-organic paresis of the lower limb. J Neurol Neurosurg Psychiatr 2004;75:121–5.

[61] Kiester PD, Duke AD. Is it malingering, or is it 'real'? Eight signs that point to nonorganic back pain. Postgrad Med 1999;106:77–80, 83.

[62] Gavin H. On feigned and factitious diseases. London: John Churchill; 1843.

[63] Collie J. Malingering and feigned sickness. London: Edward Arnold; 1913.

[64] Lezak MD. Neuropsychological assessment. 3rd edition. New York: Oxford; 1995.

[65] Frederick RI, Foster HG. The validity indicator profile. Minneapolis (MN): National Computer Systems; 1997.

[66] Powell JB, Cripe LI, Dodrill CB. Assessment of brain impairment with the Rey Auditory verbal learning test: a comparison with other neuropsychological measures. Arch Clin Neuropsychol 1991;6:241–9.

[67] Slick DJ, Hopp G, Strauss EH, et al. The Victoria Symptom Validity Test. Odessa (TX): PAR; 1997.

[68] Bruhn AR, Reed MR. Simulation of brain damage on the bender-gestalt test by college subjects. J Pers Assess 1975;39:244–55.

[69] Heaton RK, Smith HH, Lehman RA, et al. Prospects for faking believable deficits on neuropsychological testing. J Consult Clin Psychol 1978;46:892–900.

[70] Clayer JR, Bookless C, Ross MW. Neurosis and conscious symptom exaggeration: Its differentiation by the illness behaviour questionnaire. J Psychosom Res 1984;28: 237–41.

[71] Furnham A, Henderson M. Response bias in self-report measures of general health. Pers Individ Dif 1983;4:519–25.

[72] Resnick PJ. Malingered psychosis. In: Rogers R, editor. Clinical assessment of malingering and deception. 2nd edition. New York: Guilford Press; 1988. p. 47–67.

[73] Rees LM, Tombaugh TN, Gansler DA, et al. Five validation experiments of the Test of Memory Malingering (TOMM). Psychol Assess 1998;10:10–20.

[74] Strauss E, Hultsch DF, Hunter M, et al. Using intra-individual variability to detect malingering in cognitive performance. Clin Neuropsychol 2000;14:420–32.

[75] Strauss E, Slick DJ, Levy-Bencheton J, et al. Intra-individual variability as an indicator of malingering in head injury. Arch Clin Neuropsychol 2001;17:423–44.

[76] Rose FE, Hall S, Szalda-Petree AD. Portland Digit Recognition Test-Computerized: Measuring response latency improves the detection of malingering. Clin Neuropsychol 1995;9: 124–34.

[77] Greiffenstein MF, Baker WJ, Gola T. Validation of malingered amnesia measures with a large clinical sample. Psychol Assess 1994;6:218–24.

[78] Pankratz L, Binder LM. Malingering on intellectual and neuropsychological measures. In: Rogers R, editor. Clinical assessment of malingering and deception. 2nd edition. New York: Guilford Press; 1997. p. 223–38.

[79] Faust D, Ackley MA. Did you think it was going to be easy? Some methodological suggestions for the investigation and development of malingering detection techniques. In: Reynolds CR, editor. Detection of malingering during head injury litigation. New York: Plenum Press; 1998. p. 1–54.

[80] Slick DJ, Sherman EM, Iverson GL. Diagnostic criteria for malingered neurocognitive dysfunction: proposed standards for clinical practice and research. Clin Neuropsychol 1999;13:545–61.

[81] Slick DJ, Tan JE, Strauss EH, et al. Detecting malingering: A survey of experts' practices. Arch Clin Neuropsychol 2004;19:465–73.

[82] Tombaugh TN. Test of Memory Malingering (TOMM). New York: Multi-Health Systems; 1996.

[83] Greve KW, Springer S, Bianchini KJ, et al. Malingering in toxic exposure: Classification accuracy of reliable digit span and WAIS-III digit span scaled scores. Assessment 2007;14:12–21.

[84] Abubakr A, Kablinger A, Caldito G. Psychogenic seizures: clinical features and psychological analysis. Epilepsy Behav 2003;4:241–5.

[85] Cragar DE, Berry DT, Fakhoury TA, et al. Performance of patients with epilepsy or psychogenic non-epileptic seizures on four measures of effort. Clin Neuropsychol 2006;20:552–6.

[86] Huang D, Salinas P, Dougherty D. Feigned HIV in a malingering patient. Psychosomatics 2001;42:438–9.

[87] Pankratz L, Erickson RC. Two views of malingering. Clin Neuropsychol 1990;4:379–89.

[88] Adetunji BA, Basil B, Mathews M, et al. Detection and management of malingering in a clinical setting. Prim Psychiatry 2006;13:61–9.

[89] Hamilton JC, Feldman MD. Factitious disorder and malingering. In: Gabbard GO, editor. Gabbard's treatments of psychiatric disorders. 4th edition. Washington (DC): American Psychiatric Publishing, Inc.; 2007. p. 629–35.

Psychiatr Clin N Am 30 (2007) 663–676

PSYCHIATRIC CLINICS
OF NORTH AMERICA

Legal Concerns in Psychosomatic Medicine

Rebecca W. Brendel, MD, JD[a,b,*], Ronald Schouten, MD, JD[a,c]

[a]Department of Psychiatry, Massachusetts General Hospital, Harvard Medical School, 15 Parkman Street, WAC 812, Boston, MA 02114, USA
[b]Massachusetts General Hospital Psychiatry Consultation Service and Law and Psychiatry Service, Boston, MA, USA
[c]Massachusetts General Hospital Law and Psychiatry Service, Boston, MA, USA

L
egal concerns often arise in the context of medical practice, and the field of psychosomatic medicine is no exception. In the practice of psychosomatic medicine, legal issues may arise for many reasons. For example, the treatment of patients with psychiatric illness may focus particular attention on sensitive issues such as confidentiality and the limits thereof. Second, medical and surgical colleagues often consult psychiatrists for legal and quasi-legal questions such as a patient's decision-making capacity and treatment refusal, perhaps because these issues involve assessment of mental reasoning and abnormal behavior [1]. Finally, medicine is practiced in the context of an increasingly complex society with competing values and interests, and these tensions often emerge at the level of the individual patient. Examples include cases of risk of harm to third parties and malpractice liability.

The law provides a framework that affects certain aspects of how psychosomatic medicine is practiced. That framework is often invisible, yet it exerts its effect at some of the most challenging points in rendering care to patients. As a result, it is important for physicians to be familiar with the applicable laws in the jurisdictions in which they practice and the resources available to them to obtain consultation and support around complex legal issues. This article will address many of the legal issues commonly encountered in psychosomatic medicine, including confidentiality, capacity and competency, informed consent, treatment refusal, substitute decision making, and malpractice. Overall, however, it is most important for physicians to recognize that the best way to avoid entanglements with the law is through the consistent provision of sound clinical care to their patients.

*Corresponding author. Department of Psychiatry, Massachusetts General Hospital, Harvard Medical School, 15 Parkman Street, WAC 812, Boston, MA 02114. E-mail address: rbrendel@partners.org (R.W. Brendel).

0193-953X/07/$ – see front matter
doi:10.1016/j.psc.2007.07.010 © 2007 Elsevier Inc. All rights reserved.
psych.theclinics.com

CONFIDENTIALITY

Confidentiality has been a cornerstone of the doctor–patient relationship since at least 430 BC when it was codified in the Hippocratic Oath, "Whatever I see or hear, professionally or privately, which ought not to be divulged, I will keep secret and tell no one" [2]. Since the time of Hippocrates, doctor–patient confidentiality has remained an important ethical, professional, and legal requirement in the practice of medicine [3–6]. However, the ideal of absolute confidentiality between doctor and patient has come into conflict with other considerations in a complex society. Over time, a number of exceptions to the rule of confidentiality have emerged. Historically, these narrow exceptions to confidentiality occurred either where courts or legislatures determined that confidentiality would cause more harm than good, or where confidentiality would run counter to an important societal safety interest.

Tarasoff and the Duty to Protect

The duty to protect third parties from physical harm by patients is one well-known potential exception to confidentiality [1]. In the California decision of *Tarasoff v Board of Regents*, the court held that psychotherapists have a duty to act to protect third parties when the therapist knows or should know that the patient poses a threat of serious harm to the third party [7]. In reaching this conclusion, the court relied on a balancing analysis of patients' rights to privacy and the public interest, "The Court recognizes the public interest in supporting effective treatment of mental illness and in protecting the rights of patients to privacy. But this interest must be weighed against the public interest in safety from violent assault" [7].

Not all jurisdictions recognize the duty to protect [8,9]. Many states have passed statutes that address the duty to protect third parties, and others have either limited the scope of or eliminated the duty [10,11]. State statutes generally limit the circumstances in which a duty to protect arises. For example, state law may require a specific threat to an identifiable third party, a known history of violence on the part of the patient, and/or a reasonable reason to anticipate violence. In addition, state laws may also delineate the measures that may be taken to discharge the duty to warn, such as notifying police or other law enforcement agencies, hospitalizing a patient, or warning the potential victim. One state that employs this approach is Massachusetts [12].

In the context of psychiatric consultation to medical and surgical services, psychiatrists and other mental health professionals should also be aware of the scope of duty to protect laws in the jurisdictions in which they practice because these statutes may apply to psychiatrists and mental health professionals but not to physicians in general [12]. In these jurisdictions, the psychiatric consultant may have a legal obligation to warn a third party beyond that of the physician requesting the consultation. In some situations, the psychiatrist's duty to warn might even run counter to competing legal requirements for the primary treatment team [12–14]. For example, Massachusetts requires physicians, in general, to keep HIV-related information confidential, but also imposes a duty to protect on psychiatrists. In the case of an HIV-positive individual who is putting an unknowing sexual partner at risk, medical and surgical physicians are bound by the HIV confidentiality statute, whereas psychiatrists have competing obligations under the HIV and *Tarasoff*-inspired statutes.

As highlighted in the above scenario, treating patients with HIV and other infectious diseases may present a tension between confidentiality and the well-being of third parties or society at large. In fact, one of the historic precedents that the *Tarasoff* court used in its reasoning was the existence of mandated reporting of certain communicable diseases, which predated wider duties to protect third parties [7]. States and the federal government, for example, have laws regarding which communicable diseases must be reported to state authorities and/or the Centers for Disease Control. Common examples include varicella, hepatitis, severe acute respiratory syndrome, and HIV, but the list of reportable infectious diseases is generally lengthy so physicians should be aware of the requirements in the jurisdictions in which they practice [15–17]. Especially regarding HIV, jurisdictions vary regarding what information must be reported, whether reporting is anonymous, whether written permission is required to release information, and whether spousal notification is required [14,16,17]. In addition, doctors have been held civilly liable in cases both predating and since *Tarasoff* for failure to disclose a patient's infectious disease status that led to the infection of other individuals [18–21].

The tension between confidentiality and risk to third parties in the context of infectious disease, and HIV in particular, is not a new one. The Council on Ethics and Judicial Affairs of the American Medical Association recognized the need for legal guidance in this area 2 decades ago when it called for states to draft laws that provided liability protection for physicians for failure to warn contacts of their HIV-positive patients, that established clear guidelines for physician reporting to public health agencies, and that would guide public health personnel in the tracing of individuals at risk of exposure to HIV [22]. As it presently stands, the American Medical Association has called for continued efforts to address confidentiality issues that may emerge in the treatment of HIV-positive individuals. However, physicians are still left without concrete, legal guidance in many situations [14,23].

Overall, it is critical for psychiatrists to be aware of the applicable laws in the jurisdictions in which they practice and to be cognizant of available legal and risk-management resources should a complex situation arise in which the applicable laws appear to conflict with each other. As a rule of thumb, however, the starting point for practically approaching situations in which the psychiatrist may have a duty to share patient information is from the original position of doctor–patient confidentiality. Confidentiality is a cornerstone of the doctor–patient relationship and, as such, breaches for any reason should be carefully considered. Clinicians should always limit the amount of information disclosed to the minimum necessary to achieve the purpose of the disclosure and attempt to make clinical interventions, such as hospitalization of the patient or otherwise engaging the patient in a safe plan, before resorting to releasing information to any third party [24].

Abuse and Neglect

Unlike the duty to warn, there is no ambiguity about the responsibility of physicians in the United States to report child and elder abuse and neglect to state authorities; every state has legislation that mandates physicians to report child and elder abuse and neglect [25–28]. However, although federal law sets a minimum definition for what actions and/or failures to act constitute child abuse and neglect, states have interpreted the federal definition in different ways leading to jurisdictional differences in laws [25,27,28]. In general, states employ a definition of child abuse incorporating "harm or substantial risk of harm" or "serious threat or serious harm" to a person under the age of 18 [27].

Similar to child abuse, the definitions of elder abuse and neglect vary between jurisdictions, but most state laws include five common elements: infliction of pain or injury, infliction of emotional or psychologic harm, sexual assault, material or financial exploitation, and neglect [26]. Elders are also at risk for self-neglect as their mental and physical functional abilities decline [29]. As mandated reporters, physicians should familiarize themselves with both reporting requirements and available screening and investigative resources in the jurisdictions in which they practice, especially because one of the barriers to reporting elder abuse and neglect may be inadequate detection [30].

There is often concern that reporting abuse or neglect to state agencies is a breach of doctor–patient confidentiality that could leave physicians legally liable for damages. It is critical for physicians to be aware that liability attaches for failure to report, and that good-faith reporting in reliance on the law is a valid defense to a civil suit for breach of confidentiality brought by or on behalf of the patient. Finally, most jurisdictions employ a reasonable suspicion standard for reporting suspected child abuse or neglect, which means that the reporting physician or other covered provider must exercise professional judgment and good faith in making a report of suspected abuse or neglect, but need not have definitive proof or evidence that such abuse or neglect has occurred [1,26–28].

Health Insurance Portability and Accountability Act

When Congress passed the Health Insurance Portability and Accountability Act of 1996 (HIPAA) [31], physicians—and psychiatrists in particular—were concerned about the impact of this new federal legislation on the handling of confidential patient information, which was previously regulated mostly by state law. Specific concern focused on how HIPAA might alter the tradition of doctor–patient confidentiality and affect record keeping in psychiatry because the law promulgated new rules governing the management of health information that applied to physicians who perform certain electronic transactions, including billing [32]. Because hospitals perform the electronic functions covered by HIPAA, most, if not all, consultation liaison psychiatrists are covered by the provisions of HIPAA.

HIPAA governs the management of "protected health information," which includes information that identifies a patient (such as name or social security number), is about a mental or physical condition, describes services or treatment provided, or relates to payment [33]. The main provisions of HIPAA that are relevant to the practice of psychosomatic medicine relate to disclosure of medical information, patient access to information, and a new category of record established under HIPAA called "psychotherapy notes." Overall, as the following discussion will elucidate, rather than increasing the privacy of medical records, HIPAA had the opposite effect of increasing the circumstances under which protected health information could be released without specific consent from patients [25,32,34].

When lawmakers passed HIPAA, they aimed to improve the efficiency and effectiveness of the health care system [31]. In categorizing what information is considered protected health information under HIPAA, lawmakers had to recognize that although confidentiality and privacy are important considerations in medical practice, the concept of medical records as "locked files" in an office cabinet is outdated, and the functioning of a complex health care system requires sharing of information between multiple entities on a regular basis [32]. The implementation of HIPAA addressed these concerns by allowing covered entities to release protected health information for the purposes of treatment, payment, and health care operations without specific authorization or consent by the patient [32]. This decision by lawmakers to abolish the consent requirement for the release of patient medical information raised concern among advocates of medical privacy, who worried that the new era of medical information management would progressively eclipse patient confidentiality in the interest of furthering the administrative and operational needs of the modern health care system [34–36].

Of note, HIPAA does place some limits on disclosure by requiring covered entities such as hospitals to inform patients of the institution's practices under HIPAA in the form of privacy notices. In addition, patients may request records of disclosures of their protected health information. Finally, federal and state laws that grant additional protection to sensitive health information preempt HIPAA so that written informed consent may still be required for its release. Examples of these types of information include records relating to HIV status and treatment, genetic testing, records from alcohol and substance abuse treatment programs, and domestic violence and sexual assault records [25,32].

In the past, psychiatric records and medical records were often treated differently. For example, at our institution, pre-HIPAA, psychiatry notes were redacted from the general medical chart when records were released to patients. HIPAA, however, gives a broad right of access to patients for their medical records with only a narrow exception. Under HIPAA, a patient's access to records may be denied only if a licensed professional reasonably determines that releasing the record would harm, endanger the life of, or jeopardize the physical safety of the patient or another person [32]. Except in the narrow circumstance of harm avoidance, all records, medical and psychiatric, in the patient's medical chart are accessible by the patient.

HIPAA does provide a narrow exception for "psychotherapy notes," but this exception is exceedingly narrow and does not cover most documentation of psychotherapy sessions per se. Specifically, psychotherapy notes are defined in HIPAA as clinician's notes that document or analyze the contents of a conversation that occurs during a private counseling session, and are kept separate from the rest of the individual's record. Even if these notes are kept in a separate location, certain information is not subject to the psychotherapy notes provision, including medications, test results, diagnoses and prognosis, progress, and treatment plans [5,37]. Patients do not have the right to access psychotherapy notes, but there is no prohibition on access to these notes, either [37]. For these notes to be released for any purpose, specific authorization is required. Finally, even though psychotherapy notes are kept separately from the medical chart, they are considered to be part of the medical record for legal purposes should the record be subpoenaed for litigation [1].

Two additional considerations regarding HIPAA are that it sets the minimum requirements regarding the protection of health information and does not prevent the release of information in emergency settings or settings in which there are mandated reporting obligations. In other words, states are free to promulgate legislation that provides greater protection for patient information than HIPAA provides, and HIPAA continues to permit disclosure of information in situations that are already part of general practice such as emergencies and mandated reporting, in addition to 11 other circumstances [1,5]. Finally, even though HIPAA permits disclosure without consent in many situations, it is critical to use clinical judgment in determining the minimum necessary information that needs to be disclosed to fulfill the specific purpose for which it is being released [32].

TREATMENT: CONSENT AND REFUSAL

Consultation psychiatrists are often asked to assess the quality of a patient's decision-making process, especially when the patient refuses an intervention that the treating doctors believe has a favorable risk–benefit profile for the patient's condition. This threshold assessment of decision-making ability is a capacity assessment. Capacity is a clinical determination of an individual's ability to perform a task or execute a set of functions. The legal equivalent of capacity is competency, which is a judicial determination. In the eyes of the law, all adults are presumed competent [1,38–40].

Competency, or lack thereof, may be global, as in the case of a patient in a coma. More commonly, however, the assessment of capacity and competency is task specific. In the area of civil law, examples of specific competencies are testamentary capacity (the ability to make a will), decision-making capacity (the ability to consent or refuse treatment), and testimonial capacity (the ability to testify in court.) Because different tasks require different abilities, information, and levels of understanding, the first step in making a capacity determination is to ask the basic question, "Capacity for what?" An understanding of the type of decision the patient is faced with—for example, accepting or refusing a recommended procedure, refusing all treatment, refusing or accepting placement—allows the consultant to assess the degree to which the patient understands the particular information relevant to the decision.

Capacity Assessment

A patient's capacity to make a medical decision rests on an understanding of the illness, the proposed treatment, and the consequences of the treatment. Appelbaum and Grisso [41] have proposed a practical framework for capacity assessment that relies on a four-prong analysis. All four criteria must be met for the patient to demonstrate capacity. The criteria are: preference, factual understanding, appreciation of the significance of the facts presented (often referred to as a more nuanced or global understanding of risks and benefits), and rational manipulation of information.

In assessing preference, the relevant question is whether the patient is able to state a stable preference. A patient who is either unable or unwilling to express (or commit to) a preference presumptively lacks capacity. The second element, factual understanding, may be assessed by asking if the patient has attained knowledge of the nature of the illness, the treatment options, the prognosis with and without treatment, and the risks and benefits of treatment. In determining whether a patient has a factual understanding or is capable of developing one, it is critical to ascertain what efforts have been made by the treating physicians and other staff to educate the patient about the proposed treatment. A patient who has never been informed about the proposed treatment cannot be expected to know the relevant medical information. The patient must have the ability to retain the information when it is presented and use it in the decision-making process.

Third in the assessment of capacity is the determination of whether the patient appreciates the significance of the information presented. Appreciation goes beyond the facts; it requires the patient to achieve a broad perspective on the risks and benefits of accepting or refusing a proposed intervention and to demonstrate an understanding of the implications the decision will have for his or her future. Last, the patient must demonstrate that his or her decision-making process is a rational one. This element takes into account the patient's past preferences and life decisions, and focuses not on the rationality of the final decision but on the process by which the patient arrived at the final decision. For example, in the case of a Jehovah's Witness who would certainly live with a blood transfusion but certainly die without it, the decision to reject the blood transfusion might, on its face, seem irrational. However, the decision conceptualized in the context of the individual's life of faith and belief that acceptance of such treatment would be contrary to religious doctrine, would be considered a rational one.

Informed Consent

Capacity is a threshold finding for the ability to consent to or refuse medical treatment. In civil law, any unauthorized touching is considered a battery, and medical interventions are no exception. In the context of treatment, a patient must give informed consent before any medical intervention can begin [42]. Even though the term informed consent is used, patients' refusal of treatment must also be informed. The concept of informed consent has been a cornerstone of medical treatment since the 1960s, and grew out of the broader concept of autonomy before it appeared in the medical context [43,44]. Informed consent is the process by which the patient agrees to allow the physician or other treater to do something to or for him or her. Informed consent is not just signing a form; instead, the emphasis should be on the process of communication, information exchange, and acceptance or rejection of the proposed intervention by the patient [40].

The legal standard for informed consent incorporates two elements in addition to the threshold requirement of capacity. Informed consent must be knowing (or intelligent) and voluntary [42,45–48]. The standard for what information is required for consent to be knowing or intelligent varies from jurisdiction to jurisdiction. There are two general approaches to determining how much information a physician must present to a patient for consent given by that patient to meet the knowing criteria [40]. The first, known as the "reasonable professional standard," is clinician-focused. The second, known as the "reasonable patient standard," is patient-focused. The reasonable professional standard is followed by a small majority of states. This approach requires clinicians to provide the amount of information to the patient that a reasonable professional would provide under the same or similar circumstances. On the other hand, the reasonable patient standard employed by a substantial minority of states requires clinicians to provide the amount of information that would be used by a reasonable or average patient in making an informed decision. Some states employing the patient-centered approach go further, requiring an inquiry into what information the particular patient would find material or relevant in making thi sparticular decision [49]. Finally, two states use a mixed approach in determining the amount of information required [50].

From the practical perspectives of clinical practice and risk management, the general rule of thumb is that the more information provided the better. Overall, whatever the jurisdiction, clinicians will be in good stead if they provide six broad categories of information:

1. the diagnosis and the nature of the condition being treated;
2. the reasonably expected benefits from the proposed treatment;
3. the nature and likelihood of the risks involved;
4. the inability to precisely predict results of the treatment;
5. the potential irreversibility of the treatment; and,
6. the expected risks, benefits, and results of alternative, or no, treatment [50].

Overall, a process involving frank discussion and exchange of information between the doctor and the patient is seen as the ideal of informed consent [50].

Finally, there are limits to the amount of information physicians are responsible for sharing in the course of informed consent. For example, the Massachusetts Supreme Judicial Court has acknowledged the need for a balance between patients' right to know, fairness to doctors, and a more general societal interest that the law not place "unrealistic and unnecessary burdens" on clinicians [51].

Voluntariness is the second fundamental element of informed consent. Consent must be given without coercion, that is, without external forces that limit the ability of the patient to exercise a choice [42,52,53]. The distinction between a voluntary and a coerced choice is a complex inquiry [54]. For example, in general, individuals pressured by their family members to make a certain decision or to agree to a medical treatment are generally found to have acted voluntarily both from ethical and legal perspectives, although exceptions do exist [55,56]. On the other hand, although there is debate on the issue, individuals who are totally dependent on others for their care, such as residents of long-term care facilities and prisoners, are often categorically deemed unable to give voluntary consent to treatment and research because of the inherent unequal balance of power between the patient and the institutional administration or authorities [57–60].

In certain limited circumstances, informed consent is not required for the initiation of treatment. These settings, however, should be considered the exception and not the rule [61–63]. The most common of these exceptions is for emergency treatment, defined as situations in which failure to treat would result in serious and potentially irreversible deterioration of the patient's condition. Treatment under the emergency exception may only continue until the patient is stabilized, and at that time informed consent must be obtained. In addition, if the physician has knowledge that a patient would have refused the emergency treatment, if competent, the patient's prior expressed wishes cannot be overridden by the emergency.

The other generally acknowledged exceptions to the informed consent requirement are waiver and therapeutic privilege [61–63]. A patient may waive consent and opt to defer to the judgment of the clinician or another individual, but it should be well documented that the patient has the capacity to waive informed consent [42]. In the case of therapeutic privilege, a physician may proceed with a proposed intervention by getting consent from an alternate decision maker if the consent process itself would contribute to a worsening of the patient's condition [48,64]. Therapeutic privilege does not apply, however, in a situation where providing information to the patient might make the patient less likely to accept treatment. Overall, therapeutic privilege and waiver are extremely narrow categories, and represent exceptions to the doctrine of informed consent that should be used in only the most carefully considered, well-defined circumstances.

Advance Directives and Substitute Decision Making

When a patient lacks capacity and is unable to give informed consent or refusal for medical treatment, principles of law and ethics require that someone give authorization for medical intervention or nonintervention. This other person is referred to as a substitute decision maker who is charged with making decisions for the patient. In most circumstances, the substitute decision maker is required to make decisions according to what the patient would have wanted were the patient able to make his or her own decisions. This standard is known as substituted judgment. In some circumstances, especially involving guardianships and minors, the substitute decision maker may be asked to make decisions according to the patient's best interests [40].

Substitute decision makers may be appointed in several different ways. One method of appointing a substitute decision maker is through an advance directive. An advance directive is a document crafted by an individual to appoint a substitute decision maker or give instructions about how to make future decisions should the person become incapacitated and unable to make his or her own decisions in the future. Two common types of advance directives are the health care proxy and the durable power of attorney. They are both characterized by the presence of a "springing clause." That is, the documents take no effect until a future time when a patient is deemed to lack decision-making ability. When such a time comes, the documents "spring" or become active, and the terms of the advance directive are activated. Advance directives may have an instructional component directing further care in the event of future incapacity, appoint a substitute decision maker, or be a hybrid with an instructional component and appointment of a substitute decision maker.

Notwithstanding the 1990 passage of federal law that required the provision of information about advance directives, the documentation of existing directives, and the education of health care staff and the community about advance directives, most individuals still do not have advance directives [65,66]. In the absence of an advance directive, several options may exist for how to proceed in the treatment process. Some states, such as Illinois, have statutes that govern how to appoint substitute decision makers in the absence of an advance directive [67]. In Illinois, in the event that an incapacitated person has no advance directive, the law gives the highest priority to the patient's guardian, followed by spouse, adult child, and then parent as the order in which another individual should be appointed as a substitute decision maker, and then continues along progressively more distant blood relatives, ending with a close friend or the guardian of the estate [67].

In states where there is no statutory provision, the options vary by jurisdiction, the nature of the treatment, and the severity and expected duration of the incapacity. For example, in situations where the treatment is of low risk, consent is often obtained from family at the bedside. This practice may also be employed for other treatment decisions, depending on the jurisdiction [14,40]. However, as proposed treatments become increasingly intrusive, aggressive, or risky, the need for a formally designated substitute decision maker increases. State statutes and case law may determine whether a formal mechanism such as guardianship or court approval is required for a particular intervention. Depending on the jurisdiction and the proposed intervention, such formal mechanisms may be required even when the treating physician believes the intervention is routine. One example is the use of antipsychotic medications in Massachusetts [68].

MALPRACTICE

As professionals, psychiatrists owe a duty of care to their patients, both ethically and legally. Malpractice law is the area of tort law that deals with personal injuries caused by the treatment activities of medical professionals [1,69]. To establish a malpractice claim, four elements must be met. First, it must be established that a doctor–patient relationship existed, which imposed a duty of reasonable care on the physician with regard to the patient. Second, it must be shown that the physician breached that duty. Third, it must be shown that the breach, or dereliction, of the duty directly caused the patient's harm. Fourth, it must be shown that the patient suffered damage as a result of the physician's actions or inactions [1,39,52,69]. The elements of a malpractice action are often termed the four "D"s: duty, dereliction of duty, direct causation, and damages.

Malpractice is a tort of negligence. It occurs when a physician's or other professional's conduct and practice deviate from the accepted standard of care for the profession, and that deviation causes damage to the patient or recipient of care. Negligence is an unintentional tort, meaning that the deviation from the accepted level of care need not be purposeful or intended by the physician. Finally, a national standard of care is generally employed as the benchmark for whether the physician's duty was breached.

There is often confusion about the responsibility and liability of physicians acting in a consultative capacity. Treating clinicians have the primary duty of care for the patient. On the other hand, consultants do not have the same duty to the patient [62]. The duty of the consultant is to the consultee, or the requesting physician. In other words, the consultant must provide consultation with reasonable care. However, once consultants cross the boundary between advising the consultee and actually providing treatment to the patient, the consultant owes the patient the same standard of care as the treating physician. For example, if the consultant recommends that the consultee prescribe a medication to the patient, the duty is to the consultee. However, if the consultant enters the order and actually prescribes the medication to the patient, the consultant will be held to the level of care of a treating physician. It is thus important for the consultant to be aware of his or her role in the treatment of the patient, and to maintain clear division of tasks with the consultee regarding all psychiatric interventions in the care of the patient. Additionally, if the consultant does assume a treating role, then he or she should be cognizant of the need to monitor and follow-up on the patient as if he or she is the primary treating psychiatrist.

SUMMARY

In the practice of psychosomatic medicine, the psychiatric consultant is likely to be confronted with questions at the interface of psychiatry and law. These issues generally emerge around questions of confidentiality and exceptions to confidentiality, assessments of a patient's ability to consent to and refuse treatment, and concerns about malpractice liability. Overall, psychiatrists should approach the care of patients clinically, while understanding the applicable laws and regulations of the jurisdictions in which they practice. In addition, clinicians should be aware of the legal and risk management resources available to them should a complex situation arise. Finally, the psychiatric consultant should make use of consultation when complex issues emerge at the interface of psychiatry and law.

References

[1] Schouten R, Brendel RW. Legal aspects of consultation. In: Stern TA, Fricchione GL, Cassem EH, et al, editors. The Massachusetts General Hospital Handbook of General Hospital Psychiatry. 5th edition. Philadelphia: Mosby, Inc.; 2004.

[2] Hippocrates. The Oath. Translated by J Chadwick and WN Mann. In: Lloyd GER, editor. Hippocratic Writings. London: Penguin Books; 1983. p. 67.

[3] American Psychiatric Association. Position Statement on Confidentiality. Washington, DC: American Psychiatric Association; 1978.

[4] American Psychiatric Association. The principles of medical ethics with annotations especially applicable to psychiatry. Available at: http://www.psych.org/psych_pract/ethics/medicalethics2001_42001.cfm. Accessed September 26, 2007.

[5] Appelbaum PS. Privacy in psychiatric treatment. Am J Psychiatry 2002;159:1809–11.

[6] Brendel RW, Brendel DH. Professionalism and the doctor–patient relationship in psychiatry. In: Stern TA, editor. The Ten-Minute Guide to Psychiatric Diagnosis and Treatment. New York: Professional Publishing Group; 2005. p. 1–7.

[7] Tarasoff v. Board of Regents of the University of California. [17], 425. 1976. Cal.3d.

[8] Almason AL. Personal liability implications of the duty to warn are hard pills to swallow: from Tarasoff to Hutchinson v. Patel and beyond. J Contemp Health Law Policy 1997;13:471–96.

[9] Ginsberg B. Tarasoff at thirty: victim's knowledge shrinks the psychotherapist's duty to warn and protect. J Contemp Health Law Policy 2004;21:1–35.

[10] Appelbaum PS, Zonana H, Bonnie R, et al. Statutory approaches to limiting psychiatrists' liability for their patients' violent acts. Am J Psychiatry 1989;146:821–8.

[11] Kachigian C, Felthous AR. Court responses to Tarasoff statutes. J Am Acad Psychiatry Law 2004;32:263–73.

[12] Duty to warn patient's potential victims; cause of action. Ch. 123, § 36B (2005); Mass.Gen.Laws.

[13] HLTV-III test; confidentiality; informed consent. § 70F (2005); Mass. Gen. Laws Ch. 11.

[14] Brendel RW, Cohen MA. Ethical issues, advance directives, and surrogate decision-making. In: Cohen MA, Gorman J, editors. Comprehensive Textbook of AIDS Psychiatry. New York: Oxford University Press; 2008.

[15] Averhoff F, Zimmerman L, Harpaz R, et al. Varicella Surveillance Practices—United States. MMWR Morb Mortal Wkly Rep 2004;55:1126–9, 6 A.D.

[16] New York State Department of Health. HIV reporting and partner notification questions and answers, NYSDOH 2000. 2000. Available at: www.health.state.ny.us. Accessed March 26, 2006.

[17] New York State Department of Health AIDS Institute. Identification and ambulatory care of HIV-exposed and -infected adolescents, Appendix B–summary, HIV reporting and partner notification. 2003. Available at: www.hivguidelines.org. Accessed April 16, 2006.

[18] Bradshaw v. Daniel. [854], 865. 1993. S.W.2d, Supreme Court of Tennessee.

[19] Gostin LO, Webber DW. HIV infection and AIDS in the public health and health care systems—The role of law and litigation. J Am Med Assoc 1998;279:1108–13.

[20] Liang BA. Medical information, confidentiality, and privacy. Hematol Oncol Clin North Am 2002;16:1433–47.

[21] Zinn C. Wife wins case against GPs who did not disclose husband's HIV status. BMJ 2003;326:1286.

[22] American Medical Association Council on Ethical and Judicial Affairs. Ethical issues involved in the growing AIDS crisis, Report A-I-87.Available at: www.ama-assn.org. 1987. Accessed September 4, 2006.

[23] American Medical Association. Policy H-20–915: HIV/AIDS Reporting, Confidentiality, and Notification. 2003. Available at: www.ama-assn.org. Accessed September 4, 2006.

[24] Beck JC. Legal and ethical duties of the clinician treating a patient who is liable to be impulsively violent. Behav Sci Law 1998;16:375–89.

[25] Brendel RW. An approach to forensic issues. In: Stern TA, editor. The Ten-Minute Guide to Psychiatric Diagnosis and Treatment. New York: Professional Publishing Group; 2005. p. 399–412.

[26] Kazim A, Brendel RW. Abuse and neglect. In: Stern TA, Herman JB, editors. Massachusetts General Hospital Psychiatry Update and Board Preparation. 2nd edition. New York: McGraw-Hill; 2004.

[27] Milosavljevic N, Brendel RW. Abuse and neglect. In: Stern TA, Rosenbaum JF, Fava M, et al, editors. Comprehensive Clinical Psychiatry. Philadelphia: Mosby/Elsevier; 2008.

[28] Schouten R. Legal responsibilities with child abuse and domestic violence. In: Jacobson JL, Jacobson AM, editors. Psychiatric Secrets. Philadelphia: Hanley & Belfus; 2001.

[29] Abrams LC, Lachs M, McAvay G, et al. Predictors of self-neglect in community-dwelling elders. Am J Psychiatry 2002;159:1724–30.

[30] Kahan FS, Paris BE. Why elder abuse continues to elude the health care system. Mt Sinai J Med 2003;70:62–8.

[31] Health Insurance Portability and Accountability Act of 1996. Public Law 1996;104–91.

[32] Brendel RW, Bryan E. HIPAA for psychiatrists. Harv Rev Psychiatry 2004;12:177–83.

[33] HIPAA Privacy Rule. 45, 164.512. 2001. C.F.R.

[34] Feld AD. The Health Insurance Portability and Accountability Act (HIPAA): its broad effect on practice. Am J Gastroenterol 2005;100:1440–3.

[35] Friedrich MJ. Practitioners and organizations prepare for approaching HIPAA deadlines [medical news and perspectives]. J Am Med Assoc 2001;286:1563–5.

[36] Gordon S. Privacy standards for health information: the misnomer of administrative simplification. Delaware Law Review 2002;23–56.

[37] Maio JE. HIPAA and the special status of psychotherapy notes. Lippincotts Case Manag 2003;8:24–9.

[38] Appelbaum PS, Roth LH. Clinical issues in the assessment of competency. Am J Psychiatry 1981;138:1462–7.

[39] Appelbaum PS, Gutheil TG. Clinical Handbook of Psychiatry and the Law. Philadelphia: Wolters/Kluwer/Lippincott Williams & Wilkins; 2006.

[40] Schouten R, Edersheim JG. Informed consent, competency, treatment refusal, and civil commitment. In: Stern TA, Rosenbaum JF, Fava M, et al, editors. Massachusetts General Hospital Comprehensive Clinical Psychiatry. Philadelphia: Mosby/Elsevier; 2008.

[41] Appelbaum PS, Grisso T. Assessing patients' capacities to consent to treatment. N Engl J Med 1988;319:1635–8.

[42] Appelbaum PS, Lidz CW, Meisel A. Informed Consent: Legal Theory and Clinical Practice. New York: Oxford University Press; 1987.

[43] Dalla-Vorgia P, Skiadas P, Garanis-Papadatos T. Is consent in medicine a concept of only modern times? J Med Ethics 2001;27:59–61.

[44] Mohr JC. American medical malpractice litigation in historical perspective. JAMA 2000;283:1731–7.

[45] Schloendorff v. Society of New York Hospital. 92[105]. 1914. Northeast Reporter.

[46] Salgo v. Leland Stanford, Jr. University Board of Trustees. 170(317), 170–182. 1957. P.2d, California Court of Appeals.

[47] Natanson v. Kline. 1093(350), 1093–1109. 1960. P.2nd, Supreme Court of Kansas.

[48] Canterbury v. Spence. 772[464]. 1972. F.2d, D.C. Cir. *cert. denied*, 409 U.S. 1064.

[49] Iheukwumere EO. Doctor: are you experienced? The relevance of disclosure of physician experience to a valid informed consent. J Contemp Health Law Policy 2002;18:373–419.

[50] King JS, Moulton BW. Rethinking informed consent: the case for shared medical decision-making. Am J Law Med 2006;32:429–93.

[51] Precourt v. Frederick. [481], 1144. 1985. Northeast Reporter 2d, Massachusetts Supreme Judicial Court.

[52] Keeton WP, Dobbs DB, Keeton RE, et al. Prosser and Keeton on the Law of Torts. 5th edition. St. Paul: West Publishing Co.; 1984.

[53] Faden RR, Beauchamp TL. A History and Theory of Informed Consent. New York: Oxford University Press; 1986.

[54] Roberts LW. Informed consent and the capacity for voluntarism. Am J Psychiatry 2002;159: 705–12.

[55] Grisso T, Appelbaum PS. Assessing Competence to Consent to Treatment: A Guide for Physicians and Other Health Professionals. New York: Oxford University Press; 1998.

[56] Mallary SD, Gert B, Culver CM. Family coercion and valid consent. Theor Med 1986;7: 123–6.

[57] Gold JA. Kaimowitz v. Department of Mental Health: involuntary mental patient cannot give informed consent to experimental psychosurgery. Rev Law Soc Change 1974;4:207–27.

[58] National Commission for the Protection of Human Subjects of Biomedical and Behavioral Research. Report and Recommendations: Research Involving Prisoners. 1976. Washington, D.C.: U.S. Government Printing Office.

[59] National Commission for the Protection of Human Subjects of Biomedical and Behavioral Research. Research Involving Those Institutionalized as Mentally Infirm: Report and Recommendations. 1978. Washington, D.C.: U.S. Government Printing Office; Ref Type: Pamphlet.

[60] Moser DJ, Arndt S, Kanz JE, et al. Coercion and informed consent in research involving prisoners. Compr Psychiatry 2004;45:1–9.

[61] Meisel A. The "exceptions" to the informed consent doctrine: striking a balance between competing values in medical decision making. Wis L Rev 1979;1979:413–88.

[62] Schouten R, Brendel R. Legal Aspects of Consultation. In: Stern T, Fricchione G, Cassem N, et al, editors. Massachusetts General Hospital Handbook of General Hospital Psychiatry. 5th edition. Philadelphia: Mosby; 2004. p. 349–64.

[63] Sprung CL, Winick BJ. Informed consent in theory and practice: legal and medical perspectives on the informed consent doctrine and a proposed reconceptualization 43. Crit Care Med 1989;17:1346–54.

[64] Dickerson DA. A doctor's duty to disclose life expectancy information to terminally ill patients. Clevel State Law Rev 1995;43:319–50.

[65] Patient Self-Determination Act of 1990. 42, 1395 cc(a). 1990. U.S.C.

[66] Patient Self-Determination Act. 60, 123 at 33294. 1995. C.F.R.

[67] Health Care Surrogate Act. 755, 40. 2005. Ill. Comp. Stat.

[68] Rogers v. Commissioner of Department of Mental Health. Mass Rep. Mass Supreme.Judic. Court. [390], 489-513. 11-29-1983. N.E.2d.

[69] Schouten R, Brendel RW, Edersheim JG. Malpractice and boundary violations. In: Stern TA, Rosenbaum JF, Fava M, et al, editors. Comprehensive clinical psychiatry. Philadelphia: Mosby/Elsevier; 2008.

Psychiatr Clin N Am 30 (2007) 677–688

PSYCHIATRIC CLINICS
OF NORTH AMERICA

ELSEVIER
SAUNDERS

An Updated Review of Implantable Cardioverter/Defibrillators, Induced Anxiety, and Quality of Life

J. Michael Bostwick, MD, Christopher L. Sola, DO*

Department of Psychiatry and Psychology, Mayo Clinic, 200 First Street SW, Rochester, MN 55905, USA

Irrespective of its psychologic effects, the implantable cardioverter-defibrillator (ICD) has become the reference standard for treatment of potentially life-threatening ventricular arrhythmias [1]. Since the Food and Drug Administration (FDA) approved ICDs for treatment of ventricular fibrillation in 1985 [2], large-scale trials have demonstrated a survival benefit [3–9], resulting in increased use of the device in a variety of conditions and broadening FDA indications that include resistance to pharmacologic treatment and ventricular arrhythmias associated with cardiac arrest or hemodynamic compromise [10]. During the same period, technologic advances have included shrinking device size and improved firing specificity [2].

Despite overall good acceptance of ICDs [11–13], patients may experience discharges as frightening and painful. Moreover, a significant percentage of patients who have ICDs experience a shock in the first year after implantation, with estimates ranging from 10% to 54% of recipients [14,15]. Worsened quality of life may result, and a substantial proportion of patients develop psychologic disturbances [16–18].

The authors reviewed ICD-induced psychopathology in 2005 [19], concluding that the literature showed depression and anxiety to be unfortunate products of these devices in a substantial minority of patients, with recency and frequency of firing the best predictors of incipient psychopathology. Since then, coincident with the rapid increase in the use of implanted devices, dozens of studies addressing psychologic sequelae have appeared, warranting an update of that review. Using the search terms "implantable cardioverter-defibrillator," "ICD," "psychopathology," "anxiety," "depression," and "quality of life," the authors queried the MEDLINE database for articles dealing with psychologic sequelae to ICD implantation and use. Bibliographies of those articles yielded additional publications. They identified more than 50 articles of

*Corresponding author. *E-mail address:* sola.christopher@mayo.edu (C.L. Sola).

0193-953X/07/$ – see front matter
doi:10.1016/j.psc.2007.07.002
© 2007 Elsevier Inc. All rights reserved.
psych.theclinics.com

interest, most of which were published after the authors submitted their original review in late 2004.

Since then, researchers have expended considerable effort identifying potential risk factors and—to a lesser extent—mitigating factors for the development of psychopathology in ICD recipients. Commonly occurring categories of inquiry include age, gender, number of shocks experienced, predictability and perceived control of shocks, perception of support, family response, anger, anxiety, optimism, and somatization. In almost no category is there consensus on the degree of risk.

AGE

In their original review, the authors reported that youth (age less than 50 years) was a risk factor for increased anxiety, reduced quality of life, and compromised adjustment to the device. They have found six additional studies, four of which refute this conclusion, and two of which concur with it, at least in part.

The first study to disagree found neither anxiety nor depression to be increased in 20 patients aged 9 to 19 years, despite worsened physical functioning [20]. These children and adolescents do not escape unscathed, however, experiencing "a greater need for social acceptance" than the normative sample. Crossmann and colleagues [21] showed that ICD discharges, age, and gender did not predict anxiety levels in 35 ICD recipients age 35 to 65 years. In their study of 91 ICD patients, Bilge and colleagues [22] found "no significant relation between age and depression or anxiety scores." Yarnoz and Curtis [23] arrived at a similar conclusion, noting that "older patients reported a less active lifestyle, less satisfaction with their physical fitness, and more anxiety, while younger patients demonstrated improvements in the same categories."

On the other hand, Hamilton and Carroll [24] examined 70 patients aged 21 to 84 years, finding that anxiety scores in younger subjects are significantly higher than in older ones, although scores for the younger decrease at 6 months before rising again at 1 year. Although calmer than the younger subjects, the older group perceives little improvement in health and functioning, whereas the anxious younger group reports some improvement. These seemingly contradictory findings suggest a reciprocal relationship between quality of life and level of anxiety. Despite functional gains, younger adults with ICDs are thought to have "worse quality of life and more psychological distress than older adults" [25].

GENDER

Female gender has been thought to be an independent risk factor, although the literature is limited by the consistent finding that most study participants are male. Six studies update the understanding of this risk factor; like the studies of the effect of age, they either fail to achieve consensus or frankly contradict one another.

Thomas and colleagues [25] showed women reporting lower scores on the emotional subscale of the SF-36 than men. Two groups of investigators

[26,27] found women reporting clinically significant depression and anxiety nearly twice as often as men and link this distress to body image concerns and loss of social roles. Both recommend altering approaches to management of female ICD recipients. Walker and colleagues [26] propose reframing the ICD scar as "a sign of 'survivorship' and a symbol of the ability to cope with adversity." Sowell and colleagues [27] suggest reducing disfigurement by developing alternate techniques such as submammary implantation. They also recommend involving the family in preoperative decisions and encouraging ongoing psychologic support for both patient and family.

On multivariate analysis, depression and anxiety in women do not travel together reliably or increase predictably. Bilge and colleagues [22] found female gender independently to predict elevated anxiety but not depression. Luyster and colleagues [28] found the reverse. In yet another study, women experienced more pain and worse sleep but no more depression or anxiety than men [29]. Making this finding particularly robust is the relative disadvantages of the women in other respects. Compared with the men, they are younger, less functional, and less likely to have a spouse' support.

NUMBER AND FREQUENCY OF SHOCKS

Most investigators in the authors' earlier review found that increasing numbers of ICD shocks corresponded to elevated rates of psychopathology [19,25]. One such study of 167 ICD recipients revealed both increased depression and anxiety in those experiencing shock and also decreased adaptation to living with the device [15].

Although a representative early paper stated unequivocally that "multiple shocks were a clear precipitant for the psychiatric disorders" [30], more recent reports disagree partly or completely with this assertion. In their 91 subjects, Bilge and colleagues [22] found worsened anxiety but not depression in those who experienced shock, whereas Luyster and colleagues [28] observed the opposite in 100 subjects.

Three studies discern no relationship at all between shock frequency and psychopathology. Among all ICD recipients living in Iceland (44 patients), no differences in anxiety or depression occurred, regardless of shock history, and ICD and pacemaker recipients were indistinguishable in terms of anxiety, depression, and quality of life [31]. Agreeing with the Iceland study, Godemann and colleagues [32] evaluated 93 patients and ascertained no effect on quality of life from ICD discharges. Finally, even though 5 of 14 patients in another study received more than five shocks in a 24-hour period, the occurrence of shocks—appropriate or not—bore no relationship to depression or anxiety scores or quality of life [33].

When shock, or the possibility of it, does worsen quality of life, it generally does so in the context of premorbid psychologic traits. Multiple authors recommend psychologic referral for those who experience shock [34]. In general, however, patients who actually are shocked are only slightly more likely to suffer from anxiety. It is the patients who have a high level of concern about being shocked, even if they have not been, who manifest heightened anxiety [35]. Indeed, even as cardiologists interrogate devices for objective evidence of a discharge, the belief that one has experienced a shock may be more important than actually having received a shock. Of 75 ICD recipients, the 19 who experienced "phantom shocks" (a sensation of shock in the absence of verified discharge) were noted to be more anxious and depressed than the other 56, even those actually shocked [36].

For ICD recipients who have anxious temperaments, the unpredictability of the ICD shocks is likely to be associated with negative emotions [15,31]. Such patients may attempt to mitigate potential distress from shocks by trying to control their actions or environment to prevent discharges [19]. Avoidant behaviors and symptoms of hypervigilance in these patients can reach the proportions of posttraumatic stress disorder [37].

PERCEPTION OF SUPPORT AND FAMILY RESPONSE

In the authors' original review, excessive family anxiety and poor social support led to worse quality of life and emergent psychopathology. In a more recent review, Thomas and colleagues [25] reinforce this finding, stating "low anxiety, high social support and no shocks were predictive of the best quality of life." It is not necessarily the recipient's own anxiety that is the problem. Eight of 12 patients voiced frustration with "overprotective" family members, with one reportedly moving away from home to escape a parent's vigilance [38]. Although social support has been deemed "imperative in managing stress and rehabilitation," it needs to be the right kind of support [39]. Because family members also are affected by the ICD, they can benefit from education and encouragement to provide the calm and steady emotional and physical environment these patients need [35].

Marriage is considered a proxy for social support, although Walker and colleagues [26] note that the protective effects of marriage against heart disease are more marked in men than in women. Sears and colleagues [34] observe that psychologic variables such as social support "account for as much, if not more, of the variance in quality of life outcomes [than] age and ejection fraction." The lower levels of anxiety and depression reported by the married people in Bilge's cohort report did not reach statistical significance, however [22].

ANGER AND ANXIETY

The authors previously found that baseline state and traits of anger and anxiety may be higher in ICD recipients before implantation, with anxiety improving after implantation, and they noted that elevated anxiety predicts worse quality of life. ICD recipients commonly report anger and anxiety [15,40]. Thirty-five ICD recipients scored higher on the Beck Anxiety Inventory than did controls, although not as high as patients who had a full-blown anxiety disorder [21]. The authors concluded that anxiety in these patients remains "remarkably stable over a period of 2.5 years," despite their surprising finding that trait anxiety as measured by the Trait Anxiety Inventory decreases during that same period [21].

Illustrating the power of psychosomatic interactions, Burg and colleagues [41] have studied 240 ICD recipients, finding that individuals with high trait anger and anxiety are significantly more likely to experience ICD-treated ventricular arrhythmias.

One specific anxiety manifestation is avoidance. Of 143 ICD recipients in one study [40], 55% had begun to avoid activities, objects, or places they feared might cause ICD discharge, significantly diminishing quality of life. Some patients consider the price required to maintain physical health not worth the cost in mental health. Frustrated by being unable to discern whether sexual activity triggered shock, one man asked that his ICD be turned off [38]. Unwilling to give up sex and equally unwilling to risk being shocked, he states, "I just don't want to take the chance." A similar request to deactivate the ICD, although to avoid noxious memories rather than engage in pleasurable stimuli, is described in a man experiencing flashbacks of childhood physical abuse when his device fired [37].

Anxiety may also manifest as nonspecific somatic worry. Through multivariate analysis, Godemann and colleagues [32] tease out that "somatization" (defined as the summation of ratings of nonspecific physical complaints such as pain, nausea, numbness, weakness, and tingling) is the most potent contributor to poor quality of life. As seems to be case throughout the recent ICD literature, however, the findings of another research team diametrically oppose Godemann's work. In 49 patients in whom anxiety sensitivity (a measure of the intolerance of somatic symptoms of anxiety) was associated with elevations in anxiety, depression, and stress at baseline, Lemon and Edelman [42] conclude that ICDs provide reassurance, with concomitant improvement in adaptation to life with the device.

OPTIMISM AND POSITIVE HEALTH EXPECTATIONS

Just as elevated anxiety can lead to pessimism, a fundamentally optimistic outlook can generate reduced anxiety and positive health expectations. Two recent trials address this possibility. The first, looking at 88 patients who had newly implanted ICDs, demonstrated that patients who had higher baseline positive health expectations, defined as "patient beliefs specifically related to the likelihood of a positive health outcome," reported better general physical health at follow-up than patients who had lower baseline positive health expectations [43]. Additionally, patients who had high optimism ("a trait or disposition, capturing more of a generalized expectancy") reported better mental health and social functioning at follow-up. The authors concluded that these "resilience factors" warrant more attention, because they may direct eventual interventions. Trait optimism since has been suggested to be among the psychologic variables in ICD recipients "most important in predicting mental health quality of life" [34].

TREATMENT OPTIONS

Psychoeducation

In the authors' original review, as now, there is consensus as to the importance of patient education. Recent researchers would all agree with Bourke and colleagues' [30] 1997 assertion that "appropriate interventions should begin with education as to the nature and purpose of the defibrillator." Although several distinct approaches are advocated [28,44,45], commonalities include providing education about the nature of ICDs, including (1) their survival advantage over antiarrhythmic medications, (2) setting realistic expectations that shocks cannot be eliminated by avoiding such basic activities as exercise and sex, and (3) preparing a plan for dealing with the aftermath when a shock occurs. Nearly all recommend teaching relaxation techniques and problem-solving skills and encouraging rapid return to daily activities. Proposed teaching modalities range from individual therapy [38] and support groups [46] to telephone discussions [44], computer-based instruction [47], consumer newsletters such as "The Zapper" [48], and patient-centered articles [45]. Support groups are particularly favored for facilitating social interactions that help members share common experiences, normalize concerns, and exchange emotional support [28,40].

Psychotherapy

Although it has been advocated that "provision of psychological interventions to all ICD recipients presenting with known risk factors ... may be beneficial" [34], limited literature explores the efficacy of modalities other than cognitive behavioral therapy (CBT). A Cochrane review is underway to weigh CBT's benefits in ICD recepients, although results are not yet available [49]. A focus on reducing catastrophic interpretations has been recommended [19,30], as has using other techniques like cognitive reframing and changing counterproductive thoughts to reduce anxiety, improve communication skills, and teach relaxation training and stress management skills [39,47]. One case report describes a patient successfully reducing his anxiety during a 4-day intensive CBT-based program on an inpatient psychiatry unit [37].

In addition to reducing depression and anxiety, CBT also may contribute to improved physical functioning. After randomly assigning half of 70 ICD recipients to CBT and half to conventional care, Chevalier and colleagues [50] found that fewer patients receiving CBT sustained shocks. Whether improved physical functioning results from undergoing CBT or experiencing fewer instances of aversive stimuli is unknown. In either case, the difference was neither statistically significant nor persistent at 1-year follow-up. Anxiety, however, was significantly lower in the CBT group at both 3 and 12 months. A second study compares 10 ICD recipients getting conventional care and 12 ICD recipients receiving a 12-week educational program incorporating exercise, relaxation, and specific training about the cognitive modes of anxiety, phobia, and panic. The treatment group experienced decreased anxiety and depression and improved quality of life [51]. Although only 26% of the patients approached actually enrolled in the group, it was "overwhelmingly popular" among attendees. Neither study attempted to parse the proportion of benefit from CBT alone. One non-CBT study showed that prescribed exercise augmented functional capacity and quality of life in 30 ICD recipients [52].

Pharmacology

As in the authors' original review, the literature continues to offer minimal guidance on choices of psychotropic medication for this population. Noting the dearth of ICD-specific literature addressing cardiac-safe antidepressants and anxiolytics, one case report outlines a plan for short-term anxiolysis with a benzodiazepine and longer-term treatment with a serotonin reuptake inhibitor because of its relatively benign side-effect profile [37]. Tricyclic antidepressants, which prolong cardiac conduction, should be avoided, and caution should be observed with venlafaxine, which was shown in five of five subjects in one study to lower defibrillation thresholds by an order of magnitude, possibly through blocking cardiac sodium-channel activity [53].

NEW DIRECTIONS

Since the authors' original review, several areas of inquiry have emerged. Stutts and colleagues [54] note "increasing attention given to psychological factors in cardiac disease subgroups is representative of a broader trend ... in most chronic diseases." These factors include the curious experience of feeling the ICD firing when it has not, called "phantom shock" and associated with depression and anxiety [36,46]. The literature increasingly references ICD-induced posttraumatic stress disorder [36,37,46], although a formal study has yet to determine its prevalence.

Two studies have evaluated the psychologic impact of product recalls [55,56]. One suggests that not all ICD recipients are equally affected by a product recall, reminding physicians to include recall risk as part of informed consent [55]. The other highlights that pathologic anxiety risk increases in ICD recipients during a recall, with ventricular arrhythmias a potential consequence [56].

An additional line of inquiry achieving recent prominence is ICD costs, both financial and psychologic. Although implantation costs have decreased substantially, to about $30,000 currently, with average ICD-related annual health care costs ranging from $5000 to $17,000, hidden costs to ICD recipients are increasingly acknowledged [32]. These costs include worsened quality of life [57], failure to return to work [32], hesitancy to return to sexual activity [32,38], and decreased self-efficacy stemming from driving restrictions [32].

Assessment Tools

Since the authors' original review, two new scales have been introduced in response to a void in the literature regarding assessments specific to the unique experience of living with an ICD. The ICD Patient Concerns Questionnaire is a 20-item questionnaire detailing concerns about living with an ICD and addressing the number and severity of new-onset concerns patients who have ICDs may experience [58]. The Florida Shock Anxiety Scale [14] is a 10-item scale that operationalizes device-specific fears in two dimensions: consequences of device firing and triggers of discharge. The authors recommend using this instrument to identify patients at risk for emotion-triggered shock. This brief but useful instrument can recognize and track anxiety both before and after implantation.

SUMMARY

During the past 2 years the number of studies examining psychopathology and quality of life after ICD implantation has increased dramatically. Variables assessed have included recipient age, gender, and social support network. How recipients respond to having the device, particularly after experiencing firing, has been evaluated in light of new depression and anxiety disorder diagnoses as well as premorbid personality structure. Now the picture of what is known is, if anything, cloudier than it was 2 years ago, with little definitive and much contradictory data emerging in most of these categories. It still seems clear that in a significant minority of ICD recipients the device negatively affects quality of life, probably more so if it fires. Education about life with the device before receiving it remains paramount.

Reports continue to appear of patients developing new-onset diagnosable anxiety disorders such as panic and posttraumatic stress disorder. Until recently the strongest predictors of induced psychopathology were considered to be the frequency and recency of device firing. It now seems that preimplantation psychologic variables such as degree of optimism or pessimism and an anxious personality style may confer an even greater risk than previously thought.

Certainly many variables factor into the induction of psychopathology in these patients. Among these factors are age, gender, and perception of control of shocks, as well as the predictability of shocks and psychologic attributions made by the patient regarding the device. Another source of variability is this population's medical heterogeneity. Some patients receive ICDs after near-death experiences; others get them as anticipatory prophylaxis. Some have longstanding and entrenched heart disease; others were apparently healthy before sudden dangerous arrhythmias. Diagnoses as diverse as myocardial infarction in the context of advanced coronary artery disease and dilated cardiomyopathy after acute viral infection may warrant ICD placement. Moreover the course of cardiac disease after ICD placement may vary from relative stability to continuing disease progression and severe functional compromise. Unless these and other pre- and postimplantation differences are taken into account, it is almost impossible to make meaningful comparisons between studies.

Ideally, future research would consist either of large-scale, randomized, prospective studies using validated structured-interview tools to supplement a literature dominated by self-report measures, unstructured assessments, and anecdotal reports, or of smaller studies designed to focus on particular diagnostic subsets.

As ICDs become the standard of care for potentially life-threatening arrhythmias, the rate of implantations continues to increase. Because negative emotions have been linked to an increased incidence of arrhythmias, and untreated or unrecognized psychiatric illness can interfere with adaptation to an ICD, assessing and managing both pre-existing and induced psychiatric disorders becomes even more critical. Greater research attention should be paid to determining which patients meet criteria for anxiety disorders before and after implantation and what premorbid traits predispose to postimplantation psychopathology. The authors predict that psychiatrists will be involved increasingly in caring for this population, offering insights into treatment options that increase the likelihood of successful ICD acceptance and decrease the psychosocial costs of these devices.

References

[1] DiMarco JP. Implantable cardioverter-defibrillators. N Engl J Med 2003;349(19): 1836–47.
[2] Glikson M, Friedman PA. The implantable cardioverter defibrillator. Lancet 2001; 357(9262):1107–17.
[3] Moss AJ, Hall WJ, Cannom DS, et al. Improved survival with an implanted defibrillator in patients with coronary disease at high risk for ventricular arrhythmia. Multicenter Automatic Defibrillator Implantation Trial Investigators. N Engl J Med 1996;335(26): 1933–40.
[4] A comparison of antiarrhythmic-drug therapy with implantable defibrillators in patients resuscitated from near-fatal ventricular arrhythmia. The Antiarrhythmics Versus Implantable Defibrillators (AVID) Investigators. N Engl J Med 1997;337(22):1576–83.
[5] Connolly SJ, Gent M, Roberts RS, et al. Canadian Implantable Defibrillator Study (CIDS): a randomized trial of the implantable cardioverter defibrillator against amiodarone. Circulation 2000;101(11):1297–302.
[6] Kuck KH, Cappato R, Siebels J, et al. Randomized comparison of antiarrhythmic drug therapy with implantable defibrillators in patients resuscitated from cardiac arrest: the Cardiac Arrest Study Hamburg (CASH). Circulation 2000;102(7):748–54.
[7] Bokhari F, Newman D, Greene M, et al. Long-term comparison of the implantable cardioverter defibrillator versus amiodarone: eleven-year follow-up of a subset of patients in the Canadian Implantable Defibrillator Study (CIDS). Circulation 2004;110(2):112–6.
[8] Greenberg H, Case RB, Moss AJ, et al. Analysis of mortality events in the Multicenter Automatic Defibrillator Implantation Trial (MADIT-II). J Am Coll Cardiol 2004;43(8): 1459–65.
[9] Bardy GH, Lee KL, Mark DB, et al. Amiodarone or an implantable cardioverter-defibrillator for congestive heart failure. N Engl J Med 2005;352(3):225–37.
[10] U.S. Food and Drug Administration Center for Devices and Radiological Health. Available at: http://www.accessdata.fda.gov/scripts/cdrh/devicesatfda/index.cfm. Accessed June 8, 2007.
[11] Vlay SC. The automatic internal cardioverter-defibrillator: comprehensive clinical follow-up, economic and social impact—the Stony Brook experience. Am Heart J 1986;112(1): 189–94.
[12] Luderitz B, Jung W, Deister A, et al. Patient acceptance of the implantable cardioverter defibrillator in ventricular tachyarrhythmias. Pacing Clin Electrophysiol 1993;16(9): 1815–21.
[13] Eads AS, Sears SF Jr, Sotile WM, et al. Supportive communication with implantable cardioverter defibrillator patients: seven principles to facilitate psychosocial adjustment. J Cardiopulm Rehabil 2000;20(2):109–14.

[14] Kuhl EA, Dixit NK, Walker RL, et al. Measurement of patient fears about implantable cardi-overter defibrillator shock: an initial evaluation of the Florida Shock Anxiety Scale. Pacing Clin Electrophysiol 2006;29(6):614–8.

[15] Kamphuis HC, de Leeuw JR, Derksen R, et al. Implantable cardioverter defibrillator recipi-ents: quality of life in recipients with and without ICD shock delivery: a prospective study. Europace 2003;5(4):381–9.

[16] Namerow PB, Firth BR, Heywood GM, et al. Quality-of-life six months after CABG surgery in patients randomized to ICD versus no ICD therapy: findings from the CABG Patch Trial. Pac-ing Clin Electrophysiol 1999;22(9):1305–13.

[17] Irvine J, Dorian P, Baker B, et al. Quality of life in the Canadian Implantable Defibrillator Study (CIDS). Am Heart J 2002;144(2):282–9.

[18] Sears SE Jr, Conti JB. Understanding implantable cardioverter defibrillator shocks and storms: medical and psychosocial considerations for research and clinical care. Clin Cardiol 2003;26(3):107–11.

[19] Sola CL, Bostwick JM. Implantable cardioverter-defibrillators, induced anxiety, and quality of life. Mayo Clin Proc 2005;80(2):232–7.

[20] DeMaso DR, Lauretti A, Spieth L, et al. Psychosocial factors and quality of life in children and adolescents with implantable cardioverter-defibrillators. Am J Cardiol 2004;93(5): 582–7.

[21] Crossmann A, Pauli P, Dengler W, et al. Stability and cause of anxiety in patients with an implantable cardioverter-defibrillator: a longitudinal two-year follow-up. Heart Lung 2007; 36(2):87–95.

[22] Bilge AK, Ozben B, Demircan S, et al. Depression and anxiety status of patients with im-plantable cardioverter defibrillator and precipitating factors. Pacing Clin Electrophysiol 2006;29(6):619–26.

[23] Yarnoz MJ, Curtis AB. Why cardioverter-defibrillator implantation might not be the best idea for your elderly patient. Am J Geriatr Cardiol 2006;15(6):367–71.

[24] Hamilton GA, Carroll DL. The effects of age on quality of life in implantable cardioverter de-fibrillator recipients. J Clin Nurs 2004;13(2):194–200.

[25] Thomas SA, Friedmann E, Kao CW, et al. Quality of life and psychological status of patients with implantable cardioverter defibrillators. Am J Crit Care 2006;15(4):389–98.

[26] Walker RL, Campbell KA, Sears SF, et al. Women and the implantable cardioverter de-fibrillator: a lifespan perspective on key psychosocial issues. Clin Cardiol 2004;27(10): 543–6.

[27] Sowell LV, Kuhl EA, Sears SF, et al. Device implant technique and consideration of body image: specific procedures for implantable cardioverter defibrillators in female patients. J Womens Health (Larchmt) 2006;15(7):830–5.

[28] Luyster FS, Hughes JW, Waechter D, et al. Resource loss predicts depression and anxiety among patients treated with an implantable cardioverter defibrillator. Psychosom Med 2006;68(5):794–800.

[29] Smith G, Dunbar SB, Valderrama AL, et al. Gender differences in implantable cardiovert-er-defibrillator patients at the time of insertion. Prog Cardiovasc Nurs 2006;21(2): 76–82.

[30] Bourke JP, Turkington D, Thomas G, et al. Florid psychopathology in patients receiving shocks from implanted cardioverter-defibrillators. Heart 1997;78(6):581–3.

[31] Leosdottir M, Sigurdsson E, Reimarsdottir G, et al. Health-related quality of life of patients with implantable cardioverter defibrillators compared with that of pacemaker recipients. Europace 2006;8(3):168–74.

[32] Godemann F, Butter C, Lampe F, et al. Determinants of the quality of life (QoL) in pa-tients with an implantable cardioverter/defibrillator (ICD). Qual Life Res 2004;13(2): 411–6.

[33] Newall EG, Lever NA, Prasad S, et al. Psychological implications of ICD implantation in a New Zealand population. Europace 2007;9(1):20–4.

[34] Sears SF, Lewis TS, Kuhl EA, et al. Predictors of quality of life in patients with implantable cardioverter defibrillators. Psychosomatics 2005;46(5):451–7.

[35] Pedersen SS, van Domburg RT, Theuns DA, et al. Concerns about the implantable cardioverter defibrillator: a determinant of anxiety and depressive symptoms independent of experienced shocks. Am Heart J 2005;149(4):664–9.

[36] Prudente LA, Reigle J, Bourguignon C, et al. Psychological indices and phantom shocks in patients with ICD. J Interv Card Electrophysiol 2006;15(3):185–90.

[37] Hoecksel K, Bostwick J. Getting to the heart of his shocking trauma. Current Psychiatry 2007;6:84–91.

[38] Steinke EE, Gill-Hopple K, Valdez D, et al. Sexual concerns and educational needs after an implantable cardioverter defibrillator. Heart Lung 2005;34(5):299–308.

[39] Sears SF Jr, Stutts LA, Aranda JM Jr, et al. Managing congestive heart failure patient factors in the device era. Congest Heart Fail 2006;12(6):335–40.

[40] Lemon J, Edelman S, Kirkness A. Avoidance behaviors in patients with implantable cardioverter defibrillators. Heart Lung 2004;33(3):176–82.

[41] Burg MM, Lampert R, Joska T, et al. Psychological traits and emotion-triggering of ICD shock-terminated arrhythmias. Psychosom Med 2004;66(6):898–902.

[42] Lemon J, Edelman S. Psychological adaptation to ICDs and the influence of anxiety sensitivity. Psychol Health Med 2007;12(2):163–71.

[43] Sears SF, Serber ER, Lewis TS, et al. Do positive health expectations and optimism relate to quality-of-life outcomes for the patient with an implantable cardioverter defibrillator? J Cardiopulm Rehabil 2004;24(5):324–31.

[44] Dougherty CM, Lewis FM, Thompson EA, et al. Short-term efficacy of a telephone intervention by expert nurses after an implantable cardioverter defibrillator. Pacing Clin Electrophysiol 2004;27(12):1594–602.

[45] Sears SF Jr, Shea JB, Conti JB. Cardiology patient page. How to respond to an implantable cardioverter-defibrillator shock. Circulation 2005;111(23):e380–2.

[46] Prudente LA. Psychological disturbances, adjustment, and the development of phantom shocks in patients with an implantable cardioverter defibrillator. J Cardiovasc Nurs 2005; 20(4):288–93.

[47] Kuhl EA, Sears SF, Conti JB. Using computers to improve the psychosocial care of implantable cardioverter defibrillator recipients. Pacing Clin Electrophysiol 2006;29(12): 1426–33.

[48] The Zapper online newsletter. Available at: http://www.zaplife.org/. Accessed June 8, 2007.

[49] Johnson B, Francis J. Cognitive behavourial therapy for patients with implantable cardioverter-defibrillators [protocol]. The Cochrane Library, Issue 3, 2007. Available at: http://www.thecochranelibrary.com. Accessed May 29, 2007.

[50] Chevalier P, Cottraux J, Mollard E, et al. Prevention of implantable defibrillator shocks by cognitive behavioral therapy: a pilot trial. Am Heart J 2006;151(1):191.e1–191.e6.

[51] Frizelle DJ, Lewin RJ, Kaye G, et al. Cognitive-behavioural rehabilitation programme for patients with an implanted cardioverter defibrillator: a pilot study. Br J Health Psychol 2004; 9(Pt 3):381–92.

[52] Belardinelli R, Capestro F, Misiani A, et al. Moderate exercise training improves functional capacity, quality of life, and endothelium-dependent vasodilation in chronic heart failure patients with implantable cardioverter defibrillators and cardiac resynchronization therapy. Eur J Cardiovasc Prev Rehabil 2006;13(5):818–25.

[53] Carnes CA, Pickworth KK, Votolato NA, et al. Elevated defibrillation threshold with venlafaxine therapy. Pharmacotherapy 2004;24(8):1095–8.

[54] Stutts LA, Cross NJ, Conti JB, et al. Examination of research trends on patient factors in patients with implantable cardioverter defibrillators. Clin Cardiol 2007;30(2):64–8.

[55] Sears SF Jr, Conti JB. Psychological aspects of cardiac devices and recalls in patients with implantable cardioverter defibrillators. Am J Cardiol 2006;98(4):565–7.

[56] van den Broek KC, Denollet J, Nyklicek I, et al. Psychological reaction to potential malfunctioning of implantable defibrillators. Pacing Clin Electrophysiol 2006;29(9):953–6.

[57] Noyes K, Corona E, Zwanziger J, et al. Health-related quality of life consequences of implantable cardioverter defibrillators: results from MADIT II. Med Care 2007;45(5):377–85.

[58] Frizelle DJ, Lewin B, Kaye G, et al. Development of a measure of the concerns held by people with implanted cardioverter defibrillators: the ICDC. Br J Health Psychol 2006;11(Pt 2): 293–301.

Psychiatr Clin N Am 30 (2007) 689–716

PSYCHIATRIC CLINICS
OF NORTH AMERICA

Psychiatric Aspects of Infertility and Infertility Treatments

Linda Hammer Burns, PhD[a,b,*]

[a]Department of Obstetrics, Gynecology and Women's Health, University of Minnesota,
MMC 395 Mayo, 8395, 420 Delaware Street, Minneapolis, MN 55455, USA
[b]Reproductive Medicine Center, 606 24th Avenue South, Suite 500,
Minneapolis, MN 55454, USA

Throughout the history of mankind, involuntary childlessness has been a social stigma and has caused emotional trauma and relationship strain. The distress of barrenness impels individuals to seek a remedy, most typically a medical remedy, because realignment of social relationships is the least attractive alternative for individuals, couples, and communities [1].

Infertility affects between 80 million and 168 million people worldwide; approximately 1 in 10 couples experience either primary or secondary infertility. Primary infertility (involuntary childlessness) rates are 1% to 8%, whereas rates of secondary infertility (the inability to have another child) are significantly higher, at 35%. In the United States, the number of married couples who are infertile is 2.1 million, and 9.3 million American women are currently using, or have used, infertility services [2,3]. Compared with the middle of the twentieth century, when 50% of infertility was considered to be unexplained or attributable to psychosomatic disorders in the female partner (eg, conflicted feelings about motherhood, her mother, or sexuality), today, 10% of infertility is unexplained, 50% is attributable to female factors, 35% to male factors, and 5% to other factors (eg, both partners) (Fig. 1) [4]. Whatever the cause, most medical treatments for infertility are geared toward women, who bear a disproportionate share of the treatment burden.

Global rates of infertility vary dramatically, from a prevalence rate of about 5% in developed countries to more than 30% in sub-Saharan Africa [5]. The wide variance in prevalence rates contributes to the emotional experience of infertility; specifically, where infertility is experienced impacts how it is experienced. "Stratification of infertility" refers to the barriers to infertility treatment which, understandably, impact the infertility experience and include economic, social welfare, and public health issues (eg, poverty, malnutrition, obesity, smoking, and sexually transmitted diseases); ignorance of reproduction, sexual

*Reproductive Medicine Center, 606 24th Avenue South, Suite 500, Minneapolis, MN 55454. E-mail address: burns023@umn.edu

0193-953X/07/$ – see front matter
doi:10.1016/j.psc.2007.08.001
© 2007 Elsevier Inc. All rights reserved.
psych.theclinics.com

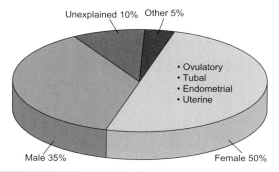

Fig. 1. Overview of medical diagnosis and treatment of infertility. (*Adapted from* Lobel M, Dunkel-Schetter C. Psychological reactions to infertility. In: Stanton AL, Dunkel-Schetter L, editors. Infertility: perspectives from stress and coping research. New York: Plenum Press; 1991. p. 29–57; with permission.)

health, or fertility preservation; or lack of availability or access to high-quality medical treatments [6]. Additionally, in many patriarchal societies (eg, Middle Eastern and African), male-factor infertility does not exist; it is an unacceptable diagnosis, thereby increasing the psychosocial stress of male-factor infertility for men (because of the increased stigma and secrecy) and for women, who have few roles in society apart from motherhood.

Today, more than 40 ways exist to have a baby without sexual intercourse (Box 1). Medical treatments facilitate parenthood through assisted reproductive technologies, such as in vitro fertilization (IVF), intrauterine inseminations (IUI), intracytoplasmic sperm injection (ICSI), and third-party (eg, donated gametes or embryos, gestational carriers, surrogates), to an ever-increasing range of individuals and couples seeking biologic parenthood (eg, married or committed couples, gay or lesbian couples, or solo parents). In addition, reproductive medicine facilitates childbearing for individuals who previously could not have biologic children because of medical conditions that impaired their fertility (eg, HIV/AIDs, azoospermia due to congenital absence of the vas deferens, and cancer). However, these new reproductive opportunities must be considered within the context of cultural, religious, economic, and legislative barriers that can, and often do, prevent couples from pursuing their procreative goals. This situation has lead to a growth industry referred to as "reproductive tourism," in which an increasing number of infertile individuals and reproductive collaborators seek treatments in other parts of their own country or internationally because it is unavailable, illegal, or too expensive where they live. Infertile patients are typically motivated to overcome treatment barriers by pursuing their preferred reproductive, family-building alternative where it is available and less costly. Some infertile patients are motivated by the belief that the level of care in other countries is better or preferable [7]. By contrast, reproductive collaborators often prefer volunteering as donors or surrogates in another part of their own country, or internationally, because they have more legal protections; they prefer the practice parameters (eg, anonymous versus identified gamete donation). Or, collaborators are drawn by financial or altruistic rewards.

With the advent of assisted and complex reproduction, the role of the mental health professional in the treatment of infertility has shifted from curative to a more complex and comprehensive role. Mental health professionals in reproductive medicine are expected to provide patient education, screening, guidance, and preparation for medical treatments; advice, support, and assistance with decision making; assessment of current mental health and marital and relationship stability; bereavement therapy; treatment of pre-existing or ongoing psychiatric diagnosis, sexual problems, or marital problems; and assistance with integration, transcendence, and recovery from the narcissistic injury and emotional crisis of infertility [8]. A few countries (eg, United Kingdom, Australia) have laws recommending counseling be offered as part of infertility treatment, whereas Canada, Greece, and Spain have laws requiring patients undergo counseling before any/all treatment or specific treatments [9]. In the United States, the American Society of Reproductive Medicine (ASRM) provides guidelines not only about medical treatment for infertility but about counseling issues (www.asrm.org) for all participants in assisted reproduction. Considerations regarding mental well-being have moved beyond those of the infertile couple alone, as the screening of and assistance with reproductive collaborators, such as donors and gestational carriers, has become an added concern for mental health professionals, in addition to the well-being of the children born as result of assisted reproduction.

PSYCHIATRIC DISORDERS IN INFERTILE INDIVIDUALS

Some degree of emotional distress in response to infertility or its treatment is expected and understandable. Reproductive failure or involuntary childlessness is a significant loss for men and women worldwide. Despite this loss, psychopathology is not a universal consequence, although some individuals experience exacerbations of pre-existing psychiatric disorders or clinically significant emotional problems. Frequent emotional responses to infertility include anger, guilt, shock, lowered self-esteem, sexual dysfunction, marital distress, and social isolation (Box 2) [10,11]. Although most infertile individuals do not experience severe or clinically significant distress, sexual problems, or psychopathology, a small portion do [12]. A recent review of the literature duplicated these findings, concluding that, although descriptive literature on the psychologic consequences of infertility presented infertility as a psychologically devastating experience, empirically sound research found no significant differences between infertile individuals and controls in terms of psychopathology or self-esteem [13]. At the same time, infertile individuals undergoing assisted reproduction do appear to be at greater risk for psychologic distress, (eg, anxiety, distress, and grief), particularly if treatment is unsuccessful [14,15]. Factors contributing to grief reaction following unsuccessful IVF/ET included a belief that the treatment is the couple's last chance at having a biologic child; pre-existing

Box 1: Methods of reproduction without sexual intercourse

Intravaginal insemination

1. Intravaginal insemination with husband or partner
2. Intravaginal insemination with ovulation stimulation or ovulation induction medication (eg, Clomid)
3. Intravaginal insemination with superovulation induction medications
4. Intravaginal insemination with donor sperm
5. Intravaginal insemination with ovulation induction medication and donor sperm
6. Intravaginal insemination with superovulation induction medications and donor sperm

Intracervical insemination

7. Intracervical insemination with husband or partner
8. Intracervical insemination with ovulation stimulation or ovulation induction medication (eg, Clomid)
9. Intracervical insemination with superovulation induction medications
10. Intracervical insemination with donor sperm
11. Intracervical insemination with ovulation induction medication and donor sperm
12. Intracervical insemination with superovulation induction medications and donor sperm

Intrauterine insemination

13. IUI with husband or partner
14. IUI with ovulation induction (eg, Clomid)
15. IUI with superovulation induction medications
16. IUI with donor sperm
17. IUI with ovulation induction (eg, Clomid) and donor sperm
18. IUI with superovulation induction medications and donor sperm

In vitro *fertilization*

19. IVF with superovulation medications
20. IVF (natural cycle)
21. IVF with donor egg (synchronized cycles)
22. IVF with donor egg (cryopreserved oocytes)

In vitro *fertilization (male-factor–related treatments)*

23. IVF with ICSI
24. IVF with microscopic epididymal sperm aspiration and ICSI
25. IVF with percutaneous epididymal sperm aspiration and ICSI

Box 1: (*continued*)

26. IVF with testicular sperm extraction and ICSI

27. IVF with donor sperm

In vitro *fertilization–related procedures*

28. Gamete intrafallopian transfer

29. Tubal embryo transfer

30. Intrauterine embryo transfer

31. Frozen embryo transfer

32. IVF with donor egg

33. Donor embryo

34. IVF with preimplantation genetic diagnosis

35. Assisted hatching

Gestational carrier or surrogacy

36. Surrogacy (surrogate donates oocyte and uterus for pregnancy)

37. Gestational carrier with intended parent's embryo

38. Gestational carrier with intended mother's oocyte and donor sperm

39. Gestational carrier with intended father's sperm and donor oocyte

40. Gestational carrier with donor embryo

Other

41. Cloning

psychologic illness; and overestimation of personal success [16–18]. Research indicates that mood (anxiety, depression, or distress) fluctuates in men and women over the course of assisted reproduction treatment cycles (anxiety and depression increase on oocyte-retrieval day, decrease on embryo-transfer day, and rise again on pregnancy-testing day), with the severity of emotional distress diminishing with repeated cycles [19,20]. In an attempt to asses the prevalence of psychiatric morbidity (pre-existing or newly emergent) in individuals attending a fertility clinic, researchers found that 69% of women and 21% of men had a psychiatric disorder [21]. Adjustment and anxiety disorders were the most common, with depression twice as prevalent in infertile women who had a history of depression [22].

Although most individuals are able to manage the experience of infertility effectively, a small portion will develop serious psychopathology requiring immediate psychiatric care (Box 3). In addition, despite a lack of prevalence or incidence studies, it must be assumed that some reproductive collaborators will also present with a current or pre-existing psychiatric disorder, or will develop one while participating in reproductive therapies. As such, it is imperative that all clinicians understand the potential effects of infertility medications, psychotropic medications, and psychopathology to provide appropriate psychiatric patient

Box 2: Observed psychologic effects of infertility

A. Emotional effects

1. Grieving and depression
2. Anger and frustration
3. Guilt
4. Shock and denial
5. Anxiety

B. Loss of control

1. Loss of control over activities, body, emotions
2. Inability to predict and plan future
3. Loss of health
4. Loss of security (about a predictable future)

C. Effects on self-esteem, identity, beliefs

1. Loss of self-esteem and self-confidence, feelings of inadequacy
2. Identity problems or shifts, loss of status or prestige
3. Changes in world views

D. Social effects

1. Effects on marital interactions and satisfaction (positive and negative)
2. Effects on sexual functioning
3. Different social network interactions, changes in relationships with network members, loneliness, embarrassment

E. Loss of a (potential) relationship

1. Loss of fantasy or hope of fulfilling an important fantasy
2. Loss of something or someone of great symbolic value
3. Loss of future and past in one person

Data from Stanton AL, Dunkel-Schetter L. Psychological reactions to infertility. In: Stanton AL, Dunkel-Schetter L, editors. Infertility: perspectives from stress and coping research. New York: Plenum Press; 1991. p. 29–57; and Mahlstedt, PP. The psychological component of infertility. Fertil Steril 1985;43:335–56.

care; consult with reproductive caregivers about the risks and benefits of reproductive treatment for individuals psychologically at-risk; and ensure the emotional well-being of infertile individuals during and after treatment.

Depression

Historically, it was thought that infertile women experienced greater levels of distress, depression, and anxiety than infertile men, except when the infertility diagnosis is male factor. Men with male-factor infertility have been reported to experience significant levels of depression, social isolation, and stigma, but were

Box 3: Psychological responses to infertility

Depression
- Dysthymia
- Bipolar Disorder
- Bereavement (complicated or delayed), pathological grief

Anxiety disorders
- Obsessive/compulsive disorder
- Panic attacks
- Phobias
- Post-traumatic stress disorder

Eating disorders

Personality disorders

Sexual dysfunction
- History of rape, trauma
- Low libido
- Infrequent or no sexual intercourse
- Anorgasmia

Addiction problems
- Alcohol
- Gambling
- Prescription medication
- Tobacco
- Recreational drugs
- Sex/pornography

Relationship problems
- Infidelity
- Sexual difficulties
- Anger management/violence
- Communication problems
- Lack of shared goals

Behavioral problems
- Noncompliance with treatment
- Occupational problems
- Identity issues
- Legal difficulties
- Impulse control issues

Religious or spiritual difficulties

Acculturation issues

Phase of life problems

Sleep disturbances

Somatization disorder

Factitious disorder

less likely to identify themselves as depressed or distressed or to seek assistance than infertile woman [23–29]. More recent research investigated patterns of suffering and social interactions in infertile men over a 12-month period after unsuccessful treatment [30]. Researchers found that over time, regardless of the source of infertility, men experienced increased social, marital, and physical stress and decreased emotional well-being. It was also found that the best predictor of psychologic well-being over time was the men's psychologic well-being before treatment had begun. These findings seem to challenge the long-held beliefs that infertile men are not as emotionally vulnerable to psychologic impairment in response to infertility (regardless of diagnosis) and, in fact, appear to have similar or comparable responses to that of infertile women.

Women with a history of depression are twice as likely to develop a recurrence of depression during infertility, reproductive treatment, and pregnancy, and postpartum. They are more likely to identify infertility treatment as the most distressing event in their lives, even more upsetting than the loss of a loved one, or divorce [31–35]. Depression among infertile women was found to be comparable to levels of depression in patients who had other chronic medical conditions (eg, hypertension and cancer) [36]. In one prevalence study, 17% of infertile women met the criteria for major depressive disorder, a significantly higher rate than controls [37]. High prevalence rates of depression in infertile women have been found to be comparable across nations and cultures [21,38–43].

Grief and bereavement in infertile individuals is common because of the myriad of losses experienced with childlessness, whether actual (eg, failed treatment cycles, miscarriages) or intangible (eg, loss of sense of self, role of parenthood) [44,45]. Rarely, infertile patients develop pathologic grief, or a major depressive episode with marked vegetative symptoms, anhedonia, suicidal ideation, cognitive impairment, or psychotic features (eg, paranoid delusions or excessive punitive thoughts). It is important that clinicians differentially diagnose the expected grief reaction to infertility from the less common, but more serious, disorders such as pathologic grief and major depressive episode [10,46].

Two forms of short-term psychotherapies have been shown to be helpful in the treatment of mild to moderate depression: interpersonal therapy and cognitive-behavioral therapy. Educating infertile women about alternatives to medications, and facilitating decisions and treatment planning about antidepressant medications before, during, and after infertility treatment, are an integral part of comprehensive infertility treatment. Optimally, decisions about psychotropic medications are best made by a psychiatrist who can facilitate individualized discussions of the pros and cons of psychotropic medications.

Bipolar Disorder

Women with bipolar disorder should receive preconception counseling that includes education about the pros and cons of pregnancy and the postpartum period, infertility, treatment failure, and issues regarding the maintenance of psychotropic medications. Whether a woman (infertile or reproductive collaborator) with bipolar disorder is undergoing infertility treatment involving hormones, pregnancy, and postpartum (or treatment failure), it is important that she be evaluated carefully in terms of psychotropic medication history; in-depth psychiatric history (eg, years of the disease, hospitalizations, medication history, history of rapid-cycling, or sensitivity to hormone changes); evidence of comorbid diagnoses and treatment; the woman's support system; and her own self-efficacy in managing her illness. Women taking mood stabilizers should be counseled about the high rates of relapse (and rapid cycling) with abrupt medication withdrawal [47,48]. Their reproductive caregivers must be aware of these risk factors for these patients who are pursuing infertility treatments and, therefore, pregnancy [49].

A psychiatric treatment plan should be developed with the woman and her partner and shared with her obstetrician and reproductive endocrinologist. Women should be aware that mood stabilizers have been associated with an increased risk of congenital malformations, so the risks of maintaining a woman on medication through infertility treatment, pregnancy, and postpartum must be weighed carefully against the risk of withdrawing the medication. Women without a history of severe illness may be tapered off psychotropic medication and followed closely in psychotherapy [46]. Women should be educated carefully about the risks of cardiac defects with lithium, which is approximately 0.1%, an estimate that is still 10 to 20 times greater than that of the general population [47,49]. Women treated with valproic acid and those with carbamazepine disorder need to be informed that first-trimester exposure of the fetus to valproic acid is associated with a 1% to 5% risk of spina bifida, whereas exposure to carbamazepine is associated with a 1% to 1.5% risk [50]. Some psychiatrists feel it is safest to switch women taking anticonvulsant mood stabilizers to lithium, whereas others prefer a regimen of frequent psychotherapy (minimum once a week) with no medications unless absolutely necessary [46,47,50]. However, women should also be informed that the postpartum period is associated with an increased risk of relapse, so they should be counseled about the benefits of resuming mood stabilizers immediately postpartum, and relinquishing breast-feeding [51–53].

For some women with bipolar disorder, particularly those facing long-term infertility treatments, the risks of childbearing are too great and they may have to consider the possibility of foregoing reproduction and considering other family-bridling options. This suggestion can be a significant emotional blow, but the risks of proceeding with infertility treatment may be too great for the reproductive collaborator or infertile woman's short- and long-term well-being, and that of any children she might have. Psychiatrists and other caregivers must acknowledge the complex and cumulative losses of these situations: chronic debilitating illness, loss of childbearing and the fulfillment of life dreams of a "normal life." For psychiatrists assessing a woman's ability to pursue infertility treatments, he/she needs to be confident that the woman is sufficiently stable to provide informed consent; be protective of her well-being despite her wish to risk it by pursuing motherhood; and not be pressured or coerced to proceed with infertility treatments if they are contraindicated.

Anxiety Disorders

Anxiety disorders (eg, phobias, obsessive-compulsive disorder) and disorders with concomitant anxiety symptoms (eg, depression) are prevalent among infertile men and women, which is understandable because anxiety symptoms typically increase during times of stress, leading to exacerbations of pre-existing conditions, triggering of phobic reactions, or an initial full-blown anxiety disorder in response to infertility diagnosis and treatment [46]. Research has reported that 23% of infertile women met the criteria for generalized anxiety disorder, a higher rate than controls [17]. Higher rates of adjustment disorder with anxiety have also been reported. Elevated anxiety levels have also been reported in both infertile men and women, often leading to increased depression following repeated treatment cycles, particularly in women (see Refs. [17,21,38,46,52,53]). The greatest levels of anxiety and distress have been reported to be in the first and last treatment cycles [54].

Infertile patients taking benzodiazepines for anxiety should be encouraged to taper off these medications gradually because therapeutic doses have been associated with an increased risk of cleft abnormalities [47]. As an alternative, tricyclic antidepressants or selective serotonin reuptake inhibitors may be substituted for anxiolytics in infertile women who are unable to manage anxiety without medications. At the same time, psychotherapeutic interventions should also be introduced (eg, cognitive-behavioral and relaxation therapies).

Obsessive-compulsive disorders affect men and women in equal numbers, typically appearing early in life. Infertile patients who have obsessive-compulsive disorders may focus on contamination obsessions and cleaning rituals associated with infertility treatments because they are expected to assume responsibility for the sterile technique associated with injections as part of various treatments for infertility [55], which can increase their unique compulsive ritualistic behaviors (eg, checking) or trigger newly emergent rituals (eg, excessive hand washing before and after injections). Needle and blood injury phobias can be especially problematic, impairing, or even impeding, treatment compliance or producing unmanageable anxiety (eg, a woman with a history of sexual abuse may be traumatized by repeated pelvic exams or inseminations). Caregivers may need to adapt treatment protocols (eg, injections given by a trained family member) and encourage or require psychologic or psychiatric care before treatment can continue (eg, anxiolytic medications for specific procedures, systematic desensitization, or relaxation training) [46]. Behavioral strategies and cognitive behavior therapies (eg, strict time limits on hand washing, thought-stopping for obsessive and intrusive thoughts) should be encouraged, although it is unrealistic to introduce an elaborate systematic desensitization or cognitive-behavioral treatment program in the midst of, or just before, infertility treatment cycles (eg, IVF) [46].

Preconception counseling should be encouraged for women with anxiety disorders to help develop a plan for managing the anxiety symptoms during infertility treatment, pregnancy, and the postpartum period. Anxiety disorders during pregnancy remain controversial, although theoretically, the increased progesterone of pregnancy may be associated with decreased anxiety [52,54,55]. Despite this, not all women with anxiety, hypervigilance, panic attacks, and obsessive-compulsive disorder symptomatology during infertility report improvement in anxiety during pregnancy. As with depressive disorder, the postpartum period appears to be a time of greatest risk for relapse or escalation of psychiatric symptomatology [56].

Stress and Posttraumatic Stress Syndrome

Posttraumatic stress syndrome is an anxiety disorder that typically develops after a terrifying experience involving an actual or perceived threat of physical harm. For most, infertility is not a discrete event but an evolving process that initially involves a potential threat or loss, which develops over time into a real threat or loss (eg, childlessness, repeated failed cycles or miscarriages) (see Refs. [15–17,20,36,57,58]). Infertility is stressful in that it is an unpredictable experience, which is negative, uncontrollable, and ambiguous.

Further, anxiety during treatment and the outcome of the treatment itself appear to be associated, with both men and women experiencing substantial distress over time, especially when treatment proves unsuccessful (see Refs. [13,30,39,59–62]). For most individuals, infertility and its treatment do not precipitate posttraumatic stress disorder (PTSD), unless they experience a particularly traumatic treatment outcome (eg, lost embryos, medical crisis during treatment). More often, men and women enter infertility treatment with a history of PTSD that impacts their ability to cope and manage in a healthy fashion the distress of infertility. An example is the individual whose prior history of sexual abuse or trauma early in life triggers anxiety during infertility treatment (eg, vaginal probe ultrasound, producing a semen specimen at the clinic). In these circumstances, caregivers may need to adapt treatment procedures, and psychiatric care may involve relaxation techniques or long-term treatment care, such as psychotherapy, to ensure that the PTSD symptoms remain manageable.

Eating Disorders and Obesity

Recently, the effects on fertility of obesity, malnutrition, and disordered eating have been given greater attention. The ideal body mass index (BMI) for reproduction ranges between 19 and 25, with lower and higher weights negatively influencing fertility in both sexes. A BMI of less than 19 or greater than 25 has been shown to reduce fertility in women by suppressing ovulation and increasing the rate of complications during infertility treatment, pregnancy, and delivery; and in men by reducing sperm production and quality [63–65]. Women with active eating disorders are not only at risk for decreased fertility, but for menstrual irregularities and increased perinatal morbidity (ie, increased incidence of miscarriage, neonatal morbidity, intrauterine growth retardation, and congenital anomalies) as well as hyperemesis gravidarum, low maternal weight gain in pregnancy, and problems with infant feeding [66–69]. One study of women attending a gynecology clinic found that 8% met the diagnostic criteria for anorexia or bulimia and 17% for an eating disorder (not specified), with 58% found to be either underweight or obese because of disordered eating [70]. Some evidence indicates that bulimia nervosa has less impact on fertility and conception in women if the woman is within the normal weight range [71]. As such, infertile women and men with an active eating disorder or weight problem (ie, BMI<19 or BMI>25) should not be treated for the fertility problem until the disordered eating is in full remission or an acceptable weight has been achieved [72,73].

Research suggests that anger triggers binge eating in men, whereas anger suppression is associated with binge eating in women. Treatment for men and women with anorexia nervosa focuses on regaining weight, normalizing eating, and stopping weight loss. Cognitive behavioral therapy is effective for men and women with bulimia. The challenge in treating infertile men and women with eating disorders is in educating them about how their disordered eating is, or may be, impacting their fertility and convincing them of the importance of treatment and behavior change. More often than not, one or both partners are opposed to interrupting their medical pursuit of parenthood, even when evidence suggests that fertility treatment is contraindicated or would be more successful if they were not under- or overweight or their disordered eating was treated.

Addictions

Alcohol dependence and abuse are associated with a broad spectrum of male- and female-factor reproductive disorders, including amenorrhea; anovulation; luteal phase dysfunction; hyperprolactinemia; increased risk of spontaneous miscarriage; impaired fetal growth and development (ie, fetal alcohol syndrome); impaired semen parameters; and risk of the impact of sexually transmitted infections such as HIV, which may be transmitted to a partner or offspring, highlighting the importance of preconception counseling [74–78]. Research on recreational drug use in women (eg, marijuana, lysergic acid diethylamide [LSD], cocaine, and amphetamines) has shown an increased risk of ovulatory abnormalities (particularly in women who had used marijuana within 1 year of trying to conceive), whereas cocaine usage contributed to increased tubal factor infertility [79,80]. Alcohol and drug abuse in men contributed to an increased risk of poor sperm morphology and motility, impotence, and low sperm count [81,82].

Approximately 30% of Americans older than age 12 use tobacco. According to one recent study, 1.7% of pregnant women used cigarettes and, among these women, 57.2% were nicotine dependent, indicating that an estimated 12.4% percent of American pregnant women are addicted to cigarettes. Smoking reduces fertility in men and women by causing impotence; poor sperm production and quality; reduced ovarian reserve; and miscarriage [83–87]; it also reduces the success rates of infertility treatments (eg, IVF) [88–91]. One study found that nicotine-dependent women were more likely to meet the criteria for at least one other mental disorder (eg, dysthymia, major depressive disorder, and panic disorder) and some evidence suggests that women who smoked during their pregnancy put their sons' fertility at risk by lowering their sperm count in adulthood [92].

Addictions also refer to psychologic, impulse-control behaviors (eg, gambling, pornography), which are less likely to be physiologically addicting. However, these behaviors can still impact fertility. An example is an individual addicted to sex or pornography resulting in frequent ejaculations or risky sexual practices that put him/her at risk of contracting sexually transmitted diseases. Further, the marital and social consequences of these behaviors, and the risk of comorbidity with other mental disorders, illustrate how these addictions can be destabilizing and can impact an individual or a couple's reproductive goals.

Approaches to addicted patients begin with education about how their addictive behavior negatively impacts their own fertility or that of their partner, and reduces the opportunity of successful outcome from treatment. Taking a collaborative approach to the treatment of addictions is imperative because deferring treatment until the addiction has been assessed and properly treated is often met with high resistance, emotional distress, or manipulative behaviors from one or both partners. However, denying or deferring further infertility treatment until the individual has attended chemical-dependency treatment or a self-help group (eg, Alcoholics Anonymous, Women for Sobriety, Gamblers Anonymous, or Narcotics Anonymous) is imperative, not only for the health and well-being of the addict but also to improve marital functioning and the long-term well-being of the child they wish to have.

Schizophrenia

Despite evidence suggesting that women with psychotic disorders (eg, schizophrenia, mania) improve during pregnancy [93–95] because of enhanced dopamine blockade with increased estrogen level [93], preconception counseling is essential for individuals with schizophrenia. Although some data suggest possible improvements during pregnancy, the reality is that the rigors of infertility treatment increase the risks of triggering a psychotic episode at any stage of the process. Psychosis is also a risk during pregnancy, or postpartum; negative interactions are possible between antipsychotic medications and fertility medications; and fetal exposure to antipsychotic medications is a concern. In addition, women with schizophrenia are at risk of substance abuse, comorbid mood disorders, and unstable lifestyles, posing further dilemmas for the caregiver, the patient, and her partner, along with significant consequences for children [96–98].

Sexual Dysfunction

The most common female sexual dysfunctions in infertile women are arousal phase disorders; orgasm phase disorders; vaginismus; and dyspareunia [99]. Sexual dysfunction in women may be due to hormonal changes, anatomic or physical factors (eg, endometriosis, ovarian cysts, or uterine fibroids), or organic conditions (eg, illness and diseases impacting general well-being and sexual health). Female sexual pain disorders can become the cause of infertility, if not the result, when pain is intense enough to limit or halt sexual intercourse [100,101]. This situation is common in conditions such as endometriosis, uterine fibroids, perimenopause, and uterine anomalies.

The most common sexual dysfunctions in men are erectile dysfunction, premature ejaculation, and retarded or inhibited ejaculation. Erectile dysfunction is the most important cause of male-factor infertility due to sexual dysfunction, although men rarely disclose this problem to caregivers [102]. Treatments for secondary erectile dysfunction have had mixed success rates, although medications (eg, sildenafil citrate or vardenafil) have been found to be effective. Additionally, sildenafil citrate has also been found to improve seminal parameters (eg, sperm motility) [103]. Sildenafil citrate was found to be helpful in increasing compliance among men using intercourse to conceive or pursuing infertility treatments that required semen collection [104].

The most common sexual problems among infertile couples are dyspareunia, progesterone-inhibited sexual desire, "sex on demand," unrealistic sexual demands, a rigid or routinized approach to sex, poor body image, depression, guilt, ambivalence, and physical conditions causing infertility (eg, endometriosis) or resulting from treatments [105]. Low libido or diminished sexual desire may also be the result of chronic health problems (eg, cystic fibrosis) or the invasiveness of medical treatment for infertility. Medications such as oral contraceptives, medroxyprogesterone contraceptive injection (Depo-Provera), GnRH agonists, ovulation-induction medications, antihypertensives, and antidepressants often interfere with sexual desire or response by changing hormone levels, affecting sexual appetite or arousal, or altering the experience of orgasm [99].

It is important to begin all infertility treatment histories (and infertility counseling interviews) with the issue of regular sexual intercourse sufficient to conceive. A small portion of couples presenting for infertility treatment are not infertile but are seeking medical treatment to avoid addressing a larger issue: they are not having sexual intercourse. Reasons may include sexual dysfunction or marital problems, or perhaps one partner is homosexual and has not acknowledged this to him/herself or partner.

As with many mental health or relationship problems, infertile couples typically ignore these problems or suggestions for psychological treatment in their single-minded pursuit of reproductive parenthood. Treatments for sexual problems range from medications, relationship therapy, individual psychotherapy, and diagnosis-specific treatments (eg, vaginal dilators for vaginismus). Careful history taking and assessments can determine the severity of the disorder, which is the best indictor of the type and length of treatment [99]. Psychiatrists working collaboratively with the reproductive team can provide patient education and treatment and valuable input into the treatment team's decision making about allowing patients to pursue infertility treatment if/when it is contraindicated.

Personality Disorders

Personality disorders and traits may have important effects on infertility patients' ability to cope and comply with treatment [106]. It is important for infertility clinicians to be aware of various personality disorders and their defensive behaviors, as outlined in Table 1. With the prevalence of personality disorders in the general population, clinicians can expect to be faced with a personality-disordered patient who can represent major challenges to the treatment team, and the patient's well-being. Individuals with Cluster A personality disorders (eg, paranoid, schizoid, and schizotypal) are rare, particularly at infertility clinics, because these individuals tend not to find interpersonal relationships rewarding and, as with schizophrenia and bipolar disorder, are often significantly disabled. Individuals with Cluster C personality disorders (avoidant, dependent, and obsessive-compulsive) are more common in the infertility clinic but their problems are easier to manage because they typically involve anxiety and the need for high levels of support and encouragement, fairly typical of infertile patients in general. However, Cluster C personality-disordered patients' expectations of caregivers may be different in that they have high dependency needs and may expect or want caregivers to be more paternalistic than collaborative.

By contrast, individuals with Cluster B disorders (ie, borderline, narcissistic, and histrionic personality disorders) are more common and problematic to the infertility treatment team. Individuals with these personality styles tend to have distorted perceptions and expectations of themselves, others, treatment success, and even clinic procedures (eg, feeling rejected and angry when phone calls are not immediately returned or having unrealistic [self-centered] expectations of success rates). Because they are already emotionally labile and frequently suffer comorbid depression, borderline patients may be especially sensitive to the effects of infertility medications on mood. The dysphoria, increased anxiety, and irritability associated with some infertility medications may be frightening to these patients. Similarly, the rollercoaster of emotions associated with infertility treatment may further destabilize these affectively labile women [46].

Table 1 Personality types and infertility	
Personality structure	Reaction to infertility
Obsessive: orderly, systematic, perfectionist, inflexible	Infertility is seen as punishment for letting things get out of control.
Narcissistic: self-involved, angry, independent, perfectionist	Infertility is seen as an attack on autonomy and perfection of self.
Borderline: demanding, impulsive, unstable	Infertility is seen as a threat of abandonment.
Dependent: long-suffering, depressed, submissive	Infertility is seen as expected punishment for worthlessness.
Avoidant: remote, unsociable, uninvolved	Infertility and its procedures are seen as a dangerous invasion of privacy.
Paranoid: wary, suspicious, blaming, hypersensitive	Infertility is seen as annihilating assault coming from everywhere outside of self.

Reproduced from Goldfarb JM, Rosenthal MB, Utian WH. Impact of psychologic factors in the care of the infertile couple. Semin Reprod Endocrinol 1985;3:97; with permission.

Individuals with borderline personality disorders can be disruptive because they react with intense, disruptive rage and splitting, causing problems for clinic staff and caregivers. Typically, they perceive the physician as the "good object" (usually because of intense, idealized transference reactions, believing the physician has the ultimate power and control over their fertility), whereas other clinic staff are perceived as the "bad object." As a result, clinic staff (eg, nurses, receptionists, and administrative personnel) suffer the brunt of these patients' angry outbursts. As such, it is important that all members of the infertility treatment team are aware of these patients' predictable pattern of behavior. Patients who have borderline personality disorder need consistent, clearly articulated, and immutable boundaries stated in a dispassionate and clinical manner and often repeated [46]. Angry rebuttals and encounters with these individuals will only fuel their projective rages and lead to even more disruptive behaviors.

PSYCHIATRIC REACTIONS AND SPECIFIC INFERTILITY CONDITIONS

Reproductive health professionals are well aware that infertility drugs are designed to have strong treatment effects, which can also mean significant side effects for their patients. However, patients are often less aware of these side effects and may not be prepared for their impact. GnRH agonists such as Lupron and triptorelin (Decapeptyl) are used to down-regulate the pituitary for extended periods (eg, 6 months) for the treatment of endometriosis. GnRH agonists lead to acute hypoestrogenism (ie, pharmacologic menopause), resulting in uncomfortable physical symptoms (eg, hot flashes, headaches, and mood changes [107]. Studies investigating the effects of GnRH agonists on mood in long-term usage found that the women developed significant depressive symptoms [107,108], although they improved with antidepressant treatment [109].

Polycystic ovary syndrome (PCOS) affects 1 in 10 women of childbearing age and is identified with high androgen levels; primary or secondary amenorrhea; ovarian cysts; and several metabolic complications (eg, insulin-resistance or type II diabetes, hypercholesteremia, and hypertension). Women with PCOS have also been found to have a characteristic difference in body composition and fat distribution patterns, when compared with healthy matched controls [68]. Some evidence indicates that women with PCOS are at significantly increased risk of anxiety and depression disorders, because of metabolic conditions or infertility. As a result, these women should be monitored carefully, not only for health complications but for risk of psychologic problems [110].

Research on animals (eg, mice and monkeys) [111,112] investigating the impact of psychosocial factors and stress have found that these factors impair reproduction. Similar findings have been in found in humans. In an investigation of women with infertility of unknown origin, researchers found that the infertile women with current depression or a history of depression experienced their first depressive episode before their infertility diagnosis. Treatment of the depression with antidepressants and psychotherapy restored ovulation and fertility in most of the women [113].

Spermatogenesis may be impacted by psychotropic medications, hypertension medications, and other medications and medical conditions (eg, heart disease and diabetes). Less investigation (and information) is known about the impact of emotional distress on male fertility [114].

PSYCHOLOGIC RESPONSES TO INFERTILITY TREATMENT MEDICATIONS

Oral birth control pills are typically used as part of the IVF treatment cycle to down-regulate the hypothalamus, to prevent premature ovulation during IVF cycles. Prevalence rates of depression in women taking oral birth control pills range from 5% to 50%, depression being most common in progesterone-dominant pills [115] (Table 2). However, because of the estrogen in oral birth control pills, some studies have reported the induction of rapid cycling mood in women with bipolar disorder when taking these pills [115].

GnRH agonists (eg, Lupron) are also typically used as a part of the IVF treatment cycle for down-regulation of the pituitary, to prevent premature ovulation during the IVF cycle. When used during an IVF treatment cycle, GnRH agonists are typically begun in the midluteal phase of the preceding cycle and continued until the stimulation phase of the treatment cycle. As noted earlier, GnRH agonists can lead to acute hypoestrogenism, triggering menopausal symptoms [107]. Research on GnRH exposure in IVF programs compared depression scores in IVF patients pretreated with the GnRH agonist triptorelin to depression scores in women undergoing IVF without down-regulation medications. Researchers found that triptorelin caused a 40% reduction in estradiol levels during the pretreatment phase, and this hypoestrogenism was associated with significantly increased symptoms of anxiety and depression, compared with controls [116]. All the subjects entering the study were euthymic, and, despite increases in mood symptoms with GnRH administration, no subject's symptoms met the criteria for major depressive or anxiety disorder [116]. Similarly, in a study in which women undergoing IVF with pretreatment

Table 2		
Psychiatric effects of infertility medications		
Drug	Use	Psychologic effects
Bromocriptine	Hyperprolactinemia	Antidepressant effects, hypomania, psychosis
Leuprolide acetate	Hypothalamic down-regulation	Depression, cognitive problems, fine motor problems
Progesterone	Endometrial support	Depression, decreased libido, irritability
Estradiol	Endometrial support	Antidepressant effects, induction of rapid cycling

From Williams KE, Zappert LN. Psychopathology and psychopharmacology in the infertile patient. In: Covington, SN, Burns LH, editors. Infertility counseling: a comprehensive handbook for clinicians. 2nd edition. New York: Cambridge University Press; 2006; with permission.

with GnRH agonist (Decapeptyl) were compared with women treated with human menopausal gonadotropin (Pergonal), ovarian suppression was associated with increased depression and anxiety scales [117]. These findings highlight the importance of recognizing that women with a current history of mood disorders and currently taking psychotropic medications may develop increased depressive or anxiety symptomatology during GnRH treatment, requiring an adjustment in psychotropic medication dosage or increased psychotherapeutic care.

Many women taking GnRH agonists complain of cognitive changes (eg, poor memory and concentration) that may or may not be accompanied by symptoms of a mood disorder [118]. Researchers found that 44% of women taking GnRH agonists reported decreased perceived memory functioning during treatment, with memory returning to normal once GnRH agonists were stopped [119]. Research has also reported significant decreased verbal memory scores in women on leuprolide [116].

Clomiphene citrate is the most commonly used fertility medication, whether to improve ovulation in women or to enhance sperm production in men. Clomiphene citrate (eg, Clomid and Serophene) is a synthetic estrogen used to induce or improve ovulation, improve luteal phase deficiency, and increase follicle number. Clomiphene is usually taken on days 3 to 5 of the menstrual cycle; however, it has a metabolite that can be found in the circulation for up to 30 days after the last dose [120]. In women, the side effects of clomiphene citrate include marked anxiety, sleep disturbance, headaches, visual disturbances, vertigo, hot flashes, mood swings, irritability, emotionality, and symptoms similar to premenstrual syndrome [121]. Clomiphene citrate may be associated with more mood changes in women who have a history of affective lability at times of hormonal change (eg, women with a history of premenstrual dysphoric disorder and postpartum depression). No psychiatric side effects have been reported in the literature in men taking clomiphene citrate to improve sperm production or quality.

Progesterone is frequently used during infertility treatment to improve luteal phase endometrial lining during ovulation induction treatment cycles and IVF treatment cycles. Progesterone in the oral birth control pill has been associated with the onset of depression in women [122]. However, some women report improvement in anxiety symptoms while on progesterone because of the sedative properties of its metabolites [47].

PSYCHOTIC EPISODES IN RESPONSE TO INFERTILITY TREATMENT

Patients most at risk for developing severe psychotic symptomatology appear to be women with pre-existing disorders, because they are more likely to experience mood shifts in response to normal hormonal changes (eg, ovulation, premenstrual period). However, psychotic episodes have also been reported in women without a pre-existing history of psychiatric disorders [123–125]. Several studies have reported women with bipolar disorder developing serious psychotic symptoms or episodes in response to clomiphene treatment. Typically, the psychosis began while clomiphene was being taken (days 2 to 7 of stimulation), indicating that the mechanism of action of the psychiatric side effect was a direct effect of clomiphene citrate on the central nervous system (rather than an indirect effect of the medication on hormone levels) [46]. Psychotic symptoms (including thought disturbances, hallucinations, and transient neurologic difficulties) appear to have abated rapidly when clomiphene treatment was terminated [126,127]. Hospitalization, psychiatric medications, and psychotherapy were required to stabilize the patient [128–130]. Bromocriptine mesylate is another infertility treatment medication that has been shown to trigger hypomania or mania, hallucinations, delusions, confusion, and behavioral changes in women with bipolar disorder on psychotropic medications [131].

Acute psychiatric episodes during various stages of IVF treatment have also been reported. One report involved an atypical response to GnRH analog. In this case, a 37-year-old woman previously diagnosed with schizophrenia developed acute schizoaffective symptoms and psychosis while taking GnRH [132]. In another case report, a 34-year-old woman with no psychiatric history suffered an acute psychotic episode, including hallucinations, dissociative amnesia, aphasia, and other neurologic disturbances, after undergoing transvaginal oocyte retrieval during an IVF cycle [133]. In another case report, a 30-year-old woman with no pre-existing psychiatric diagnosis developed ovarian hyperstimulation syndrome (OHSS) following IVF treatment, and schizoaffective symptoms during hospitalization and treatment for OHSS. In severe cases of OHSS, the patient develops anasarca, hepatic dysfunction, reduced blood volume, electrolyte imbalance, organ failure, and thromboembolic phenomena. As such, OHSS is a medical crisis requiring hospitalization and extensive medical treatment. However, the development of psychiatric symptomatology is rare. This patient was treated with haloperidol and within a week was asymptomatic for psychiatric symptoms, and within 2 weeks, OHSS was also resolved [134].

It may be that stimulation with hormone-regulating medications (eg, clomiphene citrate and GnRH analog), in connection with the physical and emotional distress of infertility treatment, may be a triggering factor for some patients, resulting in severe psychiatric episodes, even in individuals with no history of a psychiatric diagnosis. A physician giving IVF treatment to a patient who has psychiatric disorders must give special attention to her mental condition, and the patient and her partner should be fully informed about the possible mental effects of the treatment, particularly if she has a history of pre-existing psychiatric diagnoses. No psychotic episodes in men undergoing infertility treatment have been reported.

Drug Interactions

The drugs used in infertility treatment may interact with psychotropic medications, influencing their bioavailability and potentially affecting infertility and psychiatric treatment. Synthetic estrogens are metabolized by the cytochrome P-450 system in the liver; consequently, they affect psychotropic drugs that are also metabolized by the liver. Oral birth control pills stimulate the metabolism of drugs (eg, benzodiazepines, lorazepam, and oxazepam) and may be associated with decreased serum levels of these medications [115]. Oral birth control pills impair clearance of oxidatively metabolized medications (eg, alprazolam, triazolam, and imipramine), potentially leading to increased serum levels [124]. By contrast, mood stabilizers (eg, carbamazepine) may increase the metabolism of oral birth control pills, leading to failure of ovulation suppression [115]. Women taking carbamazepine and higher doses of birth control pills for down-regulation during IVF cycles may experience unacceptable interactive side-effects [47]. Bromocriptine mesylate (eg, Parlodel) is primarily used to treat women with endocrinology disorders (eg, amenorrhea with or without galactorrhea and hyperprolactinemia), resulting in infertility. Bromocriptine mesylate is a dopamine agonist, so combining it with other dopaminergic agents such as bupropion (Wellbutrin) or venlafaxine (Effexor) may lead to symptoms of dopaminergic toxicity (eg, hypertension, stereotypy, confusion, and severe psychiatric symptoms). Women taking bromocriptine mesylate who are started on tricyclic antidepressants should be warned about the increased risk of orthostatic hypotension with the combination of these two medications.

Drug interactions are always a risk factor in medicine because all individuals are at risk for developing either typical or atypical side effects to any medication. Medications used to treat infertility and psychiatric disorders are unique in that they are both metabolized by the liver and both impact pituitary functions and hormones. As such, patients with a history of pre-existing psychiatric disorders, who are currently taking psychotropic medications, and who are undergoing infertility treatment should be assessed carefully. Patients and their partners should be educated about potential medication side effects or interactions with other medications so they can self-monitor and be collaborators in their own treatment.

DENIAL OR DEFERMENT OF TREATMENT
Infertile Patients
According to the ASRM Ethics Committee Report, *Child-rearing and the Provision of Services*, fertility providers may decline to treat a patient on well-substantiated conclusions that the potential parent will not or cannot safely care for a child [135]. The ASRM recommends that infertility clinics have clear, written exclusion policies and criteria, and that a treatment team approach be used in decision making regarding denial or postponement of treatment. Disabled (mentally or physically) individuals should not be denied treatment, except when they fall within the narrowly defined parameters outlined within the recommendations, which should be applied universally to all patients.

Reproductive Collaborators (Gamete Donors, Gestational Carriers, Surrogates)
The ASRM Practice Committee has guidelines on the psychologic evaluation of gamete donors, gestational carriers, and surrogates at www.asrm.org [136–140]. These guidelines include physical criteria (eg, healthy or heritable disorder); acceptable amount of financial remuneration; and psychologic

criteria. The psychologic criteria are comprehensive and specific; however, the bottom line is that reasons for rejecting a potential collaborator include active psychiatric disorder; current psychotropic medication; history of sexual trauma; psychiatric disorder that would be exacerbated by participating as a reproductive collaborator (eg, gestational carrier volunteer with history of postpartum depression); evidence of coercion; or inability to provide informed consent. Reproductive collaborators should never be encouraged, coerced, or allowed to put their own psychosocial well-being at risk, particularly if they are on mood-stabilizing medications, have other mental health diagnoses, or are at significant risk for developing psychotic relapses or rapid cycling because of abrupt hormone changes. Careful history taking, a review of prior psychiatric records, and psychometric testing (eg, Minnesota Multiphasic Personality Inventory-2 or Personality Assessment Inventory) are recommended to help determine suitability [8].

COLLABORATION WITH THE REPRODUCTIVE MEDICINE TEAM

Some infertility clinics recommend or require that patients inform all caregivers (eg, psychiatrist or any other medicating physician) that he/she is undergoing infertility treatment. This requirement improves patient care (eg, reducing the potential for drug interactions) and reinforces a collaborative approach to infertility treatment. This collaboration is even more important when the patient also has complicating medical conditions for which he/she is being treated with other medications. Infertile individuals, however, may not be forthcoming with reproductive medicine caregivers about their current or past psychiatric problems because of ignorance (ie, lack of awareness of the potential for drug interactions); a belief that mental and physical health problems are two separate problems; embarrassment about the psychologic diagnosis; fear that infertility treatment will be denied or postponed because of the mental health problem and diagnosis; or denial, a belief that they (or their partner) does not have a mental health problem. Ideally, decisions about psychotropic medication usage and reproduction are made collaboratively and openly with the patient (and partner) as educated participants in the decision-making process with a reproductive psychiatrist [141]. With the patient's permission, these decisions should be promptly communicated to the reproductive medicine team including on staff infertility counselor(s). The plan should address setbacks, whether mental health or medical (eg, failed treatment cycle); crisis intervention; and pregnancy. Given that infertile men and women are known to be psychologically and physically vulnerable individually, as a couple, and as potential parents, it is imperative that the psychiatric needs of infertile patients be recognized and proactively addressed. Increasingly, psychiatrists work either as infertility counselors or with infertility counselors to improve the care and well-being of men and women undergoing infertility treatment. Psychiatrists, particularly those who provide primarily psychopharmacologic care, may or may not be aware that their patient is infertile; a gamete donor; a surrogate; pursuing pregnancy; or taking reproductive treatment medications.

Psychiatrists are typically called on by the reproductive medicine team to evaluate psychiatric readiness for medical procedures (eg, IVF, gamete donation); treat a patient who has an active psychiatric disorder or a history of psychopathology, or who is on psychotropic medications; and assess a patient's mental status (eg, ability to provide informed consent). Input from psychiatrists is particularly important with regard to decisions about denial of treatment or participation as a reproductive helper because of confounding mental health diagnosis or psychopharmacologic contraindications. They are in the best position to educate patients about the side effects of infertility treatment medications and the impact of hormonal shifts on psychologic well-being, particularly if the individual has pre-existing or ongoing psychopathology. They can be helpful with differential diagnosis among grief, depression, and stress; in assessing psychologic preparedness; and in determining the acceptability and suitability of gamete donation, a gestational carrier, or surrogacy as a family-building alternative for individuals, couples, and reproductive collaborators [142]. Psychiatrists can also be helpful when considering the long-term psychosocial well-being of offspring created as a result of third-party reproduction and assisted reproduction, and in treatment denial decisions. In short, infertility counseling, whether provided by a psychiatrist or other mental health professional, involves the treatment and care of various patients, not simply while they are undergoing infertility treatment but also with their long-term emotional well-being, that of their children, and that of the reproductive helpers who may assist them in achieving biologic or reproductive parenthood.

References

[1] Rosenblatt PC, Peterson P, Portner J, et al. A cross-cultural study of responses to childlessness. Behav Sci Notes 1973;8:221–31.
[2] Vayena E, Rowe P, Peterson H. Assisted reproductive technologies in developing countries: why should we care. Fertil Steril 2002;78:13–5.
[3] Butler P. Assisted reproduction in developing countries—facing up to the issues. Progress Reprod Health 2003;63:1–8.
[4] Lobel M, Dunkel-Schetter C. Psychological reactions to infertility. In: Stanton AL, Dunkel-Schetter L, editors. Infertility: perspectives from stress and coping research. New York: Plenum Press; 1991. p. 29–57.
[5] Daar A, Merali Z. Infertility and social suffering: the case of ART in developing countries. In: Vayena E, Rowe P, Griffin D, editors. Report of a meeting on medical, ethical, and social aspects of assisted reproduction. Geneva Switzerland: WHO; 2001. p. 16–21.
[6] Rutstein SO, Shah IH. Infecundity, infertility, and childlessness in developing countries. Demographic and Health Surveys (DHS) Comparative Reports 9. Baltimore (MD): ORC Marco and WHO, 2004. Available at: http://www.measuredhs.com/pubs/pdf/CR9/CR9.pdf. Accessed July 17, 2007.
[7] Palatchi C. The experience of infertility in Mexico: cross-cultural issues in infertility counseling. Symposia. American society of reproductive medicine, mental health professional group, and international infertility counseling organization. New Orleans (LA), 2006.
[8] Covington SN, Burns LH, editors. Infertility counseling: a comprehensive handbook for clinicians. 2nd edition. New York: Cambridge University Press; 2006.
[9] Haase JM, Blyth E. Global perspectives on infertility counseling. In: Covington SN, Burns LH, editors. Infertility counseling: a comprehensive handbook for clinicians. 2nd edition. New York: Cambridge University Press; 2006. p. 544–57.

[10] Mahlstedt PP. The psychological component of infertility. Fertil Steril 1985;43:335–56.

[11] Stanton AL, Dunkel-Schetter L. Psychological reactions to infertility. In: Stanton AL, Dunkel-Schetter L, editors. Infertility: perspectives from stress and coping research. New York: Plenum Press; 1991. p. 29–57.

[12] Stanton AL, Dunkel-Schetter C, editors. Infertility: perspectives from stress and coping research. New York: Plenum Press; 1991.

[13] Greil AL. Infertility and psychological distress: a critical review of the literature. Soc Sci Med 1997;45:1679–704.

[14] Boivin J, Takefman JE, Tulandi T, et al. Reactions to infertility based on extent of treatment failure. Fertil Steril 1995;63:801–7.

[15] Greenfeld D, Haseltine F. Stress in females as compared with males entering in vitro fertilization treatment. Fertil Steril 1992;57:350–6.

[16] Newton CR, Hearn MT, Yuzpe AA. Psychological assessment and follow-up after in vitro fertilization: assessing the impact of failure. Fertil Steril 1990;54:879–86.

[17] Csemiczky G, Landgren BM, Collins A. The influence of stress and state anxiety on the outcome of IVF-treatment: psychological and endocrinological assessment of Swedish women entering IVF-treatment. Acta Obstet Gynecol Scand 2000;79:113–8.

[18] Beaurepaire J, Jones M, Theiring P, et al. Psychosocial adjustment in infertility and its treatment: male and female responses at different stages of IVF/ET treatment. J Psychosom Res 1994;38:229–40.

[19] Newton CR, Sherrad W, Houle M. Preparing women for oocyte retrieval (OR): a comparison of psychological interventions. Fertil Steril 1994;S27.

[20] Kolonoff-Cohen H, Chu E, Natarajan L, et al. A prospective study of stress among women undergoing in vitro fertilization or gamete intrafallopian transfer. Fertil Steril 2001;76:75–87.

[21] Guerra D, Llobera A, Veiga A, et al. Psychiatric morbidity in couples attending a fertility service. Hum Reprod 1998;13:1733–6.

[22] Lapane KL, Zierler S, Lasater TM, et al. Is a history of depressive symptoms associated with an increased risk of infertility in women? Psychosom Med 1995;57:509–13.

[23] Nachtigall RD, Quiroga SS, Tschann JM, et al. Stigma, disclosure, and family functioning among parents with children conceived through donor insemination. Fertil Steril 1997;68:1–7.

[24] Hardy E, Makuch MY. Gender, infertility and ART. In: Vayena E, Rowe PJ, Griffin PD, editors. Current practices and controversies in assisted reproduction. Geneva: World Health Organization; 2002. p. 272–80.

[25] Berg BJ, Wilson JF, Weingartner PJ. Psychological sequelae of infertility treatment: the role of gender and sex-role identification. Soc Sci Med 1991;33:1071–80.

[26] Connolly KJ, Edelmann RJ, Cooke ID. Distress and marital problems associated with infertility. J Reprod Infant Psychol 1987;5:49–57.

[27] Mikulincer M, Horesh N, Levy-Shiff R, et al. The contribution of adult attachment style to the adjustment to infertility. Br J Med Psychol 1998;71:265–80.

[28] Daniluk JC. Gender and infertility. In: Leiblum SR, editor. Infertility: psychological issues and counseling strategies. New York: John Wiley & Sons; 1997. p. 103–25.

[29] Petok WD. The psychology of gender-specific infertility diagnoses. In: Covington SN, Burns LH, editors. Infertility counseling: a comprehensive handbook for clinicians. 2nd edition. New York: Cambridge University Press; 2006. p. 37–60.

[30] Peronace L, Boivin J, Schmidt L. Patterns of suffering and social interactions in infertile men: 12 months after unsuccessful treatment. Hum Reprod 2007;22:i86.

[31] Domar AD, Broome A, Zuttermeister PC, et al. The prevalence and predictability of depression in infertile women. Fertil Steril 1992;58:1158–63.

[32] Baram D, Tourtelot E, Muechler E, et al. Psychological adjustment following unsuccessful in vitro fertilization. J Psychosom Obstet Gynaecol 1988;9:181–90.

[33] Leiblum SR, Kemmann E, Lane MK. The psychological concomitants of in vitro fertilization. J Psychosom Obstet Gynaecol 1987;6:165–78.

[34] Laffont I, Edelmann RJ. Psychological aspects of in vitro fertilization: a gender comparison. J Psychosom Obstet Gynaecol 1994;15:85–92.

[35] Mahlstedt PP, Macduff S, Bernstein J. Emotional factors and the in vitro fertilization and embryo transfer process. J In Vitro Fert Embryo Transf 1987;4:232–6.

[36] Domar AD, Zuttermeister PC, Friedman R. The psychological impact of infertility: a comparison with patients with other medical conditions. J Psychosom Obstet Gynaecol 1993;14: 45–52.

[37] Chen T, Chang S, Tsai C, et al. Prevalence of depressive and anxiety disorders in an assisted reproductive clinic. Hum Reprod 2004;19:2313–8.

[38] Matsubayashi HT, Hosaka T, Izumi S. Emotional distress of infertile women in Japan. Hum Reprod 2001;16:966–9.

[39] Kee BS, Lee SH. A study on psychological strain in IVF patients. J Assist Reprod Genet 2000;17:445–8.

[40] Fido A. Emotional distress in infertile women in Kuwait. Int J Fertil Womens Med 2004;49: 24–8.

[41] Oddens BJ, den Tonkelaaer I, Nieuwenhuyese H. Psychological experiences in women facing fertility problems—a comparative survey. Hum Reprod 1999;14:255–61.

[42] Beutel M, Kupfer J, Kirchmeyer P, et al. Treatment-related stresses and depression in couples undergoing assisted reproductive treatment by IVF or ICSI. Andrologia 1999;31: 27–35.

[43] Dyer SJ, Abrahams N, Mokoena NE, et al. Psychological distress among women suffering from couple infertility in South Africa: a quantitative assessment. Hum Reprod 2005;20: 1938–43.

[44] Menning BE. The emotional needs of infertile couples. Fertil Steril 1980;34:313–9.

[45] Greenfeld DA, Diamond MP, Decherney AH. Grief reactions following IVF treatment. J Psychosom Obstet Gynaecol 1988;8:169–74.

[46] Williams KE, Zappert LN. Psychopathology and psychopharmacology in the infertile patient. In: Covington SN, Burns LH, editors. Infertility counseling: a comprehensive handbook for clinicians. 2nd edition. New York: Cambridge University Press; 2006. p. 97–116.

[47] Altshuler LL, Cohen L, Szuba MP, et al. Pharmacologic management of psychiatric illness during pregnancy: dilemmas and guidelines. Am J Psychiatry 1996;153:595–606.

[48] Viguera AC, Nonacs R, Cohen LS, et al. Risk of recurrence of bipolar disorder in pregnant and nonpregnant women after discontinuation of Lithium. Am J Psychiatry 2000;157: 179–84.

[49] Yonkers KA, Wisner KL, Stowe Z, et al. Management of bipolar disorder during pregnancy and the postpartum period. Am J Psychiatry 2004;16:608–20.

[50] Keck PE, McElroy SL, Tugrul KG, et al. Valproate oral loading in the treatment of acute mania. J Clin Psychiatry 1993;54:305–8.

[51] Stewart DE, Klompenhauwer JL, Kendell RE, et al. Prophylactic lithium in puerperal psychosis: the experience of three centers. Br J Psychiatry 1991;158:393–7.

[52] Cohen LS, Sichel DA, Robertson LH, et al. Postpartum prophylaxis for women with bipolar disorder. J Clin Psychiatry 1995;55:289–92.

[53] Williams KE, Casper RC. Reproduction and psychopathology. In: Casper RC, editor. Women's health: hormones, emotions and behavior. Rochester (NY): Cambridge University Press; 1997. p. 14–35.

[54] Price WA, Heil D. Estrogen induced panic attack. Psychosomatics 1988;29:433–5.

[55] Williams KE, Koran L. Obsessive compulsive disorder in pregnancy, premenstrum and postpartum. J Clin Psychiatry 1997;58:330–4.

[56] Miller LJ. Psychiatric medication during pregnancy: understanding and minimizing the risk. Psychiatr Ann 1994;24:69–75.

[57] Verhaak CM, Smeenk JM, van Minnen A, et al. A longitudinal, prospective study on emotional adjustment before, during and after consecutive fertility treatment cycles. Hum Reprod 2005;20:2253–60.

[58] Yehuda R. Biological factors associated with susceptibility to posttraumatic stress disorder. Can J Psychiatry 1999;44:69–75.

[59] Mazure CM, Greenfeld DA. Psychological studies of in vitro fertilization/embryo transfer participants. J In Vitro Fert Embryo Transf 1989;6:242–56.

[60] Wilson JF, Kopitzke EJ. Stress and infertility. Curr Womens Health Rep 2002;2:194–9.

[61] Davis DC, Dearman CN. Coping strategies of infertile women. J Obstet Gynecol Neonatal Nurs 1991;20:221–8.

[62] Peterson BD, Newton CR, Rosen KH. Examining congruence between partners' perceived infertility-related stress and its relationship to marital adjustment and depression in infertile couples. Fam Process 2003;42:59–70.

[63] Verhaak C, Burns LH. Behavioral medicine approaches to infertility counseling. In: Covington SN, Burns LH, editors. Infertility counseling: a comprehensive handbook for clinicians. 2nd edition. New York: Cambridge University Press; 2006. p. 169–95.

[64] Hammoud AO, Gibson M, Peterson CM, et al. Obesity and male reproductive potential. J Androl 2006;27:619–26.

[65] Weltzin TE, Weisensel N, Granczyk D, et al. Eating disorders in men: update. J Men's Health Gender 2005;2:186–93.

[66] Bulik CM, Sullivan PF, Fear JL, et al. Fertility and reproduction in women with anorexia nervosa: a controlled study. J Clin Psychiatry 1999;60:130–5.

[67] Stewart DE. Reproductive functions in eating disorders. Ann Med 1992;24:287–91.

[68] Kirchengast S, Huber J. Body composition characteristics and fat distribution patterns in young infertile women. Fertil Steril 2004;81:539–44.

[69] Mitchell AM, Bulik CM. Eating disorders and women's health: an update. J Midwifery Womens Health 2006;51:193–201.

[70] Stewart DE, Robinson GE, Goldbloom DS, et al. Infertility and eating disorders. Am J Obstet Gynecol 1990;163:1196–9.

[71] Crow SJ, Thuras P, Keel PK, et al. Long-term menstrual and reproductive function in patients with bulimia nervosa. Am J Psychiatry 2002;159:1048–50.

[72] Abraham S, Mira M, Llewellyn-Jones D. Should ovulation be induced in women recovering from an eating disorder or who are compulsive exercisers? Fertil Steril 1990;53:566–8.

[73] Norre J, Vandereycken W, Gordts S. The management of eating disorders in a fertility clinic: clinical guidelines. J Psychosom Obstet Gynaecol 2001;22:77–81.

[74] Mello NK, Mendelson JH, Teoh SK. Neuroendocrine consequences of alcohol abuse in women. Ann NY Acad Sci 1989;562:211–40.

[75] Eggert J, Theobald H, Engfeldt P. Effects of alcohol consumption on female fertility during an 18-year period. Fertil Steril 2004;81:379–83.

[76] Emanuele MA, Emanuele NV. Alcohol's effects on male reproduction. Alcohol Health Res World 1998;22:195–201.

[77] Muthusami KR, Chinnaswamy P. Effect of chronic alcoholism on male fertility hormones and semen quality. Fertil Steril 2005;84:919–24.

[78] Olaitan A, Reid W, Mocroft A, et al. Infertility among human immunodeficiency virus-positive women: incidence and treatment dilemmas. Hum Reprod 1996;11:2793–6.

[79] Mueller BA, Daling JR, Wiss NS, et al. Recreational drug use and the risk of primary infertility. Epidemiology 1990;1:195–200.

[80] Bracken MB, Eskenazi B, Sachse K, et al. Association of cocaine use with sperm concentration, motility, and morphology. Fertil Steril 1990;53:315–22.

[81] Ramlau-Hansen CH, Thulstrup AM, Aggerholm AS, et al. Is smoking a risk factor for decreased semen quality? A cross-sectional analysis. Hum Reprod 2007;22:188–96.

[82] Pasqualotto FF, Lucon AM, Sobreiro BP, et al. Effects of medical therapy, alcohol, smoking, and endocrine disruptors on male infertility. Rev Hosp Clin Fac Med Sao Paulo 2004;59(6):375–82.

[83] The Practice Committee of the American Society for Reproductive Medicine. Smoking and infertility. Fertil Steril 2004;81:1181–6.

[84] Vine MF, Tse CK, Hu P, et al. Cigarette smoking and semen quality. Fertil Steril 1996;65: 835–42.

[85] Said TM, Ranga GA. Relationship between semen quality and tobacco chewing in men undergoing infertility evaluation. Fertil Steril 2005;84:649–53.

[86] El-Nemr A, Shawaf T, Sabatini L, et al. Effect of smoking on ovarian reserve and ovarian stimulation in in-vitro fertilization and embryo transfer. Hum Reprod 1998;13:2192–8.

[87] Kmietowicz Z. Smoking is causing impotence, miscarriages, and infertility. BMJ 2004;328:364.

[88] Klonoff-Cohen H, Natarjan L, Marrs R, et al. Effects of female and male smoking on success rates of IVF and gamete intra-fallopian transfer. Hum Reprod 2001;16:1382–90.

[89] Crha I, Hruba D, Fiala J, et al. The outcome of infertility treatment by in-vitro fertilization in smoking and non-smoking women. Cent Eur J Public Health 2001;9:64–8.

[90] Zitzmann M, Rolf C, Nordoff V, et al. Male smokers have a decreased success rate for in vitro fertilization and intracytoplasmic sperm injection. Fertil Steril 2003;79:1550–4.

[91] Lintsen AM, Pasker de Jong PC, de Boer EJ, et al. Effects of subfertility cause, smoking and body weight on the success rate of IVF. Hum Reprod 2005;20:1867–75.

[92] Storgaard L, Bonde JP, Ernst E, et al. Does smoking during pregnancy affect sons' sperm counts? Epidemiology 2003;14:278–86.

[93] Seeman MV, Lang M. The role of estrogens in schizophrenia gender differences. Hosp Community Psychiatry 1990;16:185–94.

[94] Chang SS, Renshaw DC. Psychosis and pregnancy. Compr Ther 1986;12:36–41.

[95] McNeil TF, Kaij L, Malmquist-Larsson A. Women with non-organic psychosis: pregnancy's effect on mental health during pregnancy. Acta Psychiatr Scand 1984;75:140–8.

[96] Romans S. In the case: Karen is a 31-year-old woman who suffers from schizophrenia and has been treated with an antipsychotic medication for a number of years. Commentary. NZ Bioethic J 2001;2:34–5.

[97] Smith M. Response to Karen. NZ Bioethic J 2001;3:27–8.

[98] Ritsner M, Sherina O, Ginath Y. Genetic epidemiological study of schizophrenia: reproduction behavior. Acta Psychiatr Scand 1992;85:423–9.

[99] Burns LH. Sexual counseling and infertility. In: Covington SN, Burns LH, editors. Infertility counseling: a comprehensive handbook for clinicians. 2nd edition. New York: Cambridge University Press; 2006. p. 212–36.

[100] Binik YM, Bergeeron S, Khalife S. Dyspareunia. In: Leiblum SR, Rosen RC, editors. Principles and practice of sex therapy. 3rd edition. New York: Guilford Press; 2000. p. 154–80.

[101] Bachman GA. Dyspareunia and vaginismus. In: Sexual dysfunction: patient concerns and practical strategies. 24th annual postgraduate course of the American Fertility Society, 1991.

[102] Andrews FM, Abbey A, Halman J. Stress from infertility, marriage factors, and subjective well-being of wives and husbands. J Health Soc Behav 1991;32:238–53.

[103] Jannini EA, Lobardo F, Salacone P, et al. Treatment of sexual dysfunctions secondary to male infertility with sildenafil citrate. Fertil Steril 2004;81:705–7.

[104] Lenzi A, Lombardo F, Salacone P, et al. Stress, sexual dysfunction, and male infertility. J Endocrinol Invest 2003;25:72–6.

[105] Keye WR. The impact of infertility on psychosexual function. Fertil Steril 1980;34:308–9.

[106] Goldfarb JM, Rosenthal MB, Utian WH. Impact of psychologic factors in the care of the infertile couple. Semin Reprod Endocrinol 1985;3:97.

[107] Henzl MR. Gonadotropin-releasing hormone (GnRH) agonists in the management of endometriosis: a review. Clin Obstet Gynecol 1988;31:840–56.

[108] Warnock JK, Bundren JC. Anxiety and mood disorders associated with gonadotropin-releasing hormone agonist therapy. Psychopharmacol Bull 1997;33:311–6.

[109] Warnock JK, Bundren JC, Morris. Sertraline in the treatment of depression associated with gonadotropin releasing hormone agonist therapy. Biol Psychiatry 1998;43:464–5.

[110] Hollinrake E, Abreau A, Maifield M, et al. Increased risk of depressive disorders in women with polycystic ovary syndrome. Fertil Steril 2007;87:1369–76.

[111] Ansorge MS, Zhou M, Lira A, et al. Early life blockade of the 5HT transporter alters emotional behavior in adult mice. Science 2004;306:878–81.

[112] Williams NI, Berga SL, Cameron JL. Synergism between psychosocial and metabolic stressors: impact on reproductive function in cynomolgus monkeys. Am J Physiol Endocrinol Metab 2007;293:E270–6.

[113] Meller W, Burns LH, Crow S, et al. Major depression in unexplained infertility. J Psychosom Obstet Gynaecol 2002;23:27–30.

[114] Hendrick V, Gitlin M, Altshuler L, et al. Antidepressant medications, mood and male infertility. Psychoneuroendocrinology 2000;25:37–51.

[115] Jensvold MF. Nonpregnant reproductive age women. Part II: exogenous sex steroid hormones and psychopharmacology. In: Jensvold MF, Halbreich U, Hamilton JA, editors. Psychopharmacology and women: sex, gender and hormones. Washington DC: American Psychiatric Press; 1996. p. 171–90.

[116] Toren P, Dor J, Mester R, et al. Depression in women treated with a gonadotropin-releasing hormone agonist. Biol Psychiatry 1996;39:378–82.

[117] Weizman ES, Toren P, Dor Y, et al. Chronic GnRH agonist administration down-regulates platelet serotonin transporter in women undergoing assisted reproductive treatment. Psychopharmacologia 1996;125:141–5.

[118] Varney NR, Syrop C, Kubu CS, et al. Neuropsychologic dysfunction in women following leuprolide acetate induction of hypoestrogenism. J Assist Reprod Genet 1993;10:53–7.

[119] Newton C, Slota D, Yuzpe AA, et al. Memory complaints associated with the use of gonadotropin-releasing hormone agonists: a preliminary study. Fertil Steril 1996;65:1253–5.

[120] Glasier AF. Clomiphene citrate. Baillieres Clin Obstet Gynaecol 1990;4:491–501.

[121] Blenner J. Clomiphene-induced mood swings. J Obstet Gynecol Neonatal Nurs 1991;20: 321–7.

[122] Culberg J. Premenstrual symptom patterns and mental reactions to medication—a latent profile analysis. Acta Psychiatr Scand Suppl 1972;236:9–86.

[123] Rasgon N, Bauer M, Glenn T, et al. Menstrual cycle related mood changes in women with bipolar disorder. Bipolar Disord 2003;5:48–53.

[124] Chaudron LH, Pies RW. The relationship between postpartum psychosis and bipolar disorder: a review. J Clin Psychiatry 2003;64:1284–92.

[125] Rachman M, Garfield DA, Rachman I, et al. Lupron-induced mania. Biol Psychiatry 1999;45:243–4.

[126] Siedntopf F, Horskamp B, Stief G, et al. Clomiphene citrate as a possible cause of a psychotic reaction during infertility treatment. Hum Reprod 1997;12:706–70.

[127] Siedntopf F, Kentenich H. Future use of clomiphene in ovarian stimulation. Psychic effects of clomiphene citrate. Hum Reprod 1998;11:2986–7.

[128] Oyffe I, Lerner A, Isaacs G, et al. Clomiphene-induced psychosis. Am J Psychiatry 1997;154:1169–70.

[129] Kapfhammer HP, Messer T, Hoff P. Psychotic illness during treatment with clomifen. Dtsch Med Wochenschr 1990;115:936–9.

[130] Cashman FE. Clomiphene citrate as a possible cause of psychosis. Can Med Assoc J 1982;15:118.

[131] Altmark D, Tomaer R, Sigal M. Psychotic episode induced by ovulation-initiating treatment. Isr J Med Sci 1987;23:1156–7.

[132] Abu-Tair F, Strowitski T, Bergemann N, et al. [Exacerbation of a schizoaffective psychosis after in vitro fertilization with leuproreline acetate]. Nervenarzt 2007.

[133] Hwang JL, Kuo MC, Hsieh BC, et al. An acute psychiatric episode following transvaginal oocyte retrieval. Hum Reprod 2002;17:1124–6.

[134] Mercan S, Mercan R, Karamustafalioglu O. Case report: delirium associated with ovarian hyperstimulation syndrome. Reprod Biomed Online 2005;10:178–81.

[135] The Ethics Committee of the American Society of Reproductive Medicine. Child-rearing and the provision of services. Fertil Steril 2004;82:564–7.

[136] Thorn P. Recipient counseling for donor insemination. In: Covington SN, Burns LH, editors. Infertility counseling: a comprehensive handbook for clinicians. 2nd edition. New York: Cambridge University Press; 2006. p. 305–18.

[137] Sachs PL, Burns LH. Recipient counseling for oocyte donation. In: Covington SN, Burns LH, editors. Infertility counseling: a comprehensive handbook for clinicians. 2nd edition. New York: Cambridge University Press; 2006. p. 319–38.

[138] Applegarth LD, Kingsberg SA. The donor as a patient: assessment and support. In: Covington SN, Burns LH, editors. Infertility counseling: a comprehensive handbook for clinicians. 2nd edition. New York: Cambridge University Press; 2006. p. 339–55.

[139] Applegarth LD. Embryo donation: counseling donors and recipients. In: Covington SN, Burns LH, editors. Infertility counseling: a comprehensive handbook for clinicians. 2nd edition. New York: Cambridge University Press; 2006. p. 356–69.

[140] Hanafin H. Surrogacy and gestational carrier participants. In: Covington SN, Burns LH, editors. Infertility counseling: a comprehensive handbook for clinicians. 2nd edition. New York: Cambridge University Press; 2006. p. 370–86.

[141] Covington SN. Infertility counseling in practice: a collaborative approach. In: Covington SN, Burns LH, editors. Infertility counseling: a comprehensive handbook for clinicians. 2nd edition. New York: Cambridge University Press; 2006. p. 493–507.

[142] Mahlstedt PP, Greenfeld DA. Assisted reproductive technology with donor gametes: the need for patient preparation. Fertil Steril 1989;52L:908–14.

Psychiatr Clin N Am 30 (2007) 717–738

PSYCHIATRIC CLINICS
OF NORTH AMERICA

Psychiatric Issues in Bariatric Surgery

Lorenzo Norris, MD[a,b,*]

[a]Department of Psychiatry, Medical Faculty Associates of George Washington University Hospital, 2150 Pennsylvania Ave NW, Washington, DC 20037, USA
[b]Medical Wellness Clinic, George Washington University Hospital, Washington, DC, USA

OBESITY EPIDEMIC

Obesity is a worldwide epidemic, which is growing in strength. Obesity is defined as a body mass index (BMI) of 30 kg/m^2 or higher. Severe obesity is defined as a BMI of 40 kg/m^2 or higher or a BMI of 35 kg/m^2 or higher in the presence of high-risk conditions. With these definitions, approximately two thirds of the individuals living in the United States are overweight, and of those almost half are obese [1–4]. This number is truly staggering and equates to roughly one of every four adults, or more than 50 million people in the United States, being obese [1]. For the morbidly obese (BMI $\geq$40 kg/m^2), the state of affairs is even worse. Morbid obesity currently affects 20% of the obese population of the United States, approximately 8 million people. Notably, between 1986 and 2000 the prevalence of morbid obesity quadrupled [1–3,5]. Obesity is rising in frequency, and its greatest increases are in its most severe forms. Along with the rapid increase in the morbidly obese, approximately 15% of children and adolescents currently are considered overweight (BMI > the ninety-fifth percentile on growth charts) [1,6,7].

The rise in the prevalence of obesity is associated with an increase in the prevalence of comorbidities of obesity such as heart disease, hypertension, type 2 diabetes, obstructive sleep apnea, depression, cancer, and hyperlipidemia [2,4,8–10]. Obesity and its associated comorbidities cause a significant reduction in life expectancy. For example, a 25-year-old morbidly obese man has a 22% reduction in life expectancy, a loss of roughly 12 years [4,10,11]. Taken as a whole, these weight-related conditions account for 2.5 million deaths per year worldwide and for 400,000 deaths in the United States [4,11,12]. These data paint a picture of a chronic disease that affects multiple organ systems, that causes a substantial amount of morbidity and mortality, and whose prevalence is increasing in the young. Given these sobering facts, the prevalence of diet and weight-loss support groups is no surprise. Unfortunately, despite the

*Department of Psychiatry, Medical Faculty Associates of George Washington University Hospital, 2150 Pennsylvania Ave NW, Washington, DC 20037. E-mail address: lnorris@mfa.gwu.edu

0193-953X/07/$ – see front matter
doi:10.1016/j.psc.2007.07.011
© 2007 Elsevier Inc. All rights reserved.
psych.theclinics.com

sincere attempts of many, diet therapy, pharmaceutical treatments, and support groups have been shown to be ineffective long-term weight management strategies for the obese [9,13]. Therefore weight-loss surgery (WLS) increasingly has become the intervention of choice to treat the morbidly obese.

The treatment of a patient by WLS is a complicated matter, requiring significant expenditures of time and effort by the patient. Before patients even can see a clinician, they must find out if their health insurance covers WLS [14]. Many insurance companies now cover WLS, because it has been shown to be a proven intervention in the morbidly obese [4,9,15]. If insurance does not cover WLS, patients may be required to spend upwards of $20,000 out of pocket. Given the toll of morbid obesity on health and self-image, many patients are willing to save for the surgery if necessary. After dealing with insurance coverage, patients must select a surgeon with expertise in WLS. Qualified surgeons should have a minimum of 2 years of experience performing WLS and have adequate support staff to provide comprehensive care to patients after surgery. After selecting a surgeon, patients need to be seen by a number of clinicians for medical clearance before surgery. Because obesity is a systemic illness that affects virtually every organ system, and the surgery poses serious risks, weight-loss teams frequently advocate a multidisciplinary approach to care, in which each clinician performs his or her part of the necessary clearance with the overall care plan coordinated by a primary care physician or weight-loss surgeon.

A key component of the clearance process is the presurgical psychiatric evaluation [16–18]. This evaluation has many purposes. First, the evaluation seeks to determine the patient's capacity to understand the risk and benefits of surgery and to appreciate the consequences of surgery. Because of the comorbidity of psychiatric illness in the obese, the evaluation also screens for psychopathology, with particular attention paid to disorders of eating behavior. In the psychiatric evaluation of the WLS candidate, a robust knowledge base concerning the various aspects of WLS is essential. This knowledge allows the clinician to determine if the patient's goals for WLS are realistic, if the patient has researched the topic thoroughly, and whether the patient has taken the necessary steps to accommodate the behavioral changes that will be necessary after WLS. This article provides an update of current WLS procedures, proposed physiologic mechanisms of weight loss, elements of the presurgical psychiatric evaluation, and psychosocial predictors of outcome.

SURGICAL TREATMENT OPTIONS

A number of surgical options are available for the patient seeking WLS. The surgical procedures can be divided into two broad classes. Restrictive surgical procedures typically limit the amount of food that can be consumed by reducing the size of the stomach. Malabsorptive procedures cause food to be absorbed only partially from the gastrointestinal tract. This malabsorptive process usually is achieved by shortening the small intestine and thereby reducing the total time and surface area available for food absorption. Restrictive and malabsorptive procedures can be used separately or combined to give the WLS candidate many options. The choice of procedure depends on a number of factors, including the patient's level of obesity, desired rate of weight change, past medical history, and level of invasiveness desired.

Indications for Weight-Loss Surgery

In 1991 the National Institutes of Health (NIH) Consensus Development Panel for the Treatment of Severe Obesity established guidelines for the treatment of persons who have severe obesity. Patients should have a BMI greater than 40 kg/m^2 (be morbidly obese) and have failed numerous nonsurgical attempts to lose weight. In addition, the patient typically has a number of obesity-related comorbidities (eg, heart disease, hypertension, type 2 diabetes, obstructive sleep apnea, depression, and/or hyperlipidemia) that would benefit from WLS. If these health conditions are particularly severe, some clinicians may perform the surgery even at a BMI between 35 and 40 kg/m^2 (severe obesity).

Roux-en-Y Gastric Bypass

Roux-en-Y gastric bypass (RYGB) was the first of the procedures developed for persons who suffered from morbid obesity (BMI $\geq$ 40 kg/m^2). The operation uses both restrictive and malabsorptive elements to effect weight loss. The restrictive element is achieved by the creation of a small gastric pouch, which can measure between 15 mL and 25 mL. This small gastric pouch is formed by using staples to divide the stomach into upper and lower pouches. Food is digested in the smaller upper pouch. Because of its small capacity, the upper pouch is distended easily and contributes to the sensation of satiety that many patients report after surgery.

After the creation of the small pouch, a portion of the jejunum is attached to the small gastric pouch, forming the roux limb that bypasses a large portion of the gastrointestinal tract and thereby causing malabsorption. The degree of malabsorption can be changed by varying the length of the roux limb. Patients can expect to lose from 55% to 65% of their excess body weight (EBW). The operative mortality for RYGB has been reported to be 0.5% Operative morbidity has been reported to be about 5% [1,19]. The procedure now can be performed either laparoscopically or as an open procedure. The advantages of laparoscopic surgery include shortened hospitalization and greater postoperative comfort. Disadvantages include a higher rate of intra-abdominal complications.

Vertical Banded Gastroplasty

In a vertical banded gastroplasty a small gastric pouch is created, but there is no bypass or malabsorptive element. The small pouch is formed along the lesser curvature of the stomach and is the size of a small finger. Staples are used to create the fingerlike pouch; then the outlet for the pouch is circled by a silicone ring. This procedure can be performed laparoscopically. The weight loss associated with vertical banded gastroplasty is similar to that with RYGB, in the range of 50% to 60% of EBW [1].

Biliopancreatic Diversion and Duodenal Switch

For biliopancreatic diversion and duodenal switch, a partial gastrectomy is performed to create one gastric pouch that measures 100 to 150 mL. The pouch is roughly three to four times the size of the pouch formed by RYGB, thereby allowing increased food intake. A malabsorptive element (duodenal switch) may be added to the restrictive element by attaching the ileum to the first part of the small intestine. These surgical procedures usually are performed openly, are of long duration, and are technically more difficult. The operative mortality is 1%, and morbidity is approximately 5%. Patients can expect to lose 70% of EBW [1].

Laparoscopic Adjustable Gastric Banding

Laparoscopic adjustable gastric banding (LAGB), commonly referred to as the "lap band" procedure, forms a small gastric pouch by the placement of a band around the stomach. This band is attached to an access port secured to the abdominal wall. The size of the pouch usually is around 15 mL, but the size can be adjusted by inserting silicone into the access port. This silicone travels into the band surrounding the stomach, thereby reducing the stomach's volume. Weight loss with the adjustable banding procedure is roughly 50% of EBW. A key advantage of this procedure is that it can be reversed completely. Although a RYGB can be reversed, reversal is a complicated procedure that is rarely done.

Summary of Surgical Procedures

Table 1 summarizes the various WLS procedures.

With multiple surgical procedures available, it is imperative to match the patient with the most appropriate procedure. In general, the more invasive surgical procedures provide greater loss of EBW but at the cost of increased morbidity and mortality. The less invasive procedures can be performed laparoscopically and offer the advantages of shortened hospitalization and reversibility. All the procedures may have long- and short-term complications. The patient must be prepared to follow up with the bariatric team for successful management of complications after surgery.

Table 1
Comparison of procedures commonly used in weight-loss surgery

Procedure	Weight loss[a] (% excess body weight)	Restrictive or malabsorptive
BPDD	70	R, M
RYBG	65	R, M
VBG	60	R
LAGB	50	R

Abbreviations: BDD, biliopancreatic diversion and duodenal switch; LAGB, laparoscopic adjustable gastric banding; M, malabsorptive; R, restrictive; RYBG, roux-en-Y gastric bypass; VBG, vertical banded gastroplasty.
   [a]Weight loss is approximate amount of excess body weight, individual results may vary.

COMPLICATIONS OF WEIGHT-LOSS SURGERY

The two most common WLS procedures performed in the United States are laparoscopic RYGB and LAGB. These surgeries have significant short-term and long-term complications. It is vital that WLS candidates be aware of these potential complications so that they can make an informed decision regarding the risks and benefits of WLS. In addition, the patient's insight into the nature of postsurgical complications can inform the clinician as to the amount of research the patient has done regarding WLS and the extent of his or her planning for possible obstacles postoperatively.

A full discussion of all the possible complications of the various WLS procedures is beyond the scope of this article. Tables 2 and 3 provide an overview of the relevant complications of laparoscopic RYGB, and LAGB, the two most common WLS procedures in use today. For a more detailed discussion, the reader is referred to the recent review of complications of antiobesity surgery by Nguyen and Wilson [20].

Table 2	
Complications of laparoscopic roux-en-Y gastric bypass surgery[a]	
Complication	Description
Wound infection	Signs of infection at the wound site can include pain and purulent drainage. The incidence of wound infection has dropped with the introduction of laparoscopic RYGB
Bowel obstruction	Studies have estimated the incidence of bowel obstruction from 0.4% to 5.5%. There are a variety of causes of obstruction, but all result in symptoms of vomiting, distension, and abdominal pain. This complication can occur perioperatively or postoperatively.
Anastomotic leak	Leaks can occur at the anastomosis sites (sites where parts of bowel and stomach are joined). This complication can be potentially life threatening, and is manifested by fever, tachycardia, abdominal pain, and vomiting. Leaks can occur up to 2 weeks after surgery. Incidence of leaks initially reported to range between 2.2% and 4.4%.
Pulmonary embolism	Pulmonary embolism is a life-threatening complication that usually manifests with chest pain, tachycardia, and hypoxia. Pulmonary embolism can be responsible for up to 50% of the deaths after RYGB.
Hemorrhage	Hemorrhage can occur immediately or late (after 48 hours) after surgery, and has an incidence of 0.6% to 3.7% Signs of early hemorrhage include tachycardia, hematemesis, and bright red blood per rectum.

Abbreviation: RYGB, roux-en-Y gastric bypass.

[a]Perioperative complications occur less than 30 days after surgery. Postoperative complications are defined as occurring more than 30 days after surgery.

Adapted from Nguyen NT, Wilson SE. Complications of antiobesity surgery. Nat Clin Pract Gastroenterol Hepatol 2007;4:138–47; with permission.

Table 3
Complications of laparoscopic adjustable gastric banding[a]

Complication	Description
Erosion	Erosion usually occurs years after the initial surgery, when the band erodes and the previous restrictive element it offered becomes impaired. Erosion then can cause increased weight gain, loss of a sense of restriction, and abdominal pain. The incidence of erosion is estimated at 0.1% to 2.8%.
Perforation	Perforation is a rare complication which may occur in the first few days following surgery and present with low urine output, hypotension, and abdominal pain.
Band slippage	Band slippage is a fairly common complication with an incidence ranging from 2.3% to 12.5%. Patients can present with vomiting and failure to meet expected weight-loss goals. Band slippage usually is a late complication with symptoms occurring 30 days or more after surgery.
Infection at port site	Poet-site infection is an infrequent complication with an incidence of 0.4% to 1%. It usually resents with typical signs of infection that include induration, drainage, and redness. Infection typically is an early complication occurring within the first 30 days of surgery.

[a]Perioperative complications occur less than 30 days after surgery. Postoperative complications are defined as occurring more than 30 days after surgery.

Adapted from Nguyen NT, Wilson SE. Complications of antiobesity surgery. Nat Clin Pract Gastroenterol Hepatol 2007;4:138–47; with permission.

POSTOPERATIVE COURSE

Recovery

The length of time for recovery depends largely on the type of surgery performed and the physical condition of the patient before surgery. In general, the laparoscopic procedures have shorter hospital stays. The hospital stay for LAGB is 1 day. Laparoscopic RYGB typically requires a 2-day hospital stay, whereas open RYGB or BPDD can require a 5- to 6-day stay in the hospital. While in the hospital, most patients begin walking the same day of surgery.

Dietary Changes

Perhaps the biggest challenge postoperatively is the new diet required for the patient who has undergone WLS. Adherence to a proper diet is crucial as the patient's stomach and gastrointestinal tract heal. The patient needs to be weaned back to solid food in three main diet phases. The first phase consists of drinking clear liquids. The liquid phase usually last 1 to 2 weeks but can vary depending on the patient. After successfully completing the liquid phase, the patient transitions to purees. In the puree stage the patient usually eats 2 ounces of food three times per day. The puree phase generally lasts 2 weeks, and then the patient transitions to solid food. In this stage the patient must modify his or her eating pattern in a number of ways to facilitate the new gastric pouch (Box 1). The reality of having to give up some foods permanently

---

Box 1: Suggested changes in eating patterns during the final transition stage to solids

- Eat three meals per day.
- Chew food very thoroughly.
- Drink 30 to 45 minutes before meals, because the gastric pouch cannot accommodate liquid and solids.
- When eating, have eating be the primary focus. This focus helps the patient avoid overeating.

---

can make this phase difficult for some patients. A dietician can ease the transition by suggesting diets that meet the patient's nutritional and taste needs but adhere to the dietary restrictions imposed by the surgery.

Change in Weight-Related Diseases

Buchwald and colleagues [4,8] performed a systematic review and meta-analysis of bariatric surgery in which they looked at weight loss and comorbidity outcomes across 36 studies. There was a broad improvement in diabetes, with 76.8% of patients reporting complete resolution and subsequent changes in glycosylated hemoglobin, fasting glucose, and fasting insulin levels. In regards to hyperlipidemia, approximately 70% of patients significantly lowered their total cholesterol and low-density lipoprotein levels. This analysis, however, did not observe an increase in patents' high-density lipoprotein levels. In regards to hypertension, approximately 60% of patients experience resolution or a very significant decrease in blood pressure. Patients suffering from obstructive sleep apnea also showed a considerable improvement, with approximately 80% of patients experiencing resolution or improvement in breathing. Although this list is not inclusive, these data show that the severely obese can realize dramatic improvement in a number of weight-related medical problems.

PHYSIOLOGIC FACTORS

With the advent of RYGB, many have pushed for a better understanding of the physiologic mechanisms involved in the substantial weight loss that occurs after surgery. The factors promoting weight loss can be broken down into three broad categories: anatomic, physiologic, and behavioral. Theses categories overlap and influence each other, but different lines of research have pointed to specific mechanisms in each that may account for the weight loss. The exact role of physiologic factors still is debated, and more studies with larger sample sizes are needed to determine fully the exact physiologic mechanisms associated with WLS. The following section reviews some proposed physiologic mechanisms of weight loss after bariatric surgery.

Role of Ghrelin in Appetite Regulation

The majority of research has focused on the gastrointestinal hormones ghrelin and peptide YY (PYY). Both these hormones modulate metabolism and appetite, and the changes in their levels before and after surgery have been studied.

Ghrelin was discovered in 1999 by Kojima and colleagues [21]. Ghrelin is an orexigenic hormone that is secreted by the A cells in the oxyntic glands of the stomach fundus. Ghrelin is a strong stimulator of the growth hormone receptor and has been shown to increase food intake in animal and humans [22]. In humans the plasma levels of ghrelin rise before a meal and fall after a meal. This change in levels of ghrelin is thought to correlate with a person's urge to eat [23]. Since this discovery investigators have looked at the role of ghrelin in the pathophysiology of obesity and anorexia nervosa. Reduced levels of ghrelin have been found in obese subjects [24]. Cummings and colleagues [24] looked at the changes in plasma ghrelin levels after diet-induced weight loss in 13 obese subjects who underwent a 6-month dietary program, in 5 subjects who underwent RYGB surgery, and in 10 normal-weight controls. The authors found that ghrelin levels rose in proportion to the amount of weight loss in those who used the dietary program. The rise in ghrelin before a meal was significantly less in the subjects who underwent RYGB surgery than in their counterparts in the dietary program. The results of this study suggest that RYGB may be successful because it disrupts ghrelin secretion. Disruption of ghrelin secretion may stop the cycle of weight loss and rise in ghrelin that serves to return a patient's weight to prediet levels (Fig. 1).

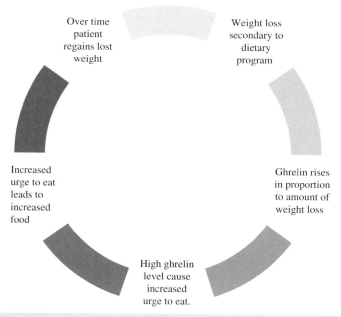

Fig. 1. The proposed relationship between ghrelin and weight loss. As patients diet, they lose weight, and their ghrelin levels rise proportionately. This increase in ghrelin counteracts the effects of the diet by increasing the patients' urge to eat. This increased urge to eat causes patients to break the diet and overeat again, re-establishing the cycle of weight gain after loss.

Role of Peptide YY in Appetite Regulation

The second gastrointestinal hormone that has been studied is PYY. PYY is secreted from L cells in the small bowel of the small bowel and colon. The secretion of PYY is triggered by protein and fat. PYY has been shown to reduce appetite and food intake when infused into normal-weight subjects [25]. This reduction is thought to be caused by the interaction of PYY with neuropeptide Y2 receptors in the hypothalamus. PYY inhibits neuropeptide Y2 receptors, triggering a series of events that leads to decreased gut motility [26,27]. Batterham and colleagues [25] looked at the effect of PYY infusion on appetite and food intake in obese subjects. They performed a double-blind, placebo-controlled crossover study with 12 lean subjects and 12 obese subjects. They found that the obese patients were responsive to the appetite-reducing effects of PYY. Following this line of research Kroner and colleagues [27] studied the effects of RYGB on fasting and postprandial concentrations of PYY, plasma ghrelin, and insulin. They found a substantial increase in postprandial PYY in patients who had undergone RYGB that may account for the reduced hunger that these patients experience.

These initial findings supporting ghrelin and PYY as potential physiologic mechanisms accounting for weight loss have been examined by a number of researchers. The conclusions have been mixed. The initial studies were limited by sample size and duration of follow-up. The results of studies with larger sample sizes and postsurgical follow-up periods of 1 to 2 years question the reported change in ghrelin and PYY levels after surgery. Nijhuis and colleagues [28] looked at changes in plasma ghrelin, leptin, and insulin levels over a period of 2 years in morbidly obese individuals who underwent RYGB surgery. This study found that plasma ghrelin levels increased after surgery. Christou and colleagues [29] looked at pre- and postprandial plasma ghrelin levels as correlates of satiety or failure to achieve a successful outcome after RYGB. Their data did not support a role for plasma ghrelin as a correlate for satiety. Couce and colleagues [30] found that weight loss after laparoscopic RYGB occurred despite the absence of significant changes in plasma ghrelin.

Taken as a whole, these results certainly suggest that a change in physiology occurs after RYGB surgery. In the short term it would seem that changes in ghrelin and PYY may support weight loss in a majority of individuals. Over the long term, however, the role of these hormones in sustained weight loss after RYGB surgery still is unclear. The direction and nature of these changes probably depend on the surgical procedure and on the nature of each individual surgery.

PSYCHOLOGIC SCREENING

Obesity is a systemic disease that has been shown to affect virtually every organ system. The etiology of obesity involves many factors, both physiologic and psychologic. For this reason, numerous organizations have advocated the use of multidisciplinary teams in the presurgical evaluation of WLS candidates. The NIH Conference on Gastrointestinal Surgery for Severe Obesity and the American Society for Bariatric Surgery [1] recommend that a psychologic evaluation be performed as part of this multidisciplinary assessment. Although psychologic evaluation is advocated, there currently is no standard evaluation protocol for patients before WLS. During the past years researchers have attempted to ascertain the necessary elements for a comprehensive psychologic evaluation of WLS candidates.

Elements of Bariatric Surgery Evaluation

Although no official standard for evaluations exists, examination of the current literature points to consensus about which broad topics should be covered [16–18,31,32]. These topics are outlined in Table 4. Many of the elements are part of a clinician's standard evaluation, but certain specific issues must be addressed in the WLS candidate. First, it is essential that the examiner and patient understand the three primary goals of WLS: reduction of weight, reduction of comorbid weight-related illness, and an improvement in the patient's quality of life. The presurgical psychiatric evaluation can contribute to all three goals rather than function simply as a "clearance for surgery." In regards to the first objective, the psychiatric evaluation can assess whether the patient has the capacity to understand the WLS procedure and has the optimal behavioral strategies in place to maximize postoperative success. The presurgical evaluation also facilitates the second and third objectives of WLS by identifying mental illness in the patient preparing for WLS. Numerous studies have documented the high prevalence of mental illness in the morbidly obese [4,32–38]. Despite the current evidence that the presence of mental illness is not a negative

Table 4
Suggested elements for a bariatric surgery evaluation

Assessment area	Key issues
Emotional/affective	Major depressive disorder
	Bipolar disorder
	Impulse control
	Coping skills
	Ability to form alliance
Capacity	Schizophrenia
	Knowledge of surgical interventions
	Baseline cognitive function
Behavioral	Eating disorder
	Substance use
	Physical activity
	Previous attempts at weight management
Developmental	History of abuse
Motivational	Rationale for surgery
Current life situation	Stressors
	Social network
	Time management

predictor of weight loss, the presence of an illness that adversely affects general health and quality of life should be reason enough for a through evaluation.

Psychiatric Comorbidity in Obese Patients

The evidence for psychiatric comorbidity in obese patients has been well established in a number of studies [13,31,34,35,39–42]. Herpertz and colleagues [13] estimated the rates of Axis I disorders among WLS candidates varies from 27.3% to 41.8%. Of the Axis I disorders, mood disorders are the most commonly diagnosed. Sarwer and colleagues [37,43] interviewed 90 candidates for WLS using several scales, including the Beck Depression Inventory-II, Lifestyles Inventory, Questionnaire on Eating and Weight Patterns. This study found that almost two thirds of patients had a psychiatric diagnosis, the most common being major depression. In addition to mood disorders, studies have shown a high prevalence of anxiety disorders including social phobia and generalized anxiety disorder [16,35,39]. Studies of the prevalence of eating disorders in candidates for WLS also found significant comorbidity. Depending on assessment methods, the prevalence of binge-eating disorder (BED) has been estimated to range from 10% to 50% [41,42,44]. If the presence of other syndromes such as night-eating syndrome or grazing are included, the prevalence rates of eating disorders increases further. Furthermore, a notable minority of patients has been diagnosed as having substance abuse disorders. The use of substances can be of particular concern, because some patients may turn to substance abuse as an alternative means of coping with stress after WLS.

Many studies also have examined Axis II pathology in the WLS candidate. Investigators using the Minnesota Multiphasic Personality Inventory (MMPI) have tried to identify personality characteristics that would be predictive of weight loss after surgery [45–49]. Duckro and colleagues [49] used the MMPI to examined the psychologic status of female candidates for WLS. Results showed that 31% of candidates could be classified as depressed and socially anxious, and another 25% could be classified as character disordered. Studies that have assessed personality using DSM-IV criteria and clinical interviews have reported passive-aggressive, schizotypal, histrionic, and borderline disorders to be the most common personality disorders [39]. Given the overall high rates of psychiatric comorbidity (particularly major depressive disorder, and BED), it is recommended that clinicians screen for serious psychopathology in addition to other psychologic factors. The following section addresses specific issues that may arise during sections of the presurgical psychologic assessment. In particular, disorders that are likely to present in a certain assessment area are highlighted.

Emotional/Affective Disorders

Depressive and anxiety disorders are the most common psychiatric disorders identified in the morbidly obese [50,51]. Onyike and colleagues [52] looked at the association between depression and obesity by examining the results from the Third National Health and Nutrition Examination Survey. This study surveyed more than 40,000 people and found that individuals who had a BMI of 40 kg/m^2 were almost five times more likely than persons of average weight to have experienced an episode of major depression in the previous year. In a recent literature review Wadden and colleagues [53] noted that nearly 25% to 30% of patients reported clinically significant symptoms of depression. Despite this level of comorbidity, preoperative depression levels have not been shown to be consistent predictors of weight loss after WLS. Nonetheless, based on their clinical experience with more than 2500 candidates for WLS, Wadden and colleagues [53,54] have suggested that presurgical screening for depression (and other disorders) is still needed, because active treatment can relieve patients' suffering. Although the prevalence of depression usually decreases after surgery, Mitchell and colleagues [55] found a subgroup of patients who remained depressed even after long-term follow-up after WLS. Furthermore Dixon and colleagues [56] reported that patients suffering form depression after surgery tend to have less weight loss and a poorer postsurgical quality of life.

Given the high prevalence of depressive symptoms in the morbidly obese, distinguishing the demoralized obese patient from a patient meeting a DSM-IV–defined mood disorder can be challenging. Obese patients may experience many physical symptoms that overlap with vegetative symptoms of depression. For example, the presence of obstructive sleep apnea can cause profound disturbances in sleep and fatigue Likewise, patients who have arthritis or other forms of joint disease frequently are unable to exercise fully or to participate in activities that previously were enjoyable. Multiple studies have also shown the effect of obesity on self-esteem and body image. The importance of accurate diagnosis is highlighted by the observation that at follow-up after WLS, the prevalence rates of Axis I psychiatric diagnosis range from one half to one third of the presurgical rates [13,16,35]. A patient who is misdiagnosed may be given a psychotropic medication that is unnecessary and could adversely effect the patient's weight. At the same time, even subsyndromal affective symptoms could impact motivation and compliance negatively.

Beyond mood, a patient should show an immature ability to cope with distress. In particular, it is important to ask how the candidate copes with both negative and positive stress. Although there is a tendency to focus on how a patient copes with setbacks, the positive benefits of weight loss often can place a patient in a new world of opportunity that poses unexpected stresses. For example, a patient may receive attention from potential suitors because of improved physical appearance. The patient's emotional reaction to the presurgical interview itself can be monitored for use of mature or immature defense mechanisms. Given that psychologic evaluation can be stressful, observing how a patient modulates himself or herself in this scenario can give the examiner crucial information.

Most studies looking at group results have not found an increased risk of suicide associated with WLS. If the focus is switched to individual patients, however, some recent findings should be noted. A study by Pories and colleagues [57] showed a higher-than-expected rate of suicide among patients followed for 8 years postoperatively. Omalu and colleagues [58] observed that three individuals who committed suicide after bariatric surgery had a history of severe depression that continued postoperatively. Although individual reports do not have the strength to establish a clear relationship between variables that could predict suicide in the WLS, they do emphasize that every patient should receive comprehensive care for comorbid mental illness.

Capacity

From a cognitive standpoint, the patient should be familiar with the various surgical options and know the difference between the two major surgeries, RYGB and LAGB. In addition, the patient should have knowledge of the risks and benefits of both procedures and how these risks apply to the patient's specific weight conditions. For example, it would be important that a patient understand the differences between restrictive procedures and malabsorptive procedures. At the very least, this knowledge would indicate that the patient understands that two different mechanisms are at work. Depending on the institution, what constitutes as adequate knowledge and insight varies. At the George Washington University Hospital, patients are shown a videotape of the procedure, and the surgeon then discusses the risks and benefits of WLS. Recommended readings are suggested to optimize patients' knowledge of WLS. Patients also meet with a nurse practitioner who helps in coordinating a variety of issues (organizes the pre-operative evaluation, helps to provide patient education, arranges for specialty consultations) and serves as a point person. At the conclusion of this education, the patient frequently can describe the surgery in words and visually. The patient also can explain in reasonable detail his or her choice of RYGB or LAGB. The patient has become familiar with all the common side effects and the potentially life-threatening side effects. Patients also should show knowledge of the expected dietary changes, the need for postsurgical follow-up, and the need for exercise. Frequently all this education takes place before the presurgical psychiatric evaluation. If the patient's knowledge base is not optimal, the deficient areas are identified, and suggestions made for the patient to improve his or her understanding of the procedure. Many clinicians would view a lack of knowledge about the surgical procedure as a possible contraindication. In addition, any form of active psychosis or severe mental retardation (IQ < 50) would be viewed as a possible contraindication [59].

Behavioral Disorders

Assessment of eating patterns and of the presence of a comorbid eating disorder is essential. BED, in which patients have recurrent subjective or objective periods of consuming food in an out-of-control fashion, has been found in up to 30% of candidates for WLS [60]. Kalarchian and colleagues [41] reported that 46% of patients who had undergone RYGB surgery more than 2 and less than 7 years previously reported binge episodes. Active binge eating is considered a contraindication to surgery. In addition to BED, the clinician should screen for grazing, night-eating syndrome, and overeating. Grazing, in particular, has been studied as a possible high-risk behavior that could predispose a patient to binge eating postoperatively [61].

A thorough history of attempted diet and exercise regimens should be obtained. There is no definitive statement on how many diets or exercise programs a patient must have undertaken; it is important to see that the patient has made an effort, has had periods in which he or she was able to endure a liquid diet, and can make time in his or her schedule to engage in exercise. Most programs advocate that a patient stop smoking before surgery. Any use of illicit drugs or heavy alcohol consumption can be considered a contraindication for surgery.

Developmental Disorders

A screen for trauma and abuse should be performed, because sexual abuse may be more common in obese patients [62,63]. This part of the assessment also should look at how the patient related to food as a child. In some patients food can play a symbolic role and is associated with ridicule, comfort, or as means of acceptance. The patient's relationship with family also should be assessed to help determine how the patient's attachment system has functioned in the past.

Motivational Problems

Patients should be motivated to obtain WLS for health reasons and not for aesthetics. It is important that patients be aware that they will still look and be overweight, even with a successful procedure, but will experience significant decreases in weight-related illnesses such as hypertension, diabetes, hyperlipidemia, and obstructive sleep apnea [4,50,55,64]. The patient's expectations of how weight change will change his or her life should be explored. The clinician should pay particular attention to patients who believe weight loss will cure most of their life problems. Additionally, patients should not wait until after surgery to begin their long-term lifestyle changes. In fact, some programs require that patients exhibit some form of dietary commitment before surgery to assess their level of motivation and their ability to comply with necessary behavior/lifestyle changes.

Current Life Situation

Current social support and financial stability should be assessed. Because WLS is a stressful procedure, a stable support network of family and friends is desirable. An assessment of current stressors also should be undertaken; areas of concern that should be included are stressors that may disrupt the patient's social support (divorce, death of loved one, moving). In general, patients should have a stable lifestyle that facilitates regular eating and dieting. Although interpersonal stress is not a contraindication, it is a point of clinical concern.

Assessment Instruments

Bauchowitz and colleagues [59] assessed the methods used for psychologic evaluation by various bariatric surgery programs. They found that the methods varied greatly, but almost half of the programs requiring an evaluation used some form of formal testing. The two most frequently used tests were the Beck Depression Inventory and the MMPI. These scales are well validated and are useful in detecting depressive disorders and personality disorders in obese and nonobese individuals. In addition to assessment methods, the authors asked the participants which psychosocial conditions could represent a contraindication to surgery. The results are shown in Table 5. Although there are no guidelines in place regarding absolute contraindications, the data gleaned from this study and others can help guide the clinician by identifying the practice patterns of other parishioners.

Summary of Possible Contraindications for Surgery

A number of scales are available to assess eating attitudes and behaviors. The Three- Factor questionnaire measures three dimensions of eating behavior: cognitive restraint of eating, disinhibition, and hunger. The Eating Disorder Examination questionnaire is a self-report questionnaire that measures the frequency of eating disorder behavior and can discriminate obese binge eaters from obese non–binge eaters. The Binge-Eating Scale was developed to diagnose binge eating in obese subjects but does not include the necessary criteria to diagnose BED and therefore is better used as a screen. Other useful screening tools include the Quality-of-Life Inventory and Binge-Eating Scale. The use of assessment measures must take into account the length of the interview and how the data will be used. No matter what assessment measure is used, almost all programs include a formal psychologic interview in addition to the assessment.

PSYCHOLOGIC PREDICTORS OF WEIGHT LOSS

Many studies have looked at possible psychologic predictors of weight loss and quality of life after surgery. Variables of interest have included past psychiatric history, presence of BED, personality traits, and eating patterns [13]. Although the idea of finding variables predictive of outcome has merit, it has proven difficult for a number of reasons. First, there are many different types of WLS; when defining predictors, it would be optimal to compare groups undergoing the same type of surgery. Also, most patients being followed over time already have been screened extensively. This screening creates a selection bias in which serious pathology probably is underrepresented in the population at study. Finally, many studies have been limited by sample size and drop-out rates, making the number of quality studies small. Despite these challenges, some preliminary conclusions can be ascertained and used to guide the clinician in screening patients.

Binge-Eating Disorder

Of principal concern to many is the patient's eating behavior before and after surgery and whether this behavior is predictive of weight loss. In two prospective studies, Busetto and colleagues [65] looked at BED, among other variables, as a predictor of weight loss. All the patients investigated underwent LAGB. The authors did not find BED to be a negative predictor of weight loss up to 3 years after surgery. The authors did find that BED was associated with more vomiting and neostoma stenosis. Mitchell and colleagues [55] performed

Table 5

Response to a survey of current the psychosocial evaluation processes in bariatric surgery programs[a]

Potential contraindication	Definite contraindication	Possible contraindication	No contraindication
Current illicit drug use	88.9	8.6	1.2
Active symptoms of schizophrenia	86.4	12.3	1.2
Severe mental retardation	81.5	13.6	3.7
Current heavy drinking	77.8	19.8	1.2
Lack of knowledge about surgery	77.8	19.8	1.2
Significant medical noncompliance	69.1	25.9	2.5
Unrealistic expectation of weight loss	61.7	35.8	1.2
Multiple suicide attempts	61.7	34.6	2.5
Active symptoms of bipolar disorder	61.7	32.1	4.9
Recent suicide attempt	60.5	34.6	2.5
Current symptoms of depression	53.1	42	3.7
Active symptoms of obsessive-compulsive disorder	51.9	42	4.9
Active binge-eating disorder	48.1	40.7	8.6
Mental retardation (IQ between 70 and 50)	45.7	46.9	6.2
History of depressive disorder	44.4	54.3	1.2
Current use of tobacco	37	35.8	25.9
Psychiatric hospitalization within the past 12 months	34.6	61.7	2.5
History of multiple psychiatric hospitalizations	32.1	61.7	4.9
No past medically supervised diet	32.1	53.1	13.6
History of chronic illicit drug use within the past 5 years	30.9	65.4	2.5
Controlled symptoms of schizophrenia	21	70.4	7.4
Antisocial personality disorder	16	71.6	11.1
Inability to diet for 3 months	14.8	64.2	19.8
Borderline personality disorder	11.1	76.5	11.1
Previous weight reduction surgery	11.1	69.1	18.5

(continued on next page)

Table 5
(continued)

Potential contraindication	Definite contraindication	Possible contraindication	No contraindication
Age < 21 years	11.1	48.1	40.7
Past criminal behavior	8.6	67.9	22.2
Distant suicide attempt (>1 year in the past)	6.2	81.5	11.1
History of binge-eating disorder	6.2	72.8	18.5
Frequent social drinking	3.7	61.7	33.3
Recent major loss (death, divorce)	3.7	69.1	25.9
Presence of another eating disorder	3.7	88.9	4.9
Poor social support	2.5	53.1	44.4
Age >55 years	2.5	38.3	59.3
Controlled symptoms of bipolar disorder	2.5	81.5	14.8
Controlled symptoms of obsessive-compulsive disorder	1.2	75.3	22.2
History of severe sexual abuse		67.9	30.9

[a]As part of the survey, respondents were asked to rate 37 potential psychosocial contraindications as definite contraindications, possible contraindications, or no contraindication.

Data from Bauchowitz AH, Gonder-Frederick LA, Olbrisch ME, et al. Psychosocial evaluation of bariatric surgery candidates: a survey of present practices. Psychosomatic Medicine 2005;67:825–32; with permission.

a retrospective study of patients after RYGB, with long-term follow-up of 13 to 15 years. In this study patients who developed BED after the surgery tended to gain more weight. Given these findings, some cautionary conclusions regarding the predictive value of BED can be stated. First, BED before surgery seems not to be necessarily predictive of ineffective weight loss. The occurrence of BED after the surgical procedure, however, is predictive of ineffective weight loss, as compared with patients who do not have BED. Although at this time BED before surgery is not a negative predictor of weight loss, it should be screened for, because it may be a predictor of increased complications after surgery. Indeed, some would argue that increased vomiting after surgery could be seen as a failed binge attempt [55,66].

Psychiatric History

Studies have looked at the predictive value of psychiatric comorbidity as a predictor of weight loss after surgery. Larsen and colleagues [35] followed 103 patients over a period of 3 years. All the patients underwent horizontal gastric banding and were interviewed and rated on DSM criteria. Those who had significant personality pathology were identified as a group with insufficient weight loss. Herpertz and colleagues [13] performed an informative systematic review of psychosocial variables affecting weight loss after WLS. They examined 18 prospective studies that assessed the effect of psychiatric symptoms on weight loss. Only four of the studies showed psychiatric comorbidity to have an impact on postsurgical weight loss. These findings suggest that psychiatric comorbidity is not a negative predictor of weight loss after surgery. Indeed some authors even have suggested that higher levels of psychologic distress may be positive correlates of weight loss, the rational being that a patient who has obesity-related dissatisfaction may be highly motivated to change. As mentioned previously, however, selection bias can influence these above findings significantly. The typical candidate for WLS usually has tried numerous diets and has gone through a multitude of logistical steps before even seeing a psychiatrist. After this process, the study population is screened by a trained professional. These conditions could create a population in which mental disorders are underrepresented.

Eating Patterns

Research on eating patterns has focused on the consumption of different foods as predictive of weight loss after surgery. In particular, authors have examined the consumption of sweet food versus nonsweet food as a predictor of weight loss. Sugerman and colleagues [67] found that sweet eaters lost less weight than nonsweet eaters 1 year after vertical banded gastroplasty. Lindroos and colleagues [68] also examined the role of sweets as a predictor of postsurgical weight loss. They followed 375 subjects who underwent vertical banded gastroplasty for 2 years and evaluated them by using questionnaires. This study found no association between the intake of sweet foods and weight loss after surgery.

In addition to the type of food eaten, studies have examined the role of stress eating as a predictor weight loss. Gentry and colleagues [17] found that stress eating may be a negative predictor for weight loss after surgery. This finding suggests that it is sensible to screen patients for their eating behavior and focus more on eating patterns rather than on what is eaten. A patient who relies on food to relive stress or who shows an irregular pattern of eating could be at risk for reduced weight loss after surgery.

SUMMARY

WLS is a proven, effective intervention for severely obese patients. There are four broad categories of surgery, but all reduce excess body weight to an extensive extent. Using surgery in the treatment of a disease with a large behavioral component may seem counterintuitive, but numerous studies have shown the ineffectiveness of diet and exercise in the morbidly obese. The ineffectiveness of these methods is the result, in part, of an alteration in hormones and peptides involved with long-term regulation of energy and weight. The WLS procedures have been shown to alter the anatomic and physiologic function of the stomach. In a motivated patient, this change in the gastrointestinal tract results in weight loss and a significant reduction in weight-related health problems.

Evaluating a patient for WLS can be challenging, and multiple organizations have suggested that a multidisciplinary approach be used. The mental health professional often is called on to assess many different domains of psychologic function. This evaluation should go beyond the standard interview and should pay attention to the patient's eating behavior, knowledge of surgery, and motivation for surgery. The use of standardized instruments will facilitate accuracy and further research in the field of WLS. Because there are few absolute psychologic contraindications to WLS, the assessment should also focus on risk management, with the goal of improving the patient's postoperative quality of life.

References

[1] 2004 American Society for Bariatric Surgery Consensus Conference on Surgery for Severe Obesity. Surg Obes Relat Dis 2005;1:297–381.

[2] Deitel M. The obesity epidemic. Obes Surg 2006;16:377–8.

[3] Deitel M. Overweight and obesity worldwide now estimated to involve 1.7 billion people. Obes Surg 2003;13:329–30.

[4] Buchwald H, Avidor Y, Braunwald E, et al. Bariatric surgery: a systematic review and meta-analysis. JAMA 2004;292:1724–37.

[5] Ogden CL, Yanovski SZ, Carroll MD, et al. The epidemiology of obesity. Gastroenterology 2007;132:2087–102.

[6] Flegal KM, Tabak CJ, Ogden CL. Overweight in children: definitions and interpretation. Health Educ Res 2006;21:755–60.

[7] Fontaine KR. Health-related quality of life among obese subgroups. Obes Res 2002;10: 854–5.

[8] Buchwald H. Consensus Conference Panel. Bariatric surgery for morbid obesity: health implications for patients, health professionals, and third-party payers. J Am Coll Surg 2005;200:593–604.

[9] Deitel M, Shikora SA. The development of the surgical treatment of morbid obesity. J Am Coll Nutr 2002;21:365–71.

[10] Fontaine KR, Redden DT, Wang C, et al. Years of life lost due to obesity. JAMA 2003;289: 187–93.

[11] Allison DB, Fontaine KR, Manson JE, et al. Annual deaths attributable to obesity in the United States. JAMA 1999;282:1530–8.

[12] Deitel M. Some consequences of the global obesity epidemic. Obes Surg 2005;15: 1–2.

[13] Herpertz S, Kielmann R, Wolf AM, et al. Do psychosocial variables predict weight loss or mental health after obesity surgery? A systematic review. Obes Res 2004;12: 1554–69.

[14] Deitel M. Bariatric surgery is a cost-saving for the healthcare system. Obes Surg 2005;15: 301–3.

[15] Buchwald H. Consensus Conference Panel. Consensus Conference statement: bariatric surgery for morbid obesity: health implications for patients, health professionals, and third-party payers. Surg Obes Relat Dis 2005;1:371–81.

[16] Gertler R, Ramsey-Stewart G. Pre-operative psychiatric assessment of patients presenting for gastric bariatric surgery (surgical control of morbid obesity). Aust N Z J Surg 1986;56: 157–61.

[17] Gentry K, Halverson JD, Heisler S. Psychologic assessment of morbidly obese patients undergoing gastric bypass: a comparison of preoperative and postoperative adjustment. Surgery 1984;95:215–20.

[18] Sogg S, Mori DL. The Boston interview for gastric bypass: determining the psychological suitability of surgical candidates. Obes Surg 2004;14:370–80.

[19] Proceedings of the American Society for Bariatric Surgery Consensus Conference on the State of Bariatric Surgery and Morbid Obesity: health implications for patients, health professionals and third-party payers. Washington, DC, May 6–7, 2004. Surg Obes Relat Dis 2005;1:105–53.

[20] Nguyen NT, Wilson SE. Complications of antiobesity surgery. Nat Clin Pract Gastroenterol Hepatol 2007;4:138–47.

[21] Kojima M, Hosoda H, Date Y, et al. Ghrelin is a growth-hormone-releasing acylated peptide from stomach. Nature 1999;402:656–60.

[22] Date Y, Kojima M, Hosoda H, et al. Ghrelin, a novel growth hormone-releasing acylated peptide, is synthesized in a distinct endocrine cell type in the gastrointestinal tracts of rats and humans. Endocrinology 2000;141:4255–61.

[23] Engstrom BE, Ohrvall M, Sundbom M, et al. Meal suppression of circulating ghrelin is normalized in obese individuals following gastric bypass surgery. Int J Obes (Lond) 2007;31: 476–80.

[24] Cummings DE, Weigle DS, Frayo RS, et al. Plasma ghrelin levels after diet-induced weight loss or gastric bypass surgery. N Engl J Med 2002;346:1623–30.

[25] Batterham RL, Cohen MA, Ellis SM, et al. Inhibition of food intake in obese subjects by peptide YY3-36. N Engl J Med 2003;349:941–8.

[26] Korner J, Inabnet W, Conwell IM, et al. Differential effects of gastric bypass and banding on circulating gut hormone and leptin levels. Obesity (Silver Spring) 2006;14:1553–61.

[27] Korner J, Bessler M, Cirilo LJ, et al. Effects of roux-en-Y gastric bypass surgery on fasting and postprandial concentrations of plasma ghrelin, peptide YY, and insulin. J Clin Endocrinol Metab 2005;90:359–65.

[28] Nijhuis J, van Dielen FM, Buurman WA, et al. Ghrelin, leptin and insulin levels after restrictive surgery: a 2-year follow-up study. Obes Surg 2004;14:783–7.

[29] Christou NV, Look D, McLean AP. Pre- and post-prandial plasma ghrelin levels do not correlate with satiety or failure to achieve a successful outcome after roux-en-Y gastric bypass. Obes Surg 2005;15:1017–23.

[30] Couce ME, Cottam D, Esplen J, et al. Is ghrelin the culprit for weight loss after gastric bypass surgery? A negative answer. Obes Surg 2006;16:870–8.

[31] Grothe KB, Dubbert PM, O'jile JR. Psychological assessment and management of the weight loss surgery patient. Am J Med Sci 2006;331:201–6.

[32] Dziurowicz-Kozlowska AH, Wierzbicki Z, Lisik W, et al. The objective of psychological evaluation in the process of qualifying candidates for bariatric surgery. Obes Surg 2006;16: 196–202.

[33] Clark MM, Balsiger BM, Sletten CD, et al. Psychosocial factors and 2-year outcome following bariatric surgery for weight loss. Obes Surg 2003;13:739–45.

[34] Fabricatore AN, Crerand CE, Wadden TA, et al. How do mental health professionals evaluate candidates for bariatric surgery? Survey results. Obes Surg 2006;16:567–73.

[35] Larsen F. Psychosocial function before and after gastric banding surgery for morbid obesity. A prospective psychiatric study. Acta Psychiatr Scand Suppl 1990;359:1–57.

[36] Rothschild M, Peterson HR, Pfeifer MA. Depression in obese men. Int J Obes 1989;13: 479–85.

[37] Sarwer DB, Wadden TA, Fabricatore AN. Psychosocial and behavioral aspects of bariatric surgery. Obes Res 2005;13:639–48.

[38] Buddeberg-Fischer B, Klaghofer R, Krug L, et al. Physical and psychosocial outcome in morbidly obese patients with and without bariatric surgery: a 4 1/2-year follow-up. Obes Surg 2006;16:321–30.

[39] Black DW, Goldstein RB, Mason EE. Prevalence of mental disorder in 88 morbidly obese bariatric clinic patients. Am J Psychiatry 1992;149:227–34.

[40] Herpertz S, Kielmann R, Wolf AM, et al. Does obesity surgery improve psychosocial functioning? A systematic review. Int J Obes Relat Metab Disord 2003;27:1300–14.

[41] Kalarchian MA, Marcus MD, Levine MD, et al. Psychiatric disorders among bariatric surgery candidates: relationship to obesity and functional health status. Am J Psychiatry 2007;164:328–34 [quiz: 374].

[42] Kalarchian MA, Marcus MD, Wilson GT, et al. Binge eating among gastric bypass patients at long-term follow-up. Obes Surg 2002;12:270–5.

[43] Sarwer DB, Cohn NI, Gibbons LM, et al. Psychiatric diagnoses and psychiatric treatment among bariatric surgery candidates. Obes Surg 2004;14:1148–56.

[44] Glinski J, Wetzler S, Goodman E. The psychology of gastric bypass surgery. Obes Surg 2001;11:581–8.

[45] Blankmeyer BL, Smylie KD, Price DC, et al. A replicated five cluster MMPI typology of morbidly obese female candidates for gastric bypass. Int J Obes 1990;14:235–47.

[46] Larsen JK, Geenen R, Maas C, et al. Personality as a predictor of weight loss maintenance after surgery for morbid obesity. Obes Res 2004;12:1828–34.

[47] Tsushima WT, Bridenstine MP, Balfour JF. MMPI-2 scores in the outcome prediction of gastric bypass surgery. Obes Surg 2004;14:528–32.

[48] Walfish S. Reducing Minnesota Multiphasic Personality Inventory defensiveness: effect of specialized instructions on retest validity in a sample of preoperative bariatric patients. Surg Obes Relat Dis 2007;3:184–8.

[49] Duckro PN, Leavitt JN Jr, Beal DG, et al. Psychological status among female candidates for surgical treatment of obesity. Int J Obes 1983;7:477–85.

[50] Karlsson J, Sjostrom L, Sullivan M. Swedish obese subjects (SOS)–an intervention study of obesity. Two-year follow-up of health-related quality of life (HRQL) and eating behavior after gastric surgery for severe obesity. Int J Obes Relat Metab Disord 1998;22:113–26.

[51] Masheb RM, White MA, Toth CM, et al. The prognostic significance of depressive symptoms for predicting quality of life 12 months after gastric bypass. Compr Psychiatry 2007;48:231–6.

[52] Onyike CU, Crum RM, Lee HB, et al. Is obesity associated with major depression? Results from the third national health and nutrition examination survey. Am J Epidemiol 2003;158:1139–47.

[53] Wadden TA, Sarwer DB, Fabricatore AN, et al. Psychosocial and behavioral status of patients undergoing bariatric surgery: what to expect before and after surgery. Med Clin North Am 2007;91:451–69.

[54] Wadden TA, Sarwer DB. Behavioral assessment of candidates for bariatric surgery: a patient-oriented approach. Obesity (Silver Spring) 2006;14(Suppl 2):53S–62S.

[55] Mitchell JE, Lancaster KL, Burgard MA, et al. Long-term follow-up of patients' status after gastric bypass. Obes Surg 2001;11:464–8.

[56] Dixon JB, Schachter LM, O'Brien PE. Sleep disturbance and obesity: changes following surgically induced weight loss. Arch Intern Med 2001;161:102–6.

[57] Pories WJ, MacDonald KG Jr, Morgan EJ, et al. Surgical treatment of obesity and its effect on diabetes: 10-y follow-up. Am J Clin Nutr 1992;55:582S–5S.

[58] Omalu BI, Cho P, Shakir AM, et al. Suicides following bariatric surgery for the treatment of obesity. Surg Obes Relat Dis 2005;1:447–9.

[59] Bauchowitz AU, Gonder-Frederick LA, Olbrisch ME, et al. Psychosocial evaluation of bariatric surgery candidates: a survey of present practices. Psychosom Med 2005;67:825–32.

[60] Spitzer RL, Yanovski S, Wadden T, et al. Binge eating disorder: its further validation in a multisite study. Int J Eat Disord 1993;13:137–53.

[61] Saunders R. "Grazing": a high-risk behavior. Obes Surg 2004;14:98–102.

[62] Felitti VJ. Childhood sexual abuse, depression, and family dysfunction in adult obese patients: a case control study. South Med J 1993;86:732–6.

[63] Gustafson TB, Gibbons LM, Sarwer DB, et al. History of sexual abuse among bariatric surgery candidates. Surg Obes Relat Dis 2006;2:369–74 [discussion: 375–6].

[64] Pories WJ, MacDonald KG. The surgical treatment of morbid obesity. Curr Opin Gen Surg 1993;195–205.

[65] Busetto L, Valente P, Pisent C, et al. Eating pattern in the first year following adjustable silicone gastric banding (ASGB) for morbid obesity. Int J Obes Relat Metab Disord 1996;20:539–46.

[66] Powers PS, Rosemurgy A, Boyd F, et al. Outcome of gastric restriction procedures: weight, psychiatric diagnoses, and satisfaction. Obes Surg 1997;7:471–7.

[67] Sugerman HJ, Londrey GL, Kellum JM, et al. Weight loss with vertical banded gastroplasty and roux-en-Y gastric bypass for morbid obesity with selective versus random assignment. Am J Surg 1989;157:93–102.

[68] Lindroos AK, Lissner L, Sjostrom L. Weight change in relation to intake of sugar and sweet foods before and after weight reducing gastric surgery. Int J Obes Relat Metab Disord 1996;20:634–43.

Psychiatr Clin N Am 30 (2007) 739–759

PSYCHIATRIC CLINICS
OF NORTH AMERICA

Hematologic Problems in Psychosomatic Medicine

Madeleine Becker, MD[a], David J. Axelrod, MD, JD[b],
Olu Oyesanmi, MD[c], Dimitri D. Markov, MD[a],
Elisabeth J. Shakin Kunkel, MD[a],*

[a]Department of Psychiatry, Thomas Jefferson University, Philadelphia, PA, USA
[b]Department of Internal Medicine, Thomas Jefferson University, Philadelphia, PA, USA
[c]ECRI Institute, Plymouth Meeting, PA, USA

The consultation psychiatrist is frequently called upon to assess patients in medical settings with primary or secondary hematologic disorders. This article addresses psychiatric issues that are specific to patients who have selected hematologic disorders, including B_{12} and folate deficiency, sickle cell disease, and hemophilia, discussing the diseases, their unique psychiatric manifestations, and approaches to management. A review of hematologic side effects of psychotropic medications is also included.

B_{12} AND FOLATE DEFICIENCY

B_{12} and folate deficiency have similar consequences on the nervous system and lead to megaloblastic anemia [1]. Both B_{12} and folate are cofactors for the conversion of homocysteine to methionine [2]. Deficiency of either B_{12} or folate correlates with high homocysteine levels [2–5], which is a risk factor for cardiovascular disease, stroke, dementia, and Alzheimer's disease [1,2,6,7]. Both high homocysteine levels and deficiencies of B_{12} and folate are also associated with depression [8].

Vitamin B_{12}
Vitamin B_{12} (cobalamin) is found in meat and dairy products. It is a necessary coenzyme and cofactor in various reactions, including DNA synthesis and the synthesis of methionine from homocysteine. Vitamin B_{12} is stored in significant amounts in the liver, and it takes years to develop a deficiency [9]. The elderly are at increased risk for B_{12} deficiency. Epidemiologic studies show a prevalence of about 20% in the general population, and the numbers of geriatric

*Corresponding author. E-mail address: elisabeth.kunkel@jefferson.edu (E.J. Shakin Kunkel).

0193-953X/07/$ – see front matter
doi:10.1016/j.psc.2007.07.006
© 2007 Elsevier Inc. All rights reserved.
psych.theclinics.com

individuals with the deficiency is even higher [2,5,9,10]. Both B_{12} and folate deficiency are common in psychiatric populations [11,12].

Pernicious anemia is the most common cause of B_{12} deficiency [2,13]. Pernicious anemia is an autoimmune disorder, resulting in the loss of parietal cells in the stomach and failure of intrinsic factor production, which is a necessary component to B_{12} absorption. Pernicious anemia is frequently associated with other autoimmune disorders, including thyroiditis, diabetes mellitus, Addison's disease, Grave's disease, vitiligo, myasthenia gravis, Lambert Eaton syndrome, and hypoparathyroidism [2,13]. Dietary B_{12} deficiency is rare but may occur in strict vegans [2]. In the elderly, deficiency is usually due to malabsorption caused by gastric atrophy or pernicious anemia [9,10,14]. Food or oral-cobalamin malabsorption may be caused by *H. pylori* infection, intestinal overgrowth caused by antibiotics, chronic use of metformin [15,16] and antacids, H-2 receptor antagonists, proton pump inhibitors [17], alcoholism, gastric surgery (including gastric bypass surgery for severe obesity), pancreatic failure, and Sjogren's syndrome. Vitamin B_{12} malabsorption results from gastrectomy, ileal diseases, bowel resection, Crohn's disease, blind loops, and infection with *Diphyllobothrium latum* or AIDS [9].

Clinical manifestations

Hematologic manifestations of B_{12} deficiency include megaloblastic anemia, macrocytosis with hypersegmented polymorphonuclear leukocytes, thrombocytopenia, leukopenia, pancytopenia and rarely, hemolytic anemia and thrombotic microangiopathy. Gastrointestinal manifestations include intestinal metaplasia, Hunter's glossitis (smooth and shiny tongue due to atrophy of the lingual papillae), diarrhea, jaundice, and increased lactate dehydrogenase and bilirubin levels. Vaginal atrophy may also occur [9,13].

Neuropsychiatric manifestations

Neuropsychiatric manifestations are common in B_{12} deficiency, especially in the elderly [9,14]. Neuropsychiatric symptoms of B_{12} deficiency may precede hematologic signs and there is frequently a disassociation between the hematologic and neuropsychiatric symptoms [1,4,12]. Symmetrical peripheral neuropathy occurs frequently with paresthesias and numbness. Subacute combined degeneration (SCD) of the spinal cord is less common [1]. SCD combines posterior column disruption, resulting in loss of vibration and position sense, and ataxia with a positive Romberg's sign with lateral column disruption, causing weakness, spasticity, and extensor plantar responses [13]. Rare manifestations of B_{12} deficiency include optic neuritis, optic atrophy, and incontinence. Psychiatric symptoms may include mood changes, psychosis, cognitive impairment, and obsessive-compulsive disorder [12,18–20]. B_{12} deficiency is a common cause of potentially reversible dementia and confusion [9,14].

Diagnosis and treatment

A low normal serum vitamin B_{12} level in the presence of megaloblastic hematopoiesis or the typical neuropsychiatric findings should lead to further investigation for B_{12} deficiency. A low normal vitamin B_{12} level is usually between 150 ng/L to 200 ng/L. When a low level is encountered, elevated serum methylmalonic acid and elevated serum total homocysteine can help establish if deficiency exists [2,9,20]. Tests for intrinsic factor antibody, serum gastrin, and a Schillings test may be helpful in diagnosing pernicious anemia. Differentiating the causes of B_{12} deficiency yields important clinical information and can guide diagnosis and treatment [2].

Treatment recommendations generally advise injections of 1000 micrograms of hydroxycobalamin or cyanocobalamin daily, for one week, then maintenance doses monthly to every three months, depending on the severity of the deficiency [13,21]. Clinical evidence suggests that oral B_{12} replacement also is effective [14]. Remission is typically achieved in weeks, but continued maintenance therapy is recommended to fully replete body stores and maintain longer periods of remission. Significant improvement of neuropsychiatric function has been shown after B_{12} administration [4,14], and the degree of recovery is correlated with symptom severity before treatment [1].

Administration of folate without B_{12} to correct macrocytic anemia (caused by unrecognized B_{12} deficiency) will reverse the hematologic abnormalities, but neurologic impairment from the B_{12} deficiency may continue to progress, sometimes leading to irreversible deficits [1,2,22].

Folic Acid

Folic acid is found in both animal products and leafy vegetables. Folate is important in mood and cognition, brain growth, differentiation, development, and repair. These mechanisms are likely mediated through nucleotide synthesis and DNA transcription and integrity [2]. Folate may protect against certain cancers, heart disease, birth defects [23], and dementia [24], presumably via the lowering of homocysteine [7].

Folate deficiency can be caused by inadequate diet, alcoholism, chronic illness, drugs (phenytoin, valproic acid, lamotrigine, barbiturates, trimethoprim/sulfamethoxazole, oral contraceptives, and methotrexate), or malabsorption [1,22]. Folate deficiency is also more common in the elderly [1]. Low folate levels are more prevalent in psychiatric inpatients when compared with patients without psychiatric illness, even when controlling for drug and alcohol abuse [12]. It has been reported in up to one third of psychiatric patients, especially with depression [8,25]. It is unclear how much of this is can be attributed to the use of psychotropic medications, especially mood stabilizers, which are known to decrease folate levels [1,12,22].

Clinical manifestations

Symptoms of folate deficiency are similar to those of B_{12} deficiency, however, SCD is specific to B_{12} deficiency and depression is more common in folate deficiency [22]. Insufficient folate during conception and early pregnancy results in neural tube defects (NTD). The megaloblastic anemia is identical to that seen in B_{12} deficiency. Folate deficiency is invariably accompanied by a raised plasma homocysteine level [3,8], which carries an increased risk of cardiovascular disease, dementia [7,26], and depression [8,11].

Since 1998, the US Food and Drug Administration has mandated fortification of grains with folate to lower the risk of NTDs in women of childbearing age. This action led to a reduction in NTD, and an improvement of blood folate status and homocysteine levels in adults in the United States [3,27–29].

Diagnosis and treatment

Low red blood cell (RBC) folate combined with high plasma homocysteine is a good standard for the diagnosis of folate deficiency and is more accurate than measuring serum folate alone. Full treatment response to folate takes many months; the delay may be partly a result of an efficient folate-blood brain barrier. Although there are no clear guidelines for the dose or duration of folate therapy for nervous system disorders, treatment is recommended for at least 6 months; clinical improvement is usually seen within the first few months [1,22]. To decrease the risk of NTDs, at least 0.4 mg of folic acid daily is recommended. For women at high risk, those with a previous child affected, or those taking anticonvulsants, 4–5 mg daily is recommended, at least one month prior to conception and through at least, the first trimester of pregnancy [30,31]. To lower the homocycsteine level, 0.8 mg daily is typically required [32]. To treat folate deficiency, 1 mg daily for at least 4 to 5 weeks or until hematologic recovery is recommended [20].

In depressed patients, low folate levels have correlated with higher levels of depression and the depression was less likely to respond to antidepressants [11,33]. Coppen [34] showed that supplementation of fluoxetine with folic acid improved antidepressant response, especially in women, although improvement was attributed to the concurrent decrease in plasma homocysteine levels and not necessarily to increased to plasma folate levels.

Recently, there has been speculation as to whether supplementation of either folate or B_{12} has any effect on cognition or the development of dementia. Multiple studies have shown that folic acid supplementation increases blood folate and decreases homocysteine [3,35]. Most studies found that higher intake of folate, but not the other B vitamins, is related to a lower risk of Alzheimer's dementia [7,36] and better cognitive functioning [35]. Other studies found no association between dietary intake of folate or B_{12} and the later development of Alzheimer's disease [37]. Several recent large reviews show that supplementation of either folic acid or B_{12} does not have a significant effect on cognition in individuals with either normal or impaired cognitive functioning [26,38].

SICKLE CELL DISEASE

Sickle cell disease (SCD) is the most common hemoglobinopathy. The disease is a classic example of a balanced polymorphism; the asymptomatic sickle cell trait provides a selective advantage against malaria, while the homozygous disease has devastating consequences. SCD includes the homozygous disease of sickle cell anemia (SCA), sickle cell-beta thalassemia, sickle cell-hemoglobin C, and other SCD variants. Sickle cell trait has no clinical consequences.

SCD occurs primarily in those of African descent, but also afflicts people of Mediterranean, Asian, and Middle Eastern origin. More than 70,000 Americans suffer from SCD. Among African Americans, the prevalence is approximately 1 in 300; 8% carry the trait. Medical advances have transformed the disease from a pediatric illness into one chronically extending into adulthood. Life expectancy over the past 35 years has increased from a mean of 14 years in the 1970s to close to 50 years today [39].

The vaso-occlusive crisis is the hallmark of SCD. These recurrent crises are the cause of acute episodes of severe pain and represent the most common reason patients seek medical care. Extremes of temperature, infectious illness, dehydration, and physical exertion may precipitate crises, but the majority of crises occur without an identifiable cause. Vaso-occlusion produces acute pain in the short term and end-organ damage in the long term. Vaso-occlusion potentially affects all organ systems, but leads to particular damage in bones, kidneys, lungs, eyes, and brain. Many patients suffer from chronic pain as a result of avascular necrosis, leg ulcers, or poorly understood chronic pain syndromes.

The neuropsychiatric manifestations of SCD can be grouped into three main categories: (1) depression and anxiety, resulting from living with a chronic stigmatizing disease associated with unpredictable painful crises and high morbidity and mortality; (2) problems with substance abuse and dependence, resulting from living with chronic and acute pain that is often under-treated; and (3) central nervous system damage, resulting from cerebral vascular accidents primarily during childhood. These issues are further complicated by the poor psychosocial circumstances and learned helplessness of many patients.

Depression and Anxiety

As with many chronic diseases, depression and anxiety are common in patients with SCD. The prevalence of depression is about 26% in SCD [40,41]. Anxiety disorders have been reported to be 7.1% [42]. Studies assessing depression and anxiety in children with SCD have yielded mixed results [43]. However, children with SCD have higher prevalence of excessive fatigue, physical complaints, impaired self-esteem, morbid ideation, and feelings of hopelessness [44,45]. These feelings arise in the context of frequent hospitalizations, absences from school, and the inability to experience a normal childhood like other children.

The stigma associated with SCD makes a significant contribution to anxiety and depression [41]. Adults with SCD face physical deformities, the stigma of addiction or mental illness, and biases related to race. The consequences of facing these stigmas include self-deprivation, self-hate, suspiciousness, depression, hostility, anxiety, bewilderment, and defensiveness. Physical deformities result from delayed growth and development as a consequence of chronic hemolysis and chronic vaso-occlusion. When compared with control subjects, pediatric SCD patients weigh less, are shorter, and have delayed puberty [46]. For adolescents, this may lead to problems with self-esteem, heightened self-consciousness, dissatisfaction with body image, and social isolation [47]. Participation in athletics is limited because of stature and fear of initiating a vaso-occlusive crisis. School performance suffers when hospitalizations lead to missing multiple school days. Accordingly, adolescents often experience hopelessness and social withdrawal [48]. In the United States, the stigma of SCD is compounded, as the disease is predominant in an ethnic minority that is already vulnerable to racial prejudice and stereotyping [49].

Chronic and Acute Pain and Opioid Use

Patients with SCD most commonly seek medical care for treatment of their pain. The average patient experiences 0.8 episodes of vaso-occlusive crises per year; however 1% of patients have more than six crises in a year [50]. Patients live with uncertainty as to when the next crisis will occur. The nature of the pain, which has been reported to be as severe as childbirth [51], and the unpredictable onset of pain can be psychologically debilitating.

Over the last 15 years, opioid treatment has gained mainstream acceptance for the treatment of SCD pain. Opioids help control pain, improve functional capacity, and decrease hospitalizations in patients with SCD [52]. Chronic opioid use may result in tolerance, physiologic dependence, substance dependence, and abuse. There is concern among investigators that cognitive deficits may occur with opioid use in patients with chronic pain; however, studies have not revealed consistent evidence to support this claim [53].

Substance dependence and addiction behaviors are difficult to define in any chronic pain condition. The few studies that address addiction in SCD report a low prevalence, yet despite this lack of evidence in the medical literature for addiction in SCD, medical practitioners often overestimate addiction [54]. Studies demonstrate that 63% of nurses believe addiction is prevalent in SCD [55] and that 53% of emergency department physicians and 23% of hematologists thought more than 20% of SCD patients were addicted [56]. Some of this misconception results from failure to understand the difference between physiologic tolerance and opioid dependence.

Because of skepticism and fear of introducing iatrogenic addiction, medical practitioners may under treat pain in patients with SCD [54]. As a result of under treatment, patients may develop a pseudo-addiction, where addiction-like behaviors occur as a result of inadequate pain management [57]. Some SCD patients may seek illegal narcotics as a way to manage their painful crises. This behavior can lead to long-term problems with true addiction and illicit substance abuse [58]. Some patients may inappropriately use opioids to help with nonpain symptoms, such as insomnia, depression, and anxiety. In a recent study looking at alcohol abuse, 31.4% of adult SCD patients were found to abuse alcohol [59].

Central Nervous System Damage

Brain disease from SCD complications begins early in life and often herald a neurocognitive dysfunction. An estimated 25% to 33% of children with SCD have central nervous system (CNS) effects from the disease [60]. Seizures occur in 12% to 14% of patients with SCD, and often lead to stroke [61,62]. Cerebral vascular accidents occur in 10% to 15% of children with SCA. These children demonstrate intellectual deficits, ranging from borderline to moderate mental retardation, reduced language function, and problems with adjustment [63]. Cognitive deficits in children with SCD can lead to educational problems, intellectual impairment, verbal problems, problems with attention and concentration, and dementia later in life [44]. As early as kindergarten, SCD patients had lower scores in language skills and auditory discrimination that could not be attributed to school absence [64].

A significant problem with obtaining psychiatric treatment in patients with SCD is that African Americans, in general, are often reluctant to obtain help for mental illness and may attempt to overcome mental health problems through self-reliance and determination [65]. Even in milder cases, lack of psychosocial resources may put SCD patients at higher risk for poor adaptation to SCD [40]. There may be additional barriers to accessing care in patients with lower socioeconomic status.

In conclusion, psychological and psychiatric complications in patients with SCD are common and contribute to impairment in function and quality of life. Psychologic and psychiatric care improves outcomes and should be a routine component of comprehensive SCD care.

HEMOPHILIA

Hemophilia is a bleeding disorder caused by a deficiency of the coagulation factors essential for blood clotting. Hemophilia A (factor VIII deficiency) and hemophilia B (factor IX deficiency) are the most well known inherited bleeding disorders. Hemophilia A and B are X-linked and mainly affect males. Female carriers can experience excessive bleeding, as they may have half the normal amount of clotting factors. Hemophilia A and B are clinically, indistinguishable from one another.

Disease severity is related to the plasma concentrations of the clotting factors. Classification into severe, moderate, and mild hemophilia is useful for predicting bleeding tendency and prognosis, as well as for guiding treatment [66–68]. Patients with severe hemophilia (less than 1% clotting factor) typically bleed spontaneously into joints, muscles, soft tissues, and body cavities. During the neonatal period, especially during the first week of life, the risk of intracranial hemorrhage is estimated to be between 1% and 4%. Most children are asymptomatic until they start crawling or walking. Affected children may bruise easily and bleed following minor injuries. Families of these children may inappropriately be suspected of child abuse. By the age of 4 years, most children experience a bleed into a joint. Adults with severe hemophilia used to experience recurrent (sometimes weekly) bleeds into large joints and muscles. Joint bleeding caused severe acute pain; repeated bleeds led to destruction of cartilage and bone, muscle wasting, and chronic pain. Inadequately treated patients suffered from arthritis, immobility, and chronic pain [66–68]. Moderate hemophilia (1%–5% clotting factor) is typically diagnosed by the age of 5; bleeding episodes in patients with moderate hemophilia occur less frequently. Mild hemophilia (greater than 5% clotting factor) is usually diagnosed later following trauma, tooth extraction, or surgery. Bleeding episodes in these patients typically occur secondary to trauma; spontaneous bleeding is rare [66,68,69].

Since the 1960s, the availability of purified factor VIII has allowed for home-based infusions, improved quality of life, and increased life expectancy of patients with severe hemophilia. In the early 1980s, more than 80% of patients with severe hemophilia who were over the age of 10 were infected with viral illnesses, including HIV, and hepatitis B and C. Beginning in the 1990s, the use of recombinant clotting factors eliminated the risk of transmitting viral infections. Advances in the treatment of hemophilia have resulted in effective prevention and control of bleeding. Today, patients with severe hemophilia are much less likely to experience bleeding and its associated complications [66,68].

The extent of psychiatric disorders in patients with hemophilia is unknown. In children and adolescents higher rates of anxiety disorders have been reported in hemophiliacs than in asthmatics. Children with hemophilia must achieve developmental milestones while being confronted with chronic disease, and face different disease-related stressors at different ages of development. While facing chronic pain, disability, social ostracism, and job and insurance discrimination, adults living with hemophilia strive for a healthy identity, autonomy, and a good quality of life [70].

Physicians, who fear inducing drug dependence with opiates, are reluctant to prescribe opiates, despite the severe pain associated with joint bleeds. Even adults without drug dependence report concern about narcotic addiction [71]. In actual practice, opiate analgesics may be used safely in patients with hemophilia. It is important to address patient concerns about becoming opiate dependent to provide adequate analgesia [20].

Individual, group, and family psychotherapy are useful psychotherapeutic modalities. Caution is needed in prescribing psychotropic agents to hemophiliacs. Doses of antidepressants, antipsychotics, and opiate analgesics should be reduced to compensate for hepatic impairment. Several psychotropic agents may increase the risk of bleeding, and caution must be exercised when prescribing those agents to hemophiliacs [67,72].

Hemophiliacs who developed AIDS face many additional stressors: opportunistic infections, physical wasting, declining health, chronic pain, CNS complications, frequent monitoring of viral load and CD4+ cell counts, medication side effects, and disclosure of HIV status, resulting in further social ostracism and insurance discrimination. Regardless of their HIV status, most boys with hemophilia show remarkable resilience and cope well with psychologic and physical stressors caused by the disease. Some children have neuropsychologic deficits and lower academic achievement. Mothers of HIV seropositive hemophiliacs are more distressed than mothers of HIV negative hemophiliacs [73–75].

After death from AIDS, bereaved families may need extensive psychologic counseling and support. A study in Japan found that 7 to 9 years after their loved one's death, bereaved family members reported continuing deep sorrow and grief about their loss, as well as resentment, regret, anger, guilt, and anxiety over discrimination. Additionally, up to 70% of bereaved family members reported restricting their daily activities because of the stigma of HIV or fear of discrimination, and up to half of bereaved family members continue suffering from mental health problems [76].

When caring for HIV-infected hemophiliacs, health care workers may experience anxiety about exposure to HIV and guilt about having unknowingly administered hepatitis and HIV-infected clotting factors to patients in the 1980s (before safe clotting factors became available). Health care providers are faced with complex ethical and medical dilemmas when caring for HIV-infected hemophiliacs. Examples include whether to disclose HIV status to an HIV-positive child or teenager when the patient's parents oppose the disclosure, and whether to breach the confidentiality of a sexually active hepatitis or HIV-positive hemophiliac to inform their sexual partners of potential risk of contracting hepatitis or HIV [77].

HEMATOLOGIC SIDE EFFECTS AND DRUG INTERACTIONS OF PSYCHOTROPIC AGENTS

Antipsychotics

Various psychotropics and their potential hematologic side effects are listed in Table 1 and their interactions with anticoagulants are listed in Table 2. Antipsychotic agents that do not have any reported hematologic side effects include aripiprazole and ziprasidone.

Agranulocytosis is rare, except with clozapine, but is the most common and most serious (less than 0.1%) hematologic side effect of the antipsychotics [78–80]. Low-potency antipsychotics have a higher frequency of agranulocytosis than high-potency ones. Clozapine causes agranulocytosis in 0.8% of patients [81]. The highest risk of clozapine-induced agranulocytosis is in the first 6 months of treatment and then decreases significantly. The case fatality rate of clozapine-induced agranulocytosis is estimated as 4.2% to 16%, depending on whether a growth stimulating factor (GSF) is used [82]. A weekly white blood cell (WBC) count is necessary to detect and manage clozapine-induced agranulocytosis, and a WBC count less than $2000/mm^3$ or an absolute neutrophil count less than $1000/mm^3$ are indications for immediate cessation of clozapine. Stopping clozapine usually leads to recovery in WBC counts in three weeks [83]. The mortality risk associated with agranulocytosis is significantly increased if infection occurs while still on the drug [84,85]. As clozapine causes bone marrow suppression, GSFs may help restore normal bone marrow production [85–87].

Other potential hematologic adverse effects of antipsychotics include aplastic anemia, neutropenia, eosinophilia, and thrombocytopenia.

Antidepressants

Serotonin reuptake inhibitors (SSRIs) inhibit platelet function and have been associated with bruising and bleeding, especially with concomitant use of aspirin or nonsteroidal anti-inflammatory drugs (NSAIDs) [88–93]. SSRIs increase

Table 1
Psychotropics and hematologic side effects

Antipsychotics
  Conventional antipsychotic agents
    Chlorpromazine

agranulocytosis
anemia (aplastic, hemolytic)
eosinophilia
leukopenia
thrombocytopenia

    Mesoridazine

agranulocytosis
disorder of hematopoietic structure
leukopenia
thrombocytopenia

    Fluphenazine

agranulocytosis
eosinophilia
pancytopenia
leukocytosis
leukopenia
thrombocytopenia

    Haloperidol

agranulocytosis
leukocytosis
leukopenia
lymphomonocytosis
minimal changes in red blood cell counts

    Loxapine

agranulocytosis
leukopenia
thrombocytopenia

  Atypical antipsychotic agents
    Clozapine

agranulocytosis (1%–2%)
eosinophilia
leukocytosis
leukopenia
thrombocytopenia

    Risperidone

anemia
leukocytosis
leukopenia
thrombocytopenia

    Olanzapine

leukocytosis
thrombocytopenia

Antidepressants
  Tricyclic antidepressants
    Amitriptyline

agranulocytosis
eosinophilia
leukopenia
thrombocytopenia

(continued on next page)

Table 1
(*continued*)

Nortriptyline	agranulocytosis
	eosinophilia
	thrombocytopenia
Imipramine	agranulocytosis
	eosinophilia
	leukopenia
	thrombocytopenia
Clomipramine	agranulocytosis
	neutropenia
	leukopenia
	pancytopenia
	thrombocytopenia
Doxepin	eosinophilia
Serotonin/Norepinephrine/Reuptake inhibitors	
Duloxetine	unusual bleeding or bruising
Venlafaxine	anemia
	leukocytosis
	leukopenia
Monoamine oxidase inhibitors	
Phenelzine	anemia
Tranylcypromine	agranulocytosis
	anemia
	leukopenia
	thrombocytopenia
Selective serotonin reuptake inhibitors	
Citalopram	anemia
	impaired platelet aggregation
	leukocytosis
	leukopenia
Fluoxetine	disseminated intravascular coagulation
	impaired platelet aggregation
Fluvoxamine	impaired platelet aggregation
Paroxetine	impaired platelet aggregation
Sertraline	anemia
	impaired platelet aggregation
	thrombocytopenia
Serotonin-2 receptor antagonism with serotonin reuptake blockade	
Trazodone	agranulocytosis
	anemia
	eosinophilia
	leukocytosis
	neutropenia
	thrombocytopenia

(*continued on next page*)

Table 1
(continued)

Alpha-2 antagonism plus Serotonin-2 and Serotonin-3 antagonism	
Mirtazapine	anemia
	eosinophilia
	agranulocytosis
	leukopenia
	pancytopenia
	thrombocytopenia
Norepinephrine and dopamine reuptake inhibition	
Bupropion	leukopenia
Antianxiety agents	
Chlordiazepoxide	anemia
	agranulocytosis
	thrombocytopenia
Clonazepam	thrombocytopenia
Clorazepate	anemia
Diazepam	anemia
	agranulocytosis
	pancytopenia
	thrombocytopenia
Flurazepam	leukopenia
	granulocytopenia
Lorazepam	leukopenia
Oxazepam	leukopenia
Mood stabilizers	
Carbamazepine	agranulocytosis
	anemia
	eosinophilia
	leukocytosis
	leukopenia
	pure red cell aplasia
	thrombocytopenia
Gabapentin	leukopenia
	neutropenia
Lamotrigine	agranulocytosis
	neutropenia
	anemia
	pancytopenia
	pure red cell aplasia
	thrombocytopenia
Lithium	leukocytosis
	thrombocytosis

(continued on next page)

Table 1 (continued)	
Phenytoin	agranulocytosis
	granulocytopenia
	pancytopenia (with or without bone marrow suppression)
	leukopenia
	thrombocytopenia
Tigabine	ecchymosis
Topimarate	anemia
	increase prothrombin
	purpura
	thrombocytopenia
Valproic acid	pure red cell aplasia
	thrombocytopenia
Zonisamide	anemia
	leukopenia

Data from LEXiDrug. Available at: www.lexidrug.com. Accessed May 11, 2007; Stahl SM. Basic psychopharmacology of antidepressants, part 1: Antidepressants have seven distinct mechanisms of action. J Clin Psychiatry 1998;59(Suppl 4):5–14; Physicians' Desk Reference. 61st ed. Montvale, NJ: Medical Economics Co, Inc.; 2007; Cimo PL, Pisciotta AV, Desai RG, et al. Detection of drug-dependent antibodies by the 51Cr platelet lysis test: Documentation of immune thrombocytopenia induced by diphenylhydantoin, diazepam, and sulfisoxazole. Am J Hematol 1977;2:65–72; Damiani JT, Christensen RC. Lamotrigine-associated neutropenia in a geriatric patient. Am J Geriatr Psychiatry 2000;8:346; Derbyshire E, Martin D. Neutropenia occurring after starting gabapentin for neuropathic pain. Clin Oncol 2004;1:575–6; and Refs. [120–123].

Adapted from Shakin EJ, Thompson TL. Psychiatric aspects of hematologic disorders. In: Stoudemire A, Fogel BS, eds. Medical-Psychiatric Practice. Vol 1. Washington, DC: American Psychiatric Press, Inc.; 1991. p. 193–242; Shakin EJ, Thompson TL. Hematologic disorders. In: Stoudemire A, Fogel BS, eds. New York, NY: Oxford University Press; 1993. p. 691–712; and Kunkel EJS, Thompson TL, Oyesanmi O: Hematologic disorders. In: Psychiatric Care of the Medical Patient. 2nd Edition. Edited by Stoudemire A, Fogel BS, and Greenberg D, New York, NY: Oxford University Press; 2000. p. 835–56.

central nervous system 5-hydroxytryptamine (5-HT; serotonin), and reduce 5-HT in platelets (leading reduced platelet aggregation). Platelets normally release serotonin at the site of a vascular tear, leading to further platelet aggregation and vasodilatation, and permitting the sealing of the tear without thrombosis of the vessel [94].

Upper gastrointestinal bleeding may occur at a frequency ranging from 1 in 100 to 1 in 1,000 patient-years of exposure to high-affinity drugs with SSRIs, especially in the elderly [90]. The magnitude of this effect is modest, similar to low dose NSAIDs [95]. Caution is advised in patients at high risk of gastrointestinal bleeding, for whom clinicians may consider prescribing an antidepressant with low serotonin reuptake inhibition. Patients taking high-serotonin reuptake inhibition antidepressants should generally use smaller doses or avoid aspirin and NSAIDs [96–98]. The risk of gastrointestinal bleeding is highest among patients on both SSRIs and NSAIDs [95]. While the evidence to date indicates that SSRIs do not cause intracranial bleeding [99], there is a report that patients taking SSRIs along with statins had a higher risk for subarachnoid hemorrhage-related vasospasm [100]. Pharmacovigilance is prudent in the use

Table 2
Psychotropics and their interactions with anticoagulants

Psychotropic agent	Interaction with anticoagulant
Antidepressants	
TCAs	Increased bleeding with warfarin anticoagulants
SSRIs	Increased INR with warfarin (especially, fluvoxamine and fluoxetine)
MAOIs	Increased INR with anticoagulants
Bupropion	Unknown
Mirtazapine	Unknown
Mood stabilizers	
Carbamazepine (CBZ)	Oral anticoagulants: reduces INR; CBZ increases metabolism of warfarin agents by inducing hepatic metabolism
	Coumarin decreases effect of CBZ
Divalproex & valproic acid	Increases bleeding with anticoagulation therapy
	Aspirin can induce valproic acid toxicity
Lithium	Unknown
Antipsychotics	
Neuroleptics	Increased bleeding with warfarin
	Decreased bleeding with phenindione
Atypicals	Unknown

Abbreviations: INR, international normalized ratio; MAOI, monoamine oxidase inhibitor; SSRI, Serotonin reuptake inhibitor; TCA, tricylic antidepressant.

Data from Jenkins SC, Hansen MR. A Pocket Reference for Psychiatrist. 2nd ed. Washington, DC: American Psychiatric Press; 1995; Rosse RB, Giese AA, Deutsch SI, et al. Hematological measure of potential relevance to psychiatrists. In: Laboratory Diagnostic Testing in Psychiatry. Washington, DC: American Psychiatric Press; 1989. p. 31–5; Physicans' Desk Reference. 61st ed. Montvale, NJ: Medical Economics Co, Inc.; 2007; and Ref. [79].

Adapted from Shakin EJ, Thompson TL. Psychiatric aspects of hematologic disorders. In: Stoudemire A, Fogel BS, eds. Medical-Psychiatric Practice. Vol 1. Washington, DC: American Psychiatric Press, Inc.; 1991. p. 193–242; Shakin EJ, Thompson TL. Hematologic disorders. In: Stoudemire A, Fogel BS, eds. New York, NY: Oxford University Press; 1993. p. 691–712; and Kunkel EJS, Thompson TL, Oyesanmi O. Hematologic disorders. In: Stoudemire A, Fogel BS, and Greenberg D, eds. Psychiatric Care of the Medical Patient. 2nd Edition. New York, NY: Oxford University Press; 2000. p. 835–56.

of SSRIs in patients at high-risk for hemorrhagic and vasoconstrictive stroke [99].

While some reviews have concluded there is no increased risk of combining SSRIs with warfarin [101], there have been case reports of bleeding with concomitant use of warfarin and the SSRIs. Among the SSRIs, fluoxetine is the most commonly reported offending agent [102]. The interactions between warfarin and antidepressants can have potentially serious consequences, resulting from enhanced or reduced anticoagulant activity. The possible mechanisms are considered with particular reference to the cytochrome p450 system. Fluoxetine, fluvoxamine, and paroxetine appear to have the highest potential of the antidepressants for interactions [103]. Newer antidepressants, such as citalopram, nefazodone, and sertraline may be relatively less likely to interact with warfarin [103].

Agranulocytosis due to the tricyclic antidepressants is a rare, idiosyncratic condition caused by bone marrow toxicity, with a lower frequency than is reported for neuroleptics [104]. Agranulocytosis has been associated with imipramine [105,106], clomipramine [106–108], and desipramine [109,110]. Clomipramine-induced agranulocytosis may be treated with recombinant granulocyte colony-stimulating factor [111].

Benzodiazepines
Agranulocytosis has rarely been reported with the benzodiazepines, but no causal relationship has been established. There is no relationship between the daily dose or total cumulative dose and the occurrence of hematological side effects [102,112].

Lithium
Lithium stimulates leukocytosis with a true proliferative response. Lithium-induced leukocytosis has been used to ameliorate leukopenia associated with other agents and disorders. In patients on lithium therapy for cluster headaches, Medina and colleagues documented increases, in the number of platelets and in platelet serotonin and histamine levels [105,113]. Lithium-induced hematologic side effects can be used to manage hematologic toxicities associated with other agents and disorders. Patients with persistent leucopenia and thrombocytopenia, following chemotherapy or radiotherapy, can be treated with lithium [114].

Anticonvulsants and Mood Stabilizers
Carbamazepine should be avoided in patients with a history of bone marrow depression. Carbamazepine produces a transient reduction in WBCs in approximately 10% of patients during the first 4 months of treatment [115]. Very rarely it causes potentially fatal agranulocytosis and aplastic anemia. Agranulocytosis results from direct toxicity to the bone marrow [86]. A baseline complete blood cell count is always advised before starting carbamazepine. Carbamazepine should be discontinued if the WBC count drops to below $3500/mm^3$. Administration of lithium and carbamazepine concurrently may lower the risk of carbamazepine-induced neutropenia, because lithium stimulates WBC production, predominantly neutrophils [116]. Carbamazepine stimulates its own metabolism. Thus, after being taken for a period of time, the amount of carbamazepine in the blood will suddenly decrease. As carbamazepine induces hepatic metabolism, it reduces the anticoagulant effect of warfarin, so both the carbamazepine level and the international normalized ratio will need to be monitored frequently when both drugs are used [117].

Valproate-induced increases in red blood cell mean corpuscular volume and mean corpuscular hemoglobin concentration have been postulated to result from alterations in erythrocyte membrane phospholipids [118]. Sometime fatal, hematopoietic complications, such as neutropenia, thrombocytopenia, and macrocytic anemia have been associated with valproate [119,120]. Lamotrigine may also cause agranulocytosis [120]. All anticonvulsants should be discontinued when the WBC count drops below 3,000/mm^3 [122].

Acetylcholinesterase Inhibitors

Donepezil is associated with anemia, thrombocythemia, thrombocytopenia, ecchymosis (4%), and eosinophilia. The mechanism for the hematologic side effects is unknown. Purpura occurs in up to 2% of patients on tacrine. Only one case of agranulocytosis has been reported with tacrine [123]. Rivastigmine has been reported to cause anemia and galantamine to cause epistaxis, purpura, and thrombocytopenia [124].

SUMMARY

Vitamin B$_{12}$ deficiency is associated with problems in cognition, mood, psychosis, and less commonly, anxiety. Folate deficiency primarily is associated with problems in mood. Patients who have sickle cell disease, a disease of chronic pain, experience difficulties with depression, anxiety, stigma, and are at risk for substance abuse and dependence. Patients with hemophilia have benefited from advances in treatment; however, their morbidity and mortality were compounded in those who received blood products contaminated with HIV, or hepatitis B and C. Psychiatrists who practice psychosomatic medicine should expect to encounter patients with the above problems, as they are frequently seen in medical settings. Finally, most of the commonly used psychotropic medications have uncommon but potentially important hematologic side effects or may interact with the anticoagulants used in medically ill patients.

References

[1] Reynolds E. Vitamin B12, folic acid, and the nervous system. Lancet Neurol 2006;5: 949–60.

[2] Carmel R, Green R, Rosenblatt DS, et al. Update on cobalamin, folate, and homocysteine. Hematology Am Soc Hematol Educ Program 2003;1:62–81.

[3] Jacques PF, Selhub J, Bostom AG, et al. The effect of folic acid fortification on plasma folate and total homocysteine concentrations. N Engl J Med 1999;340:1449–54.

[4] Lindenbaum J, Healton EB, Savage DG, et al. Neuropsychiatric disorders caused by cobalamin deficiency in the absence of anemia or macrocytosis. N Engl J Med 1988;318: 1720–8.

[5] Loikas S, Koskinen P, Irjala K, et al. Vitamin B12 deficiency in the aged: a population-based study. Age Ageing 2007;36:177–83.

[6] Seshadri S, Beiser A, Selhub J, et al. Plasma homocysteine as a risk factor for dementia and Alzheimer's disease. N Engl J Med 2002;346:476–83.

[7] Ravaglia G, Forti P, Maioli F, et al. Homocysteine and folate as risk factors for dementia and Alzheimer disease. Am J Clin Nutr 2005;82:636–43.

[8] Bottiglieri T, Laundy M, Crellin R, et al. Homocysteine, folate, methylation, and monoamine metabolism in depression. J Neurol Neurosurg Psychiatry 2000;69:228–32.

[9] Andres E, Loukili NH, Noel E, et al. Vitamin B12 (cobalamin) deficiency in elderly patients. CMAJ 2004;171:251–9.

[10] Selhub J, Bagley LC, Miller J, et al. B vitamins, homocysteine, and neurocognitive function in the elderly. Am J Clin Nutr 2000;71:614S–20S.

[11] Fava M, Borus JS, Alpert JE, et al. Folate, vitamin B12, and homocysteine in major depressive disorder. Am J Psychiatry 1997;154:426–8.

[12] Lerner V, Kanevsky M, Dwolatzky T, et al. Vitamin B12 and folate serum levels in newly admitted psychiatric patients. Clin Nutr 2006;25:60–7.

[13] Toh BH, van Driel IR, Gleeson PA. Pernicious anemia. N Engl J Med 1997;337: 1441–8.

[14] Andres E, Affenberger S, Vinzio S, et al. Food-cobalamin malabsorption in elderly patients: clinical manifestations and treatment. Am J Med 2005;118:1154–9.

[15] Liu KW, Dai LK, Jean W. Metformin-related vitamin B12 deficiency. Age Ageing 2006;35: 200–1.

[16] Bauman WA, Shaw S, Jayatilleke E, et al. Increased intake of calcium reverses vitamin B12 malabsorption induced by metformin. Diabetes Care 2000;23:1227–31.

[17] Valuck RJ, Ruscin JM. A case-control study on adverse effects: H2 blocker or proton pump inhibitor use and risk of vitamin B12 deficiency in older adults. J Clin Epidemiol 2004;57: 422–8.

[18] Lerner V, Kanevsky M. Acute dementia with delirium due to vitamin B12 deficiency: a case report. Int J Psychiatry Med 2002;32:215–20.

[19] Durand C, Mary S, Brazo P, et al. Psychiatric manifestations of vitamin B12 deficiency: a case report. Encephale 2003;29:560–5.

[20] Kunkel EJ, Thompson TL, Abdelgheni MB, et al. Hematologic disorders. In: Stoudemire A, Fogel BS, Greenberg DB, editors. Psychiatric care of the medical patient. 2nd edition. Oxford (NY): Oxford University Press; 2000. p. 833–56.

[21] Sadock BJ, Sadock VA. Kaplan and Sadock's synopsis of psychiatry. 9th edition. Philadelphia: Williams and Wilkins; 2003.

[22] Reynolds EH. Folic acid, ageing, depression, and dementia. BMJ 2002;324:1512–5.

[23] Lucock M. Is folic acid the ultimate functional food component for disease prevention? BMJ 2004;328:211–4.

[24] Wang HX, Wahlin A, Basun H, et al. Vitamin B(12) and folate in relation to the development of Alzheimer's disease. Neurology 2001;56:1188–94.

[25] Carney MW, Chary TK, Laundy M, et al. Red cell folate concentrations in psychiatric patients. J Affect Disord 1990;19:207–13.

[26] Malouf M, Grimley EJ, Areosa SA. Folic acid with or without vitamin B12 for cognition and dementia. Cochrane Database Syst Rev 2003;4:CD004514.

[27] Dietrich M, Brown CJ, Block G. The effect of folate fortification of cereal-grain products on blood folate status, dietary folate intake, and dietary folate sources among adult non-supplement users in the United States. J Am Coll Nutr 2005;24:266–74.

[28] Choumenkovitch SF, Jacques PF, Nadeau MR, et al. Folic acid fortification increases red blood cell folate concentrations in the Framingham study. J Nutr 2001;131:3277–80.

[29] Choumenkovitch SF, Selhub J, Wilson PW, et al. Folic acid intake from fortification in United States exceeds predictions. J Nutr 2002;132:2792–8.

[30] US Preventative Services Task Force. Guide to Clinical Preventative Services. 2nd edition. Baltimore (MD): Williams & Williams; 1996.

[31] Wilson RD, Davies G, Desilets V, et al. The use of folic acid for the prevention of neural tube defects and other congenital anomalies. J Obstet Gynaecol Can 2003;25:959–73.

[32] Homocysteine Lowering Trialists' Collaboration. Dose-dependent effects of folic acid on blood concentrations of homocysteine: a meta-analysis of the randomized trials. Am J Clin Nutr 2005;82:806–12.

[33] Papakostas GI, Petersen T, Mischoulon D, et al. Serum folate, vitamin B12, and homocysteine in major depressive disorder, part 2: predictors of relapse during the continuation phase of pharmacotherapy. J Clin Psychiatry 2004;65:1096–8.

[34] Coppen A, Bailey J. Enhancement of the antidepressant action of fluoxetine by folic acid: a randomised, placebo controlled trial. J Affect Disord 2000;60:121–30.

[35] Durga J, van Boxtel MP, Schouten EG, et al. Effect of 3-year folic acid supplementation on cognitive function in older adults in the FACIT trial: a randomised, double blind, controlled trial. Lancet 2007;369:208–16.

[36] Luchsinger JA, Tang MX, Miller J, et al. Relation of higher folate intake to lower risk of Alzheimer disease in the elderly. Arch Neurol 2007;64:86–92.

[37] Morris MC, Evans DA, Schneider JA, et al. Dietary folate and vitamins B-12 and B-6 not associated with incident alzheimer's disease. J Alzheimers Dis 2006;9:435–43.

[38] Balk EM, Raman G, Tatsioni A, et al. Vitamin B6, B12, and folic acid supplementation and cognitive function: a systematic review of randomized trials. Arch Intern Med 2007;167: 21–30.

[39] Platt OS, Brambilla DJ, Rosse WF, et al. Mortality in sickle cell disease. Life expectancy and risk factors for early death. N Engl J Med 1994;330:1639–44.

[40] Burlew K, Telfair J, Colangelo L, et al. Factors that influence adolescent adaptation to sickle cell disease. J Pediatr Psychol 2000;25:287–99.

[41] Jenerette C, Funk M, Murdaugh C. Sickle cell disease: a stigmatizing condition that may lead to depression. Issues Ment Health Nurs 2005;26:1081–101.

[42] Levenson JL, McClish DK, Dahman BA, et al. Depression and anxiety in adults with sickle cell disease: the PiSCES. Psychosom Med, in press.

[43] Benton TD, Ifeagwu JA, Smith-Whitley K. Anxiety and depression in children and adolescents with sickle cell disease. Curr Psychiatry Rep 2007;9:114–21.

[44] Anie KA. Psychological complications in sickle cell disease. Br J Haematol 2005;129: 723–9.

[45] Yang YM, Cepeda M, Price C, et al. Depression in children and adolescents with sickle-cell disease. Arch Pediatr Adolesc Med 1994;148:457–60.

[46] Cepeda ML, Allen FH, Cepeda NJ, et al. Physical growth, sexual maturation, body image and sickle cell disease. J Natl Med Assoc 2000;92:10–4.

[47] Morgan SA, Jackson J. Psychological and social concomitants of sickle cell anemia in adolescents. J Pediatr Psychol 1986;11:429–40.

[48] Hurtig AL, Park KB. Adjustment and coping in adolescents with sickle cell disease. Ann N Y Acad Sci 1989;565:172–82.

[49] Jacob E. American Pain Society. Pain management in sickle cell disease. Pain Manag Nurs 2001;2:121–31.

[50] Platt OS, Thorington BD, Brambilla DJ, et al. Pain in sickle cell disease. Rates and risk factors. N Engl J Med 1991;325:11–6.

[51] Ballas SK. Sickle Cell Pain. Progress in pain research and management, Vol. 11. Seattle (WA): IASP Press; 1998.

[52] Brookoff D, Polomano R. Treating sickle cell pain like cancer pain. Ann Intern Med 1992;116:364–8.

[53] Chapman SL, Byas-Smith MG, Reed BA. Effects of intermediate- and long-term use of opioids on cognition in patients with chronic pain. Clin J Pain 2002;18:S83–90.

[54] Labbe E, Herbert D, Haynes J. Physicians' attitude and practices in sickle cell disease pain management. J Palliat Care 2005;21:246–51.

[55] Pack-Mabien A, Labbe E, Herbert D, et al. Nurses' attitudes and practices in sickle cell pain management. Appl Nurs Res 2001;14:187–92.

[56] Shapiro BS, Benjamin LJ, Payne R, et al. Sickle cell-related pain: perceptions of medical practitioners. J Pain Symptom Manage 1997;14:168–74.

[57] Weissman DE, Haddox JD. Opioid pseudoaddiction—an iatrogenic syndrome. Pain 1989;36:363–6.

[58] Alao AO, Westmoreland N, Jindal S. Drug addiction in sickle cell disease: case report. Int J Psychiatry Med 2003;33:97–101.

[59] Levenson JL, McClish DK, Dahman BA, et al. Alcohol abuse in sickle cell disease: the PiSCES project. Am J Addict, in press.

[60] Schatz J, McClellan CB. Sickle cell disease as a neurodevelopmental disorder. Ment Retard Dev Disabil Res Rev 2006;12:200–7.

[61] Adams RJ. Neurological complcations. In: Mohandas N, Steinberg MH, editors. Sickle cell disease: basic principles and clinical practice. New York: Raven Press; 1994. p. 599–621.

[62] Liu JE, Gzesh DJ, Ballas SK. The spectrum of epilepsy in sickle cell anemia. J Neurol Sci 1994;123:6–10.

[63] Hariman LM, Griffith ER, Hurtig AL, et al. Functional outcomes of children with sickle-cell disease affected by stroke. Arch Phys Med Rehabil 1991;72:498–502.

[64] Steen RG, Hu XJ, Elliott VE, et al. Kindergarten readiness skills in children with sickle cell disease: evidence of early neurocognitive damage? J Child Neurol 2002;17:111–6.

[65] Snowden LR. Barriers to effective mental health services for African Americans. Ment Health Serv Res 2001;3:181–7.

[66] Bolton-Maggs PH, Pasi KJ. Haemophilias A and B. Lancet 2003;361:1801–9.

[67] Casey RL, Brown RT. Psychological aspects of hematologic diseases. Child Adolesc Psychiatr Clin N Am 2003;12:567–84.

[68] Manco-Johnson M. Hemophilia management: Optimizing treatment based on patient needs. Curr Opin Pediatr 2005;17:3–6.

[69] White GC 2nd, Rosendaal F, Aledort LM, et al. Definitions in hemophilia. Recommendation of the scientific subcommittee on factor VIII and factor IX of the scientific and standardization committee of the international society on thrombosis and haemostasis. Thromb Haemost 2001;85:560.

[70] Spilsbury M. Models for psychosocial services in the developed and developing world. Haemophilia 2004;10(Suppl 4):25–9.

[71] Elander J, Barry T. Analgesic use and pain coping among patients with haemophilia. Haemophilia 2003;9:202–13.

[72] Gerstner T, Teich M, Bell N, et al. Valproate-associated coagulopathies are frequent and variable in children. Epilepsia 2006;47:1136–43.

[73] Bordeaux JD, Loveland KA, Lachar D, et al. Hemophilia growth and development study: caregiver report of youth and family adjustment to HIV disease and immunologic compromise. J Pediatr Psychol 2003;28:175–83.

[74] Loveland KA, Stehbens JA, Mahoney EM, et al. Declining immune function in children and adolescents with hemophilia and HIV infection: effects on neuropsychological performance. Hemophilia growth and development study. J Pediatr Psychol 2000;25:309–22.

[75] Nichols S, Mahoney EM, Sirois PA, et al. HIV-associated changes in adaptive, emotional, and behavioral functioning in children and adolescents with hemophilia: results from the hemophilia growth and development study. J Pediatr Psychol 2000;25:545–56.

[76] Mizota Y, Ozawa M, Yamazaki Y, et al. Psychosocial problems of bereaved families of HIV-infected hemophiliacs in Japan. Soc Sci Med 2006;62:2397–410.

[77] Kulkarni R, Scott-Emuakpor AB, Brody H, et al. Nondisclosure of human immunodeficiency virus and hepatitis C virus coinfection in a patient with hemophilia: medical and ethical considerations. J Pediatr Hematol Oncol 2001;23:153–8.

[78] Rajagopal S. Clozapine, agranulocytosis, and benign ethnic neutropenia. Postgrad Med J 2005;81:545–6.

[79] Sedky K, Shaughnessy R, Hughes T, et al. Clozapine-induced agranulocytosis after 11 years of treatment. Am J Psychiatry 2005;162:814.

[80] Buckley PF, Meltzer HY. Treatment of schizophrenia. In: Schatzberg AF, Nemeroff CB, editors. Textbook of psychopharmacology. 1st edition. Washington (DC): American Psychiatric Press; 1995. p. 627.

[81] Guzelcan Y, Scholte WF. Clozapine-induced agranulocytosis: genetic risk factors and an immunologic explanatory model. Tijdschr Psychiatr 2006;48:295–302 [Dutch].

[82] Schulte PF. Risk of clozapine-associated agranulocytosis and mandatory white blood cell monitoring. Ann Pharmacother 2006;40:683–8.

[83] Folkenberg J. Balancing hope with safety. Available at: http://www.fda.gov/bbs/topics/CONSUMER/CON00055.html. Accessed June 12, 2007.

[84] McEvoy JP, Lieberman JA, Stroup TS, et al. Effectiveness of clozapine versus olanzapine, quetiapine, and risperidone in patients with chronic schizophrenia who did not respond to prior atypical antipsychotic treatment. Am J Psychiatry 2006;163:600–10.

[85] Gerson SL, Meltzer H. Mechanisms of clozapine-induced agranulocytosis. Drug Saf 1992;7(Suppl 1):17–25.

[86] Sedky K, Lippmann S. Psychotropic medications and leukopenia. Curr Drug Targets 2006;7:1191–4.

[87] Lieberman JA, Alvir JM. A report of clozapine-induced agranulocytosis in the United States. Incidence and risk factors. Drug Saf 1992;7(Suppl 1):1–2.

[88] Turner MS, May DB, Arthur RR, et al. Clinical impact of selective serotonin reuptake inhibitors therapy with bleeding risks. J Intern Med 2007;261:205–13.

[89] Mort JR, Aparasu RR, Baer RK. Interaction between selective serotonin reuptake inhibitors and nonsteroidal antiinflammatory drugs: review of the literature. Pharmacotherapy 2006;26:1307–13.

[90] de Abajo FJ, Montero D, Rodriguez LA, et al. Antidepressants and risk of upper gastrointestinal bleeding. Basic Clin Pharmacol Toxicol 2006;98:304–10.

[91] Andreasen JJ, Riis A, Hjortdal VE, et al. Effect of selective serotonin reuptake inhibitors on requirement for allogeneic red blood cell transfusion following coronary artery bypass surgery. Am J Cardiovasc Drugs 2006;6:243–50.

[92] Wessinger S, Kaplan M, Choi L, et al. Increased use of selective serotonin reuptake inhibitors in patients admitted with gastrointestinal haemorrhage: a multicentre retrospective analysis. Aliment Pharmacol Ther 2006;23:937–44.

[93] Goldberg RJ. Selective serotonin reuptake inhibitors: infrequent medical adverse effects. Arch Fam Med 1998;7:78–84.

[94] Hourani SM, Cusack NJ. Pharmacological receptors on blood platelets. Pharmacol Rev 1991;43:243–98.

[95] Weinrieb RM, Auriacombe M, Lynch KG, et al. Selective serotonin re-uptake inhibitors and the risk of bleeding. Expert Opin Drug Saf 2005;4:337–44.

[96] Mansour A, Pearce M, Johnson B, et al. Which patients taking SSRIs are at greatest risk of bleeding? J Fam Pract 2006;55:206–8.

[97] Serebruany VL. Selective serotonin reuptake inhibitors and increased bleeding risk: are we missing something? Am J Med 2006;119:113–6.

[98] Weinrieb RM, Auriacombe M, Lynch KG, et al. A critical review of selective serotonin reuptake inhibitor-associated bleeding: balancing the risk of treating hepatitis C-infected patients. J Clin Psychiatry 2003;64:1502–10.

[99] Ramasubbu R. Cerebrovascular effects of selective serotonin reuptake inhibitors: a systematic review. J Clin Psychiatry 2004;65:1642–53.

[100] Singhal AB, Topcuoglu MA, Dorer DJ, et al. SSRI and statin use increases the risk for vasospasm after subarachnoid hemorrhage. Neurology 2005;64:1008–13.

[101] Kurdyak PA, Juurlink DN, Kopp A, et al. Antidepressants, warfarin, and the risk of hemorrhage. J Clin Psychopharmacol 2005;25:561–4.

[102] Skop BP, Brown TM. Potential vascular and bleeding complications of treatment with selective serotonin reuptake inhibitors. Psychosomatics 1996;37:12–6.

[103] Duncan D, Sayal K, McConnell H, et al. Antidepressant interactions with warfarin. Int Clin Psychopharmacol 1998;13:87–94.

[104] Oyesanmi O, Kunkel EJ, Monti DA, et al. Hematologic side effects of psychotropics. Psychosomatics 1999;40:414–21.

[105] Albertini RS, Penders TM. Agranulocytosis associated with tricyclics. J Clin Psychiatry 1978;39:483–5.

[106] Gravenor DS, Leclerc JR, Blake G. Tricyclic antidepressant agranulocytosis. Can J Psychiatry 1986;31:661.

[107] Alderman CP, Atchison MM, McNeece JI. Concurrent agranulocytosis and hepatitis secondary to clomipramine therapy. Br J Psychiatry 1993;162:688–9.

[108] Souhami RL, Ashton CR, Lee-Potter JP. Agranulocytosis and systemic candidiasis following clomipramine therapy. Postgrad Med J 1976;52:472–4.

[109] Hardin TC, Conrath FC. Desipramine-induced agranulocytosis. A case report. Drug Intell Clin Pharm 1982;16:62–3.

[110] Crammer JL, Elkes A. Agranulocytosis after desipramine. Lancet 1967;1:105–6.

[111] Hunt KA, Resnick MP. Clomipramine-induced agranulocytosis and its treatment with G-CSF. Am J Psychiatry 1993;150:522–3.

[112] Moss RA. Drug-induced immune thrombocytopenia. Am J Hematol 1980;9:439–46.

[113] Medina JL, Fareed J, Diamond S. Lithium carbonate therapy for cluster headache. Changes in number of platelets, and serotonin and histamine levels. Arch Neurol 1980;37:559–63.

[114] Hager ED, Dziambor H, Hohmann D, et al. Effects of lithium on thrombopoiesis in patients with low platelet cell counts following chemotherapy or radiotherapy. Biol Trace Elem Res 2001;83:139–48.

[115] Rall TW, Schleifer LS. Drugs effective in the therapy of epilepsys. In: Gilman AG, Goldman LG, Gilman A, editors. The pharmacological basis of therapeutics. 6th edition. New York: Macmillan; 1980. p. 448–74.

[116] Kramlinger KG, Post RM. Addition of lithium carbonate to carbamazepine: hematological and thyroid effects. Am J Psychiatry 1990;147:615–20.

[117] Herman D, Locatelli I, Grabnar I, et al. The influence of co-treatment with carbamazepine, amiodarone and statins on warfarin metabolism and maintenance dose. Eur J Clin Pharmacol 2006;62:291–6.

[118] Ozkara C, Dreifuss FE, Apperson Hansen C. Changes in red blood cells with valproate therapy. Acta Neurol Scand 1993;88:210–2.

[119] Dulcan MK, Bregman JD, Weller BE, et al. Treatment of childhood and adolescent disorders. In: Schatzberg AF, Nemeroff CB, editors. Textbook of psychopharmacology. 1st edition. Washington, DC: American Psychiatric Press; 1995. p. 680.

[120] Acharya S, Bussel JB. Hematologic toxicity of sodium valproate. J Pediatr Hematol Oncol 2000;22:62–5.

[121] Fadul CE, Meyer LP, Jobst BC, et al. Agranulocytosis associated with lamotrigine in a patient with low-grade glioma. Epilepsia 2002;43:199–200.

[122] Ramsay RE. Clinical efficacy and safety of gabapentin. Neurology 1994;44:S23–30 [discussion: S31–2].

[123] Micromedex. 2007. Healthcare Series Integrated Index.

[124] Mosby drug consult. St. Louis (MO): Mosby, Inc.; 2007.

Psychiatr Clin N Am 30 (2007) 761–780

PSYCHIATRIC CLINICS
OF NORTH AMERICA

Psychiatric Considerations in Pulmonary Disease

Ganesh Shanmugam, MD[a], Sumit Bhutani, MD[a],
David A. Khan, MD[a], E. Sherwood Brown, MD, PhD[b],*

[a]Division of Allergy and Immunology, Department of Internal Medicine,
University of Texas Southwestern Medical Center, 5323 Harry Hines Boulevard, Dallas,
TX 75390–8849, USA
[b]Department of Psychiatry, University of Texas Southwestern Medical Center,
5323 Harry Hines Boulevard, Dallas, TX 75390–8849, USA

L ung disease is a prominent cause of morbidity and mortality worldwide. When a patient has a common lung disease, such as asthma, or a less prevalent one, such as idiopathic pulmonary fibrosis (IPF), psychiatric issues should be considered as an integral part of the care plan for each patient. There have been many studies of psychologic factors and psychiatric syndromes in various lung diseases and their treatment. In this article, the authors focus on an evidence-based approach to reviewing this clinical literature.

It is often difficult to distinguish whether symptoms are attributable to lung disease or the psychiatric conditions related to the lung disease. For example, dyspnea and fatigue are common in pulmonary diseases but may also represent mood or anxiety disorders. Additionally, mood and anxiety symptoms may be caused by medications used to treat pulmonary illness. The authors' main aims in this article are (1) to discuss psychiatric conditions associated with the major lung diseases most commonly seen in clinical practice, (2) to discuss psychiatric syndromes that mimic respiratory diseases, and (3) to discuss psychiatric considerations in the pharmacologic therapy of pulmonary diseases. Unless specified otherwise, the content of this review applies to adult patients.

ASTHMA

Asthma is a chronic respiratory disease with a global economic burden of greater than $30 billion yearly [1]. The prevalence of asthma seems to be increasing in recent decades, and it is now estimated that more than 300 million people worldwide have the disease [2]. A variety of psychiatric conditions have been evaluated in patients who have asthma, including depression, anxiety, and substance use disorders.

*Corresponding author. E-mail address: sherwood.brown@utsouthwestern.edu (E.S. Brown).

0193-953X/07/$ – see front matter © 2007 Elsevier Inc. All rights reserved.
doi:10.1016/j.psc.2007.07.008

Depression and Asthma

Depressive symptoms are more common in patients who have asthma than in the general population in nearly all studies examining this topic [3]. The prevalence of depressive symptoms in asthma has been reported to be as high as 50% [4]. Depressive symptoms occur more commonly in individuals who have asthma than with other severe illnesses. One study found higher depression symptom scores in patients who have asthma (n = 35) as compared with healthy controls and seven other medically ill populations on the Scale of Anxiety and Depression [5]. Only patients who have rheumatoid arthritis had higher scores than patients who have asthma. It should be noted that these studies looked at depressive symptoms and did not use *Diagnostic and Statistical Manual of Mental Disorders, Fourth Edition* (DSM-IV) criteria to diagnose major depressive disorder (MDD) in the study subjects.

Some data examining the prevalence of MDD and other depressive syndromes in asthmatics are available, however. MDD seems to be more common in patients who have asthma than in the general population. One small study found a point prevalence of MDD in adults who had asthma of 25% and a lifetime prevalence of 47% [3]. A more recent international large-scale study involving 17 countries and several thousand patients also revealed that MDD (odds ratio [OR] = 1.6, 95% confidence interval [CI]: 1.4–1.8) was significantly associated with asthma [6]. The diagnosis of depression in this study was made using the World Mental Health Composite International Diagnostic Interview (WMH-CIDI) administered by trained lay interviewers. Adolescent asthmatics aged 11 to 17 years who are smokers seem to have higher rates of MDD (20.7% versus 6.7%) and anxiety disorders (29.7% versus 12.2%) compared with nonsmokers of the same age [7]. It is unknown whether or not MDD is more common in patients who have asthma than in those who have other chronic illnesses, such as diabetes or cardiovascular disease [3].

Patients who have depressive symptoms and severe asthma seem to be more likely to use health care resources, including visits to the emergency room and primary care physicians. This observation may be attributable to a link between stress, emotions, and asthma; specific psychologic features seen in patients with suboptimal asthma control, including denial, panic-fear, and inappropriate coping skills, could lead to frequent visits to health care providers [8].

The presence of depression may be associated with an increased risk for sudden death related to asthma [3]. The pathophysiologic link for this observation is not fully understood. It has been suggested that depressed patients have an impaired voluntary drive to breathe when compared with nondepressed patients [9]. Additionally, poor compliance with therapy for asthma among depressed patients may contribute to this elevated rate of sudden death [10].

The treatment of depression in patients who have asthma seems to have a favorable impact on their asthma. A small, double-blind, placebo-controlled study evaluated the effect of tricyclic antidepressant therapy in depressed patients who had asthma and found moderate improvement in some patients receiving tricyclics [11]. It is possible that these beneficial effects may have been attributable to the anticholinergic effects of tricyclics, however. More recently, Brown and colleagues [12] studied the effects of citalopram versus placebo given to patients who had asthma and MDD. Although no significant difference was found in the primary outcome measure of change in depressive symptoms, citalopram was associated with improvement on some secondary measures, including a reduction in need for oral corticosteroids. Improvement in depressive symptoms was associated with improvement in asthma symptoms and asthma-related quality of life (QOL). Despite the prevalence and morbidity and mortality associated with depression in patients who have asthma, these two studies represent the only controlled trial data examining the treatment of depression with antidepressants in patients who have asthma.

Although the association between asthma and depression has been established, the pathophysiologic link is unclear. Reduced functioning and QOL secondary to asthma may lead to depression. Furthermore, there may be two separate subsets of patients who have asthma. Severe asthmatics with concomitant depression may have poor compliance and increased morbidity and mortality. In contrast, patients who have milder asthma and depressive symptoms may tend to use health care resources more often because of heightened perceptions of their disease [3].

Anxiety Disorders and Asthma

Dyspnea, chest tightness, and sensations of choking are symptoms common to patients who have anxiety disorders and asthma. Anxiety disorders seem to be more common in patients who have asthma than in the general population, with an OR of 1.5 (95% CI: 1.4–1.7) based on a large international study [6]. Another recent large study found that generalized anxiety disorder (GAD; OR = 5.51, 95% CI: 2.29–13.22), panic disorder (OR = 2.61, 95% CI: 1.29–5.25), and panic attacks (OR = 2.84, 95% CI: 1.66–4.89) were significantly more common among lifetime severe asthmatics [13].

Anxiety disorders in asthmatics seem to compromise patient outcomes. Increased subjective perceptions of dyspnea in anxious individuals have been reported despite the absence of objectively measured physiologic changes in the airways [14]. This may lead to increased use of asthma medication for anxiety symptoms, along with other unnecessary treatments.

Regarding treatment of anxiety disorders in asthmatics, Deshmukh and colleagues [15] suggest that anxiety-reducing medications are not preferred therapy in patients who have asthma with comorbid anxiety because they do not affect the root cause of the problem. The authors recommend that anxiolytic agents should be used to treat anxiety disorders in patients who have asthma but that anxiolytics as monotherapy should not be relied on or expected to control asthma symptoms in patients who have comorbid anxiety. Relaxation therapies, including hypnotherapy, biofeedback techniques, and mental and muscle relaxation therapies, have all been studied in asthmatics in general, but there is not evidence to support their unselective prescription in asthma [16].

The pathophysiologic link between asthma and anxiety disorders is not clear. One theory linking these comorbidities is the dyspnea-fear theory [17].

In this model, hyperventilatory panic attacks arise from an innate emotional response to severe breathlessness; the panic experienced by the individual is actuated by fear because of physiologic responses to hyperventilation. Another possibility is that bronchoconstriction is attributable to some combination of vagal input and inflammation. Symptoms of stress may trigger bronchoconstriction through vagal mechanisms, and some individuals may be particularly susceptible to this phenomenon [18]. This was first shown by McFadden and colleagues [19] in 1969 when they studied 29 asthmatics who were told that they were inhaling an allergen known to cause their asthma attacks when they were actually inhaling nebulized physiologic saline. Fifteen patients exhibited increased airway resistance measured by whole-body plethysmography, suggesting bronchoconstriction to the nebulized saline. Intravenous atropine sulfate, 1 to 2 mg, prevented this bronchoconstriction response to suggestion, intimating a vagally mediated cholinergic phenomenon responsible for this conditioned bronchospasm.

Substance Abuse and Asthma

Alcohol abuse or dependence has been significantly associated with asthma (OR = 1.7, 95% CI: 1.4–2.1) [6]. Adolescents with chemical dependence also exhibit a higher prevalence of physician-diagnosed asthma when compared with age-matched controls (15.6% versus 12%; OR = 1.37, 95% CI: 1.01–1.84) [20]. Studies addressing causal relations and treatment effects of asthma and alcohol and chemical dependence have yet to be performed, however.

Psychiatric Considerations in the Asthma Caregiver

Psychiatric symptoms are also common in caregivers of children who have asthma. Approximately 50% of caregivers of inner-city children who have asthma have significant psychiatric symptom severity on the Brief Symptom Inventory scale [21]. Brown and colleagues [22] have shown that depression and anxiety disorders were much more common among asthma caregivers than in the general public. Additionally, depression in the caregiver was associated with a 58% increase in unscheduled clinic visits by the child, and an anxiety disorder in the caregiver was associated with a 31% increase in asthma-related hospitalizations for the child.

CHRONIC OBSTRUCTIVE PULMONARY DISEASE

Chronic obstructive pulmonary disease (COPD) is characterized by chronic bronchitis or emphysema, with smoking being the major risk factor. The number of patients who have this disease is estimated at 24 million in the United States [23] and 600 million worldwide [24]. The psychiatric illnesses that have been studied in COPD include depression, anxiety, and psychosis.

Chronic Obstructive Pulmonary Disease and Depression

Much like asthma, there is a higher prevalence of depression in patients who have COPD than in the general population. Multiple studies have shown that approximately 40% of patients who have COPD have lifetime MDD [23].

Patients who have COPD with comorbid depression have lower QOL and have greater objective impairment in functional performance when compared with nondepressed patients who have COPD [23]. Depression also seems to account for more of the deficits in functional performance than COPD severity itself [25,26]. These data illustrate the importance of identifying and managing depression in COPD.

An effective treatment algorithm for managing depression in patients who have COPD has not been established. One study, a placebo-controlled trial of nortriptyline, has demonstrated an improvement in depression symptoms with the use of antidepressants in patients who have COPD [27]. The treatment group also reported improvement in anxiety and better functional status compared with placebo-treated subjects. As previously mentioned in regard to asthma, the anticholinergic effects of nortriptyline may have contributed to the benefits seen.

Whether selective serotonin reuptake inhibitors (SSRIs) are beneficial in COPD is even less clear [23]. Limitations in studies to date include low power, inadequate treatment duration, dependence on patient-report instruments to measure outcome measures of treatment effect, and low maximal doses of medications [23]. In perhaps the most well designed of the SSRI studies, 28 patients who had COPD and psychiatrist-diagnosed MDD were given paroxetine, 20 mg/d, or placebo for 6 weeks [28]. All subjects were then given paroxetine in an unblinded fashion for 3 more months. Paroxetine was associated with improvement in depression scores and 6-minute walking distances after 18 weeks of therapy as compared with placebo. The improvement was noted only after the first 6 weeks of the study, however, when all subjects were unblinded and taking paroxetine.

The pathophysiologic relation between COPD and depression is complex. Patients who are depressed have higher rates of smoking, increasing the risk for COPD. Derangement of cerebral microvascular circulation and chronic hypoxemia in COPD have been proposed to lead to comorbid depression [23]. Chronic hypoxemia has been shown in rats to disrupt the synthesis, release, and replenishment of noradrenergic and dopaminergic neurotransmitters in the brain [29], which may lead to depression.

Chronic Obstructive Pulmonary Disease and Anxiety Disorders

As mentioned previously, the sensation of dyspnea is shared by obstructive lung diseases (including COPD) and anxiety disorders. The prevalence of GAD may be as high as 15.8% in patients who have COPD, which is more than three times the prevalence in the general US population [30]. Panic attacks also seem to be more frequent in patients who have COPD than in the general population. In one small study, 37% of outpatients who had COPD reported symptoms of a panic attack in the preceding 3 weeks [31].

Much like the negative impact of depression on COPD outcomes, patients who have COPD and anxiety disorders seem to have increased morbidity compared with patients who have COPD and do not have anxiety [30].

This elevated morbidity includes greater disability, poorer functional status, and decreased lung function. Increased rates of hospitalization may be associated with anxiety disorders in patients who have COPD as well. A study examining rates of hospitalization in geriatric patients who had COPD showed that the presence of anxiety had a statistically significant association with hospital admission in the previous 12 months [32].

Pharmacologic therapy for anxiety disorders in patients who have COPD seems to be beneficial based on limited data. Benzodiazepines are often avoided as first-line therapy in COPD because of their potential respiratory drive depressive effects. Clinically, this is primarily a concern in patients who have COPD, who retain carbon dioxide (CO_2). In a small study, buspirone, which does not have the same sedating effect as benzodiazepines, was associated with decreases in anxiety and dyspnea as compared with placebo and with improved exercise tolerance in patients who had COPD [33]. SSRIs are considered to be first-line therapies for anxiety disorders. Small trials involving fewer than 10 patients have been performed assessing the use of SSRIs, specifically sertraline, in patients who have COPD. These limited results suggest that SSRIs are well tolerated by patients who have COPD and may reduce their anxiety symptoms [30].

Nonpharmacologic therapies have also been studied in patients who have COPD and anxiety disorders, including progressive muscle relaxation, cognitive behavioral therapy, and pulmonary rehabilitation. Overall, these therapies in anxious patients who have COPD may improve anxiety symptoms, decrease dyspnea, and, in some trials, even improve lung function [30].

Mechanisms of association between COPD and anxiety disorders have been theorized. When a patient who has COPD and is anxious has dyspnea, he or she may misconstrue the severity of breathlessness. This leads to a heightened state of physiologic arousal, which leads to additional misperception of the sensations of dyspnea and an exaggerated feeling of breathlessness [30]. Patients who have COPD with panic disorder have increased perceptions of dyspnea compared with patients who have COPD without panic disorder, despite a lack of measured differences in pulmonary function tests [34]. This incorrect perception may be attributed to the dyspnea-fear theory discussed previously.

Chronic Obstructive Pulmonary Disease and Schizophrenia

Subjects with schizophrenia seem to be more likely to have COPD according to a large retrospective chart review analysis (adjusted OR = 2.11, 95% CI: 1.36–3.28) [35] comparing 1074 patients who had schizophrenia with 726,262 controls over a 6-year period. The increased COPD rate is attributed to the increased smoking rates among schizophrenics, suggesting a "self-medication" hypothesis that stimulation of central nervous system (CNS) nicotinic cholinergic receptors may improve the negative symptoms of schizophrenia [36].

CYSTIC FIBROSIS

Cystic fibrosis (CF) is an autosomal recessive multisystem disorder beginning in early childhood. CF is the most common fatal hereditary disease in the white population. Worldwide, CF affects 1 in 2500 live births [37]. With CF, several complications can arise, including airway obstruction with chronic infection, pancreatic exocrine insufficiency, pansinusitis, sterility, and insulin-dependent diabetes.

In recent years, the life expectancy of patients who have CF has dramatically increased because of earlier diagnosis and treatment advances provided by multidisciplinary CF centers. In the United States, the median survival age doubled between 1969 and 1990 from 14 to 28 years [38]. Despite advances in survival, CF continues to be a chronic debilitating illness with burdensome and expensive therapeutic regimens. Although the physiologic and therapeutic aspects of CF have been extensively researched, few reports have assessed the psychologic aspects of this life-limiting disease.

Overview of Psychologic Function in Patients Who Have Cystic Fibrosis

Psychologic functioning has been assessed in children and adults who have CF, with variable results. Some investigators have suggested that the psychologic development of children who have CF is not significantly different than that of healthy controls, whereas others have found increased depression, eating disorders, and anxiety [39]. Several studies have suggested that emotional disturbance increases in adult patients who have CF as they age [39,40]. Rather than reflecting age per se, the increased psychopathologic findings may be more a manifestation of disease progression [41]. Overall, the evidence suggests that young adult patients who have CF generally have psychologic functioning similar to their healthy counterparts [42]. Several studies have examined lung function and disease severity correlated with psychologic function in patients who have CF, although there has been little study of psychologic function of critically ill patients who have CF [39,41,43].

Age and Gender Effects

Studies from the 1960s and 1970s of psychosocial problems in children who had CF revealed significant emotional disturbances [44]. At that time, however, early death in CF was much more common. In a recent study by Bregnballe and colleagues [44], the investigators evaluated psychosocial problems in children between the ages of 7 and 14 years. These investigators found that children who had CF did not differ from healthy controls with respect to depression, self-concept, and disruptive behavior. Younger children (ages 7–10 years) tended to have more anxiety than the control children. Increased anxiety in younger children has been shown in other studies as well [45,46].

Overall, studies examining psychologic health of adult patients who have CF have shown that these patients generally do not have significant disturbances in their emotional well-being. Shepard and colleagues [47] found that emotional support and overall life satisfaction were similar in adult patients who have CF compared with healthy controls. Anderson and colleagues [41] found that adults who have CF have some subclinical elevated hypochondriasis and hysteria scores on the Minnesota Multiphasic Personality Inventory. They did not demonstrate significant levels of depression, anxiety, or other psychopathology, however, and such subclinical elevations are common in other chronic illnesses. One study reported a trend in older patients toward lower self-esteem and increased frustration, leading to decreased compliance with therapies [42].

With regard to gender and mortality in CF, female patients have lower survival rates. Although older publications suggested that women were more likely to experience more severe emotional disturbance [39,48], more recent publications have not supported this finding [42]. One study even found higher scores for depression and anxiety in men who had CF than in women who had CF [41].

Eating Disorders in Cystic Fibrosis

The nature of CF as a disease involves frequent malabsorption, and thus concern about food and weight; therefore, the disease in itself may be a risk factor for eating disorders. Chronic issues of malabsorption with resultant poor weight gain are secondary to the pancreatic effects of CF. The prevalence of distorted body image and eating disorders in CF is largely unknown [49]. Pearson and colleagues [39] found in their comparison of children and adults who had CF that younger patients were significantly more likely to display significant eating disturbances than older patients. A study of 55 adolescents who had CF found that none of the patients met criteria for anorexia nervosa (AN) or bulimia nervosa (BN), however [50]. Although there is no evidence of an increased incidence of AN or BN in adolescent patients who have CF, eating disturbances do occur, including food avoidance and aversions, marked weight loss, and body image distortions.

Psychiatric Interventions

There have been limited studies on the utility of psychiatric interventions in patients who have CF. A meta-analysis assessed four different psychologic interventions in children and adults who had CF [37]. These interventions (eg, massage therapy, biofeedback, behavioral therapies) were mainly directed at improving physical outcomes and treatment compliance. The investigators concluded that there was no evidence that these measures improved clinical outcomes [37]. There have been no studies of the effectiveness aimed at the use of psychotherapy or psychotropic medications in patients who have CF with emotional or behavioral problems [45].

RESPIRATORY FAILURE

Every year, more than 1 million people in the United States are admitted to the intensive care unit (ICU) with acute respiratory failure. With mechanical ventilation, there is an associated high rate of mortality regardless of the patient's underlying condition. Therefore, psychiatric complications after mechanical ventilation are common. Psychiatric symptoms that can occur after ICU discharge include depression, substance withdrawal, anxiety, and unwanted recall of unpleasant experiences [51].

Posttraumatic Stress Disorder

Posttraumatic stress disorder (PTSD) affects a significant proportion of patients after critical illness, including respiratory failure (Box 1). As with experiences like combat and natural disasters, the stress experienced during critical illnesses may invoke symptoms that persist well beyond physical recovery. Although few studies have assessed the long-term outcomes of post-ICU PTSD, Kapf-hammer and colleagues [52] conducted a long-term follow-up (median of 8 years) of 46 patients who had previously been placed on mechanical ventila-tion secondary to acute respiratory distress syndrome (ARDS). They found that greater than 50% (11 of 20 survivors) still had from PTSD at follow-up. The reported incidence of PTSD after critical illness varies anywhere between 4% and 25% [53], which is considerably higher than the rate of 1.3% to 12% reported in community samples [54]. Little is known about risk factors for PTSD after critical illness. The significance of gender as a risk factor for PTSD in the critically ill is not known [55]. One prospective study of 43 me-chanically ventilated patients found that 14% had high levels of PTSD symp-toms, with a higher proportion of women than men [55].

There are varying beliefs regarding the effects of sedation of mechanically ventilated patients on the future development of PTSD. There is no evidence that the use of sedative drugs curtails the development of PTSD [56]. Schelling and colleagues [57] found a correlation between current PTSD symptoms and the number of ICU symptoms that patients recalled, however. These results might suggest a beneficial role of total amnesia achieved by means of sedation in the prevention of PTSD after critical illness. In contrast, Kress and col-leagues [56] found that interruption of daily sedation in mechanically ventilated patients led to fewer subsequent symptoms of PTSD. Another study asserted that delusional memories of the ICU experience led to a higher likelihood of

---

Box 1: PTSD risk factors in the ICU

ICU length of stay (longer duration)

Hospital stay (longer duration)

Length of mechanical ventilation

Greater levels of sedation

Female gender

Younger age

Preexisting psychiatric history

Greater number of traumatic memories/frightening recollections

Presence of delusional memories

Data from Jackson JC, Hart RP, Gordon SM, et al. Post-traumatic stress disorder and post-traumatic stress symptoms following critical illness in medical intensive care unit patients: as-sessing the magnitude of the problem. Crit Care 2007;11(1):R27.

later PTSD-related symptoms than those with factual memories [58], suggesting that sedation might be counterproductive.

Another controversy regarding PTSD and critical illness is the role of stress hormones (ie, cortisol). Patients who have established PTSD have lower baseline levels of cortisol than controls [51]. Two small, randomized, placebo-controlled trials (one in patients who had ARDS and the other in patients after cardiac surgery) have shown that hydrocortisone use may decrease the frequency of PTSD in the critically ill [59,60]. Given these studies' methodologic limitations, the use of corticosteroids to reduce PTSD in mechanically ventilated patients in the ICU requires further study [59].

Depression in Respiratory Failure

Rates of depression after prolonged respiratory failure vary depending on the assessment method used and time of evaluation after recovery. Depression of moderate or greater severity affects 12% to 43% of ICU survivors [61]. No clear risk factors have been determined for increased incidence of post-ICU depression.

Kress and colleagues [56] found in their follow-up of 32 ICU survivors (mean time from discharge of 381 days) that the incidence of moderate to severe depression on the Beck Depression Inventory (BDI) was 34%. Jackson and colleagues [62] followed 33 previously ventilated patients, with assessment by the Geriatric Depression Scale (GDS), and found a 16% incidence of depression at hospital discharge, which increased to 25% at 6 months.

Although several studies have assessed the prevalence of depression in post-ventilated patients, there have been few studies regarding the treatment of depression in this same population. Weinert and Meller [61] conducted interviews of patients recovering from ARDS syndrome 2 months after their acute illness. These investigators found that more than one third of patients had been prescribed new antidepressants even though the prevalence of MDD in their survey was only 15%. Jones and colleagues [63] conducted a randomized trial in 126 patients in the ICU to evaluate the effectiveness of a rehabilitation program on physical and psychologic recovery. Their intervention group received a booklet explaining psychologic and physical impairments to be expected during recovery and a 6-week self-directed exercise program. At 8 weeks, only 12% of the intervention group versus 25% of the nonintervention group had evidence of depression, but this did not reach statistical significance. Despite the suggestion of decreased incidence of depression with physical rehabilitation and widespread antidepressant use in the post-ICU population, no intervention has been shown to have proved specific effectiveness.

OTHER CHRONIC PULMONARY DISEASES

Most of the literature on the psychiatric effects of chronic pulmonary diseases addresses asthma, COPD, and CF, and few studies have evaluated other chronic pulmonary diseases, probably because these other diseases are far less prevalent than asthma and COPD. Nonetheless, there is some relevant literature regarding IPF and sarcoidosis.

Idiopathic Pulmonary Fibrosis

IPF is a chronic fibrotic disorder of the lower respiratory tract that usually affects adults older than the age of 40 years [64]. IPF is the most common of the interstitial lung diseases, with an incidence rate of 15 cases per 100,000 population per year [65]. Overall, the disease carries a high mortality rate and there is no known cure, although patients are often treated with immunosuppressive agents to curb disease progression. Progressive dyspnea is the most debilitating feature of this disease.

Few studies have assessed QOL in patients who have IPF. The available data suggest a correlation between worsening QOL scores with lower lung volumes, regardless of the instrument used to assess QOL [65–67]. De Vries and colleagues [66] found that approximately one quarter of patients who have IPF had significant depressive symptoms. Another small study in IPF found that scores for depression and anxiety were higher than in healthy controls but were not high enough to suggest clinically significant depression or anxiety [67]. Finally, there has been a single study using diagnostic criteria to determine the true incidence of depression in IPF. A single case report of bipolar disorder in a patient who had IPF has suggested a possible genetic link between the two disorders [68].

Sarcoidosis

Sarcoidosis primarily affects the respiratory tract but also often involves other organs (skin, eyes, liver, heart, and nervous system). The prevalence of sarcoidosis is much higher in the African-American population than in whites. Although sarcoidosis can be a mild self-limited disease, between 10% and 30% of patients may experience chronic debilitating disease with profound effects on QOL [69]. The primary chronic symptoms that affect QOL include fatigue, night sweats, cough, dyspnea, and chest pain [70]. A few studies have examined the effects of the disease on patients' QOL and the incidence of depression.

Wirnsberger and colleagues [71] reported that patients who have symptomatic sarcoidosis had significantly higher BDI scores (greater than twofold on average) than patients without sarcoidosis. They found no relation between the results of pulmonary function tests and QOL. Chang and colleagues [70] found that 60% of patients who have sarcoidosis were depressed per the Center of Epidemiologic Studies Depression Scale (CES-D). Female gender, lack of ability to access or pay for medical care, and increased number of affected organ systems were all factors associated with increased likelihood of depression.

Although these studies do indicate an increased incidence of depression in patients who have sarcoidosis, the psychiatric effects of the disease may include more than simply adverse outcomes on QOL associated with sarcoidosis' chronic symptoms. Sarcoidosis affects the CNS in 5% to 10% of patients, with the cranial nerves, hypothalamus, and pituitary glands most commonly involved [72]. Neurosarcoidosis is often unrecognized and may be the source of depressive symptoms [73]. Other reported psychiatric manifestations of neurosarcoidosis include dementia and psychosis [9,74]. Sarcoidosis can also cause neuropsychiatric symptoms by means of its associated hypercalcemia.

A summary of evidence on psychiatric syndromes and their treatment in respiratory illnesses is given in Table 1.

PSYCHIATRIC SYNDROMES THAT MIMIC RESPIRATORY DISEASES

Respiratory disorders can present with several nonspecific manifestations, including cough, dyspnea, and wheeze. Several nonasthmatic conditions are often misdiagnosed as asthma, and many of these conditions have a relatively minor physiologic component. Some of these asthma mimickers seem to be largely, but not necessarily entirely, psychogenic in cause. These conditions (sighing dyspnea, vocal cord dysfunction [VCD], hyperventilation syndrome [HVS], and habit cough) are often grouped under the category of functional respiratory disorders.

Psychogenic Cough

Coughing has important physiologic benefits in terms of clearing the airways of debris and preventing infection. There are several physiologic mechanisms that

Table 1
Evidence for association of psychiatric disorders in pulmonary diseases

Lung disease	Psychiatric disorder	Level of evidence for association	Level of evidence for pharmacologic therapy
Asthma	MDD	IIa	Doxepin-Ib Citalopram-Ib
	Anxiety disorders	IIa	None
	Substance abuse	IIa	None
COPD	MDD	IIa	Nortriptyline-Ib SSRIs-IV
	Anxiety disorders	IIa	Buspirone-Ib SSRIs-IIb
	Schizophrenia	IIa	None
CF	MDD	IIa	None
	Eating disorders	IIa	None
	Anxiety	IIa	None
Respiratory failure	PTSD	IIa	Corticosteroids-Ib
	MDD	IIa	None
IPF	MDD	III	None
Sarcoidosis	MDD	III	None

Key to level of evidence: Ia, evidence from meta-analysis of randomized controlled trials; Ib, evidence from at least one randomized controlled trial; IIa, evidence from at least one controlled study without randomization; IIb, evidence from at least one other type of quasiexperimental study; III, evidence from nonexperimental descriptive studies, such as comparative studies; IV, evidence from expert committee reports or opinions or clinical experience of respected authorities or both.

Key to level of evidence *adapted from* Shekelle PG, Woolf SH, Eccles M, et al. Clinical guidelines: developing guidelines. BMJ 1999;318(7183):593–6.

can induce cough, which include airway/vocal cord irritation and anatomic injuries to the chest or chest wall. In addition to the common physiologic causes of cough (ie, postnasal drip, gastroesophageal reflux, asthma), there are some patients who have cough primarily attributable to psychologic causes.

Psychogenic cough is also commonly referred to as habit cough and is defined as a chronic cough without any physiologic cause. There are no specific diagnostic criteria, and other physiologic diseases associated with cough should be ruled out first, including tic disorders, such as Tourette syndrome. Kravitz and colleagues [75] were the first to identify this entity in 1969, describing nine patients who had "psychogenic cough tics." The disease is much more common in children than in adults, with the diagnosis being made in 3% to 10% of children with cough of unknown origin persisting greater than 1 month [76]. In most cases, the cough tends to be a dry, repetitive, "honking" cough that does not occur during sleep [77]. A distinguishing factor between psychogenic cough and the cough of asthma is that during exacerbations, asthmatics are often awakened with cough. Also, asthmatics typically state that their cough originates from their chest, whereas patients who have habit cough tend to localize their symptoms to the throat. Although the cough can be socially disruptive and can result in school absenteeism [78], there is no associated morbidity. Objective evaluation measures (ie, physical examination, laboratory tests, chest radiographs, pulmonary function testing) are normal in the patients who present with psychogenic cough [79].

Treatment of psychogenic cough involves reassurance to the patient and family [80]. For more resistant cases, biofeedback, suggestion therapy, and aversion techniques have been used with varying success [78].

Vocal Cord Dysfunction

VCD is caused by the paradoxical adduction of the vocal cords on inspiration. VCD has also been referred to misleadingly as Munchausen stridor, episodic laryngeal dyskinesia, factitious asthma, psychosomatic stridor, and emotional laryngeal asthma [77]. Some of these terms are misleading, because VCD is rarely factitious. Like other functional disorders, its cause is best considered idiopathic at present, although it is recognized that psychologic factors are frequently important in VCD. VCD is frequently misdiagnosed as asthma, leading to extensive and costly diagnostic and therapeutic measures.

The prevalence of VCD among children and adults is unknown, but it is more common in girls and women. Sexual abuse in women seems to be a predisposing factor for VCD, and there is a higher prevalence of the disease in health care workers [81].

The inappropriate vocal cord apposition can induce wheezing, shortness of breath, and cough. Other confounding factors that lead to confusion with asthma are that patients who have VCD report improvement with bronchodilators. In some patients who have VCD, as with asthma, the symptoms are provoked by exercise. It is also not uncommon for a patient to have asthma and VCD. Newman and colleagues [82] found that in 95 of the patients they studied who had VCD, 53 (46%) also had asthma. Unique aspects of asthma that are not seen in patients who have VCD alone include nighttime symptoms, presence of hyperinflation of lungs on chest radiographs, and the possible presence of hypoxemia. In addition, patients who have VCD often improve with distraction, whereas patients who have asthma do not.

Some psychiatric disorders seem to be associated with VCD. Newman and colleagues [82] found that 73% of patients who had pure VCD had an axis I psychiatric diagnosis. Stress, mood, and anxiety disturbances may exacerbate VCD. A recent study by Doshi and Weinberger [83] found that only 11% of their patient population had symptoms of anxiety or depression, however.

The diagnosis of VCD is best established by flexible rhinolaryngoscopy [84]. The laryngoscopy should be performed during an attack, because vocal cord appearance is completely normal when asymptomatic. Provocative maneuvers, such as having the patient perform breathing maneuvers or repetitive sounds, can help to induce the paradoxical vocal cord adduction seen in VCD.

Treatment of VCD involves reassurance and relaxation techniques. Excellent results have been reported with speech therapy [85]. Patients are taught to concentrate on the expiratory phase of breathing and how to use their abdominal muscles in their breathing to distract them from the VCD. Another useful technique is to have patients maximally open the glottis and breathe in and out. Patients who have underlying psychiatric disorders should have appropriately targeted treatment. In terms of long-term prognosis, the condition is thought to be self-limiting with no significant long-term sequelae.

Hyperventilation Syndrome

The term *hyperventilation syndrome* was first introduced by Kerr and colleagues [86] in 1937 to describe a syndrome of hyperventilation, anxiety, and physical signs. In this disorder, patients have tachypnea, which leads to respiratory alkalosis, which, in turn, can induce tetany or syncope in some cases. Although the symptoms of HVS clearly overlap with panic disorder, they are not synonymous.

The incidence of this syndrome varies from 6% to 11%, with a female predominance [87]. The syndrome tends to occur in the third and fourth decades but can affect patients at any age. The duration of HVS attacks can vary from a few minutes up to several hours.

Although the disease is relatively benign, failure to recognize it can lead to inappropriate therapies. A cycle can develop in which these panic symptoms are addressed by unnecessary measures that increase the likelihood of future attacks being mismanaged by intensive or invasive approaches [77]. Acute symptoms can be treated with a rebreathing bag, which helps to terminate acute attacks. Sedatives are not usually required. As with other functional respiratory disorders, reassurance and education are the primary treatment. Overall, the prognosis for recovery is good, except in children and adolescents; 40% of such patients show persistent symptoms into adulthood [88].

Sighing Dyspnea

"Sighing dyspnea" refers to patients who have deep sighing respirations and shortness of breath in the absence of an increased respiratory rate [89]. Although first described at the beginning of the twentieth century, this entity is not frequently diagnosed in recent times. The exact prevalence of this symptom pattern is unknown, but the authors' own experience suggests that it is not rare. Sighing dyspnea usually affects patients in the second to fourth decade of life and tends to be more common in girls and women [78].

Patients who have sighing dyspnea may present with "attacks" similar to asthma but may also complain of baseline shortness of breath. Associated anxiety is one of the principal components of this syndrome. Although patients may seem to be distressed and episodes can last up to several hours, patients have no change in their respiratory rate. Another classic feature that helps to distinguish sighing dyspnea from asthma is that patients who have sighing dyspnea often exhibit yawning and sighing even outside of acute episodes [78]. No underlying cause of this syndrome has been proven. Treatment has focused on reassurance by the physician and on instruction on relaxation techniques.

PSYCHIATRIC SYMPTOMS ASSOCIATED WITH PHARMACOTHERAPY OF PULMONARY DISEASE

Corticosteroids

Systemic corticosteroids are frequently used in the treatment of various pulmonary diseases, especially asthma and COPD. The psychiatric side effects of corticosteroids have been well chronicled and include mood disturbances (ie, mania, mood lability, depression), cognitive changes, and, less commonly, "steroid psychosis" with hallucinations and delusions [90]. Psychiatric disturbances seem to occur most frequently within the first 2 weeks of therapy [90] and seem to be dose related, with patients receiving prednisone at a dose between 40 and 80 mg/d at moderate risk (4.6%) and those receiving more than 80 mg/d at high risk (18.4%) of psychiatric side effects [91]. The treatment response, like the symptoms, seems to be similar to that of bipolar disorder, with improvement reported with lithium, anticonvulsants, or antipsychotics [90]. Cognitive side effects of short-term therapy with systemic corticosteroids typically disappear with the discontinuation of the steroid [90].

Severe psychiatric disturbance seems to be uncommon with inhaled corticosteroid use. Although there are published case reports of severe mania in adults and children after the addition of an inhaled corticosteroid [90], it is unlikely for inhaled corticosteroids to cause any psychotic symptoms, because systemic absorption is so minimal.

Theophylline

Although its use has declined with the introduction of better long-acting bronchodilators with fewer side effects, theophylline remains an important adjunctive treatment in certain patients who have obstructive lung disease. Side effects, such as impaired memory, decreased attention, and restlessness, may occur with theophylline use even at therapeutic levels, especially in children [92]. Theophylline also has many well-described potential drug interactions.

β₂-Receptor Agonists

β₂-receptor agonists are important medications in patients who have COPD and asthma. There have been several isolated reports of psychotic events related to systemic β₂-receptor agonist use [92]. Inhaled β₂-receptor receptor agonists do not seem to have any significant psychiatric side effects whether used short or long term.

Anticholinergics

Inhaled anticholinergic agents, such as ipratropium and tiotropium, are frequently used as part of the treatment regimen for patients who have COPD and asthma. No psychiatric side effects have been reported with the use of inhaled anticholinergic drugs.

References

[1] Braman SS. The global burden of asthma. Chest 2006;130(Suppl 1):4S–12S.

[2] Masoli M, Fabian D, Holt S, et al. The global burden of asthma: executive summary of the GINA Dissemination Committee report. Allergy 2004;59(5):469–78.

[3] Zielinski TA, Brown ES, Nejtek VA, et al. Depression in asthma: prevalence and clinical implications. Prim Care Companion J Clin Psychiatry 2000;2(5):153–8.

[4] Mancuso CA, Peterson MG, Charlson ME. Effects of depressive symptoms on health-related quality of life in asthma patients. J Gen Intern Med 2000;15(5):301–10.

[5] Lyketsos CG, Lyketsos GC, Richardson SC, et al. Dysthymic states and depressive syndromes in physical conditions of presumably psychogenic origin. Acta Psychiatr Scand 1987;76(5):529–34.

[6] Scott KM, Von Korff M, Ormel J, et al. Mental disorders among adults with asthma: results from the World Mental Health Survey. Gen Hosp Psychiatry 2007;29(2):123–33.

[7] Bush T, Richardson L, Katon W, et al. Anxiety and depressive disorders are associated with smoking in adolescents with asthma. J Adolesc Health 2007;40(5):425–32.

[8] ten Brinke A, Ouwerkerk ME, Zwinderman AH, et al. Psychopathology in patients with severe asthma is associated with increased health care utilization. Am J Respir Crit Care Med 2001;163(5):1093–6.

[9] Allen GM, Hickie I, Gandevia SC, et al. Impaired voluntary drive to breathe: a possible link between depression and unexplained ventilatory failure in asthmatic patients. Thorax 1994;49(9):881–4.

[10] Bosley CM, Fosbury JA, Cochrane GM. The psychological factors associated with poor compliance with treatment in asthma. Eur Respir J 1995;8(6):899–904.

[11] Sanger MD. The treatment of anxiety and depression in the allergic patient. Ann Allergy 1969;27(10):506–10.

[12] Brown ES, Vigil L, Khan DA, et al. A randomized trial of citalopram versus placebo in outpatients with asthma and major depressive disorder: a proof of concept study. Biol Psychiatry 2005;58(11):865–70.

[13] Goodwin RD, Jacobi F, Thefeld W. Mental disorders and asthma in the community. Arch Gen Psychiatry 2003;60(11):1125–30.

[14] Steptoe A, Vogele C. Individual differences in the perception of bodily sensations: the role of trait anxiety and coping style. Behav Res Ther 1992;30(6):597–607.

[15] Deshmukh VM, Toelle BG, Usherwood T, et al. Anxiety, panic and adult asthma: a cognitive-behavioral perspective. Respir Med 2007;101(2):194–202.

[16] Huntley A, White AR, Ernst E. Relaxation therapies for asthma: a systematic review. Thorax 2002;57(2):127–31.

[17] Ley R. Dyspneic-fear and catastrophic cognitions in hyperventilatory panic attacks. Behav Res Ther 1989;27(5):549–54.

[18] Lehrer PM, Isenberg S, Hochron SM. Asthma and emotion: a review. J Asthma 1993;30(1): 5–21.

[19] McFadden ER Jr, Luparello T, Lyons HA, et al. The mechanism of action of suggestion in the induction of acute asthma attacks. Psychosom Med 1969;31(2):134–43.

[20] Mertens JR, Flisher AJ, Fleming MF, et al. Medical conditions of adolescents in alcohol and drug treatment: comparison with matched controls. J Adolesc Health 2007;40(2):173–9.

[21] Wade S, Weil C, Holden G, et al. Psychosocial characteristics of inner-city children with asthma: a description of the NCICAS psychosocial protocol. National Cooperative Inner-City Asthma Study. Pediatr Pulmonol 1997;24(4):263–76.

[22] Brown ES, Gan V, Jeffress J, et al. Psychiatric symptomatology and disorders in caregivers of children with asthma. Pediatrics 2006;118(6):e1715–20.

[23] Norwood R, Balkissoon R. Current perspectives on management of co-morbid depression in COPD. COPD 2005;2(1):185–93.

[24] World Health Organization. The world health report 1997—conquering suffering, enriching humanity. Available at: http://www.who.int/whr/1997/en/. Accessed May 3, 2007.

[25] Kim HF, Kunik ME, Molinari VA, et al. Functional impairment in COPD patients: the impact of anxiety and depression. Psychosomatics 2000;41(6):465–71.

[26] Felker B, Katon W, Hedrick SC, et al. The association between depressive symptoms and health status in patients with chronic pulmonary disease. Gen Hosp Psychiatry 2001;23(2):56–61.

[27] Borson S, McDonald GJ, Gayle T, et al. Improvement in mood, physical symptoms, and function with nortriptyline for depression in patients with chronic obstructive pulmonary disease. Psychosomatics 1992;33(2):190–201.

[28] Eiser N, Harte R, Spiros K, et al. Effect of treating depression on quality-of-life and exercise tolerance in severe COPD. COPD 2005;2(2):233–41.

[29] Miwa S, Fujiwara M, Inoue M, et al. Effects of hypoxia on the activities of noradrenergic and dopaminergic neurons in the rat brain. J Neurochem 1986;47(1):63–9.

[30] Brenes GA. Anxiety and chronic obstructive pulmonary disease: prevalence, impact, and treatment. Psychosom Med 2003;65(6):963–70.

[31] Porzelius J, Vest M, Nochomovitz M. Respiratory function, cognitions, and panic in chronic obstructive pulmonary patients. Behav Res Ther 1992;30(1):75–7.

[32] Yohannes AM, Baldwin RC, Connolly MJ. Depression and anxiety in elderly outpatients with chronic obstructive pulmonary disease: prevalence, and validation of the BASDEC screening questionnaire. Int J Geriatr Psychiatry 2000;15(12):1090–6.

[33] Argyropoulou P, Patakas D, Koukou A, et al. Buspirone effect on breathlessness and exercise performance in patients with chronic obstructive pulmonary disease. Respiration 1993;60(4):216–20.

[34] Moore MC, Zebb BJ. The catastrophic misinterpretation of physiological distress. Behav Res Ther 1999;37(11):1105–18.

[35] Carney CP, Jones L, Woolson RF. Medical comorbidity in women and men with schizophrenia: a population-based controlled study. J Gen Intern Med 2006;21(11):1133–7.

[36] Dalack GW, Healy DJ, Meador-Woodruff JH. Nicotine dependence in schizophrenia: clinical phenomena and laboratory findings. Am J Psychiatry 1998;155(11):1490–501.

[37] Glasscoe CA, Quittner AL. Psychological interventions for cystic fibrosis. Cochrane Database Syst Rev 2003;3:CD003148.

[38] FitzSimmons S. The changing epidemiology of cystic fibrosis. J Pediatr 1993;122(1):1–9.

[39] Pearson DA, Pumariega AJ, Seilheimer DK. The development of psychiatric symptomatology in patients with cystic fibrosis. J Am Acad Child Adolesc Psychiatry 1991;30(2): 290–7.

[40] Blair C, Cull A, Freeman CP. Psychological functioning of young adults with cystic fibrosis and their families. Thorax 1994;49:798–802.

[41] Anderson DL, Flume PA, Hardy KK. Psychological functioning of adults with cystic fibrosis. Chest 2001;119(4):1079–84.

[42] Pfeffer PE, Pfeffer JM, Hodson ME. The psychosocial and psychiatric side of cystic fibrosis in adolescents and adults. J Cyst Fibros 2003;2(2):61–8.

[43] Britto MT, Kotagal UR, Hornung RW, et al. Impact of recent pulmonary exacerbations on quality of life in patients with cystic fibrosis. Chest 2002;121(1):64–72.

[44] Bregnballe V, Thastum M, Schiotz PO. Psychosocial problems in children with cystic fibrosis. Acta Paediatr 2007;96(1):58–61.

[45] Elgudin L, Kishan S, Howe D. Depression in children and adolescents with cystic fibrosis: case studies. Int J Psychiatry Med 2004;34(4):391–7.

[46] Thompson RJ Jr, Gustafson KE, George LK, et al. Change over a 12-month period in the psychological adjustment of children and adolescents with cystic fibrosis. J Pediatr Psychol 1994;19(2):189–203.

[47] Shepherd SL, Hovell MF, Harwood IR, et al. A comparative study of the psychosocial assets of adults with cystic fibrosis and their healthy peers. Chest 1990;97:1310–6.

[48] Strauss GD, Wellisch DK. Psychological assessment of adults with cystic fibrosis. Int J Psychiatry Med 1980;10(3):265–72.

[49] Duff AJ. Psychological interventions in cystic fibrosis and asthma. Paediatr Respir Rev 2001;2(4):350–7.

[50] Shearer JE, Bryon M. The nature and prevalence of eating disorders and eating disturbance in adolescents with cystic fibrosis. J R Soc Med 2004;97(Suppl 44):36–42.

[51] Weinert C. Epidemiology and treatment of psychiatric conditions that develop after critical illness. Curr Opin Crit Care 2005;11(4):376–80.

[52] Kapfhammer HP, Rothenhäusler HB, Krauseneck T, et al. Posttraumatic stress disorder and health-related quality of life in long-term survivors of acute respiratory distress syndrome. Am J Psychiatry 2004;161(1):45–52.

[53] Jones C, Bäckman C, Capuzzo M, et al. Precipitants of post-traumatic stress disorder following intensive care: a hypothesis generating study of diversity in care. Intensive Care Med 2007;33(6):978–85.

[54] Cuthbertson BH, Hull A, Strachan M, et al. Post-traumatic stress disorder after critical illness requiring general intensive care. Intensive Care Med 2004;30(3):450–5.

[55] Girard TD, Shintani AK, Jackson JC, et al. Risk factors for post-traumatic stress disorder symptoms following critical illness requiring mechanical ventilation: a prospective cohort study. Crit Care 2007;11(1):R28.

[56] Kress JP, Gehlbach B, Lacy M, et al. The long-term psychological effects of daily sedative interruption on critically ill patients. Am J Respir Crit Care Med 2003;168(12):1457–61.

[57] Schelling G, Stoll C, Haller M, et al. Health-related quality of life and posttraumatic stress disorder in survivors of the acute respiratory distress syndrome. Crit Care Med 1998;26(4):651–9.

[58] Jones C, Griffiths RD, Humphris G, et al. Memory, delusions, and the development of acute posttraumatic stress disorder-related symptoms after intensive care. Crit Care Med 2001;29(3):573–80.

[59] Schelling G, Kilger E, Roozendaal B, et al. Stress doses of hydrocortisone, traumatic memories, and symptoms of posttraumatic stress disorder in patients after cardiac surgery: a randomized study. Biol Psychiatry 2004;55(6):627–33.

[60] Schelling G, Roozendaal B, Krauseneck T, et al. Efficacy of hydrocortisone in preventing posttraumatic stress disorder following critical illness and major surgery. Ann N Y Acad Sci 2006;1071:46–53.

[61] Weinert C, Meller W. Epidemiology of depression and antidepressant therapy after acute respiratory failure. Psychosomatics 2006;47(5):399–407.

[62] Jackson JC, Hart RP, Gordon SM, et al. Six-month neuropsychological outcome of medical intensive care unit patients. Crit Care Med 2003;31(4):1226–34.

[63] Jones C, Skirrow P, Griffiths RD, et al. Rehabilitation after critical illness: a randomized, controlled trial. Crit Care Med 2003;31(10):2456–61.

[64] American Thoracic Society. Idiopathic pulmonary fibrosis: diagnosis and treatment. International consensus statement. American Thoracic Society (ATS), and the European Respiratory Society (ERS). Am J Respir Crit Care Med 2000;161(2 Pt 1):646–64.

[65] Martinez TY, Pereira CA, dos Santos ML, et al. Evaluation of the short-form 36-item questionnaire to measure health-related quality of life in patients with idiopathic pulmonary fibrosis. Chest 2000;117(6):1627–32.

[66] De Vries J, Kessels BL, Drent M. Quality of life of idiopathic pulmonary fibrosis patients. Eur Respir J 2001;17(5):954–61.

[67] Tzanakis N, Samiou M, Lambiri I, et al. Evaluation of health-related quality-of-life and dyspnea scales in patients with idiopathic pulmonary fibrosis. Correlation with pulmonary function tests. Eur J Intern Med 2005;16(2):105–12.

[68] Bhandari S, Samellas D. Bipolar affective disorder and idiopathic pulmonary fibrosis. J Clin Psychiatry 2001;62(7):574–5.

[69] Cox CE, Donohue JF, Brown CD, et al. Health-related quality of life of persons with sarcoidosis. Chest 2004;125(3):997–1004.

[70] Chang B, Steimel J, Moller DR, et al. Depression in sarcoidosis. Am J Respir Crit Care Med 2001;163(2):329–34.

[71] Wirnsberger RM, de Vries J, Breteler MH, et al. Evaluation of quality of life in sarcoidosis patients. Respir Med 1998;92(5):750–6.

[72] Hoitsma E, Faber CG, Drent M, et al. Neurosarcoidosis: a clinical dilemma. Lancet Neurol 2004;3(7):397–407.

[73] Curtis JR, Borson S. Examining the link between sarcoidosis and depression. Am J Respir Crit Care Med 2001;163(2):306–8.

[74] Sabaawi M, Gutierrez-Nunez J, Fragala MR. Neurosarcoidosis presenting as schizophreniform disorder. Int J Psychiatry Med 1992;22(3):269–74.

[75] Kravitz H, Gomberg RM, Burnstine RC, et al. Psychogenic cough tic in children and adolescents. Nine case histories illustrate the need for re-evaluation of this common but frequently unrecognized problem. Clin Pediatr (Phila) 1969;8(10):580–3.

[76] Irwin RS, Glomb WB, Chang AB. Habit cough, tic cough, and psychogenic cough in adult and pediatric populations: ACCP evidence-based clinical practice guidelines. Chest 2006;129(Suppl 1):174S–9S.

[77] Powell C, Brazier A. Psychological approaches to the management of respiratory symptoms in children and adolescents. Paediatr Respir Rev 2004;5(3):214–24.

[78] Butani L, O'Connell EJ. Functional respiratory disorders. Ann Allergy Asthma Immunol 1997;79(2):91–9, quiz 99–101.

[79] Shuper A, Mukamel M, Mimouni M, et al. Psychogenic cough. Arch Dis Child 1983;58(9):745–7.

[80] Lavigne JV, Davis AT, Fauber R. Behavioral management of psychogenic cough: alternative to the "bedsheet" and other aversive techniques. Pediatrics 1991;87(4):532–7.

[81] Bahrainwala AH, Simon MR. Wheezing and vocal cord dysfunction mimicking asthma. Curr Opin Pulm Med 2001;7(1):8–13.

[82] Newman KB, Mason UG 3rd, Schmaling KB. Clinical features of vocal cord dysfunction. Am J Respir Crit Care Med 1995;152(4 Pt 1):1382–6.

[83] Doshi DR, Weinberger MM. Long-term outcome of vocal cord dysfunction. Ann Allergy Asthma Immunol 2006;96(6):794–9.

[84] Wood RP 2nd, Milgrom H. Vocal cord dysfunction. J Allergy Clin Immunol 1996;98(3):481–5.

[85] Christopher KL, Wood RP II, Eckert RC, et al. Vocal-cord dysfunction presenting as asthma. N Engl J Med 1983;308(26):1566–70.

[86] Kerr WJ, Dalton JW, Gliebe PA. Some physical phenomena associated with anxiety states and their relationship to hyperventilation. Ann Intern Med 1937;11:961–92.

[87] Brashear RE. Hyperventilation syndrome. Lung 1983;161(5):257–73.

[88] Niggemann B. Functional symptoms confused with allergic disorders in children and adolescents. Pediatr Allergy Immunol 2002;13(5):312–8.

[89] Wong KS, Huang YS, Huang YH, et al. Personality profiles and pulmonary function of children with sighing dyspnoea. J Paediatr Child Health 2007;43(4):280–3.

[90] Brown ES, Khan DA, Nejtek VA. The psychiatric side effects of corticosteroids. Ann Allergy Asthma Immunol 1999;83(6 Pt 1):495–503, quiz 503–4.

[91] Drug-induced convulsions. Report from Boston Collaborative Drug Surveillance Program. Lancet 1972;2(7779):677–9.

[92] Bender B, Milgrom H. Neuropsychiatric effects of medications for allergic diseases. J Allergy Clin Immunol 1995;95(2):523–8.

Psychiatr Clin N Am 30 (2007) 781–802

PSYCHIATRIC CLINICS
OF NORTH AMERICA

Psychiatric Aspects of Epilepsy

Michael J. Marcangelo, MD[a],*, Fred Ovsiew, MD[b]

[a]Department of Psychiatry and Behavioral Medicine, Medical College of Wisconsin,
8701 Watertown Plank, Milwaukee, WI 53226, USA
[b]Department of Psychiatry, MC 3077, University of Chicago Medical Center,
5841 S. Maryland Ave, Chicago, IL 60637, USA

Patients who have epilepsy frequently have psychiatric illnesses, but often their psychiatric symptoms are overlooked. Long-held beliefs about the psychosocial difficulties of having epilepsy led to low rates of psychiatric evaluation and treatment. Duirng the past 20 years, awareness of the importance of psychiatric illness in epilepsy has led to increased research attention and better treatment. These advances include an enhanced understanding of the link between psychiatric disorders and seizures and safer, more effective treatments. Some of these factors are reviewed here.

EPIDEMIOLOGY

Epilepsy has a prevalence estimated between 0.4% and 0.8%; a population-based study in Minnesota suggested a prevalence of 0.68% in 1980 [1]. In rural Ecuador, the prevalence of active epilepsy was measured as being between 0.67% and 0.80% [2]. Prevalence rises with age, probably because of the impact of cerebrovascular disease and head trauma on the development of new seizure disorders. Risk factors for the development of epilepsy in adults include a family history of epilepsy and a personal history of depression, mental retardation, head trauma, and brain tumor [3]. Among children and adolescents, a history of psychiatric disorder is a risk factor for the development of seizures [4]. The risks are highest among boys aged 6 to 12 years who have psychiatric diagnoses [4].

Psychiatric illness is an important predictor of health status in epilepsy. Patients who had psychiatric disorders scored 21% lower on the SF-36, a measure of overall physical and mental health with low scores indicating worse status, than did patients who had only epilepsy; posttraumatic stress disorder was the most disabling comorbid illness, followed by depression [5]. Quality-of-life ratings are consistently lower in patients who have higher levels of depression [6], regardless of the severity of their epilepsy [7].

*Corresponding author. E-mail address: mmarcang@mcw.edu (M.J. Marcangelo).

0193-953X/07/$ – see front matter
doi:10.1016/j.psc.2007.07.005 © 2007 Elsevier Inc. All rights reserved.

MOOD DISORDERS

Mood disorders are more common in patients who have epilepsy than in the general population. The lifetime prevalence of depression in the general population was estimated as 16.2% in the National Comorbidity Survey Replication [8], but in a different study the prevalence of depression was 32.6% in people who had been told they had epilepsy and 39.7% in people who had active epilepsy [9]. A United Kingdom–based population survey found a similar prevalence of depression (36.5%) in patients who had epilepsy [10]. Patients who were younger, female, and reported greater levels of disability were more likely to be depressed [10].

Although depression clearly is common in epilepsy, epilepsy also is more common in depression [11,12]. Depression itself may be a risk factor for epilepsy. A population-based study suggests that people who have depression develop epilepsy more often, but the authors note that this finding may result from comorbid substance abuse leading to new-onset seizures [13]. Alterations in neurotransmitter function, including changes in serotonin, norepinephrine, and dopamine, are common to both disorders [14] and may help explain the high comorbidity between the disorders. Other biologic factors that may contribute to this comorbidity include structural changes to the limbic system [15] and hypometabolism of the frontal lobe [16].

Risk factors for depression in epilepsy may differ from those in the general population. Complex partial epilepsy has been proposed as a risk factor for depression, and a recent analysis of epilepsy and depression confirmed that patients who had depression and epilepsy were more likely to have complex partial epilepsy than patients who were not depressed [17]. Postpartum depression may be more common in epilepsy; one recent pilot study found that 29% of epileptic women developed postpartum depression [18], a rate significantly higher than in the general population.

In spite of the high prevalence of depression in epilepsy, screening is not routine in neurology clinics. A complicating factor in diagnosing depression in epilepsy is that many depressed epileptic patients do not have classic major depression. In a study of 1339 patients who had epilepsy, 50% of those diagnosed as having depression had a diagnosis of "depression not otherwise specified" [19]. Based on ideas of Kraepelin, Blumer and colleagues [20] proposed a construct of "interictal dysphoric disorder," a type of depression specific to patients who have epilepsy. This syndrome features variable or labile dysphoric mood, irritability, and intermittent euphoria. Pain complaints, anergy, and insomnia also are seen. To the general psychiatrist the description is reminiscent of a bipolar mixed state. The proposal has met with some confirmation [21], but the existence of this syndrome and its specificity to epilepsy remain controversial [22,23]. Because standard screening tools for depression may prove inadequate in epilepsy, a brief screen for depression in epilepsy that can be administered rapidly has been developed (Box 1) [24]. Elevated scores had a specificity of 90% and a sensitivity of 81%; the positive predictive value was 0.62. Tools such as this may increase the detection and treatment of depression.

Box 1: Brief screen for depression in epilepsy

Everything is a struggle

Nothing I do is right

I feel guilty

I'd be better off dead

I feel frustrated

I have difficulty finding pleasure

Depression can be ictal, preictal, postictal, or interictal. Ictal depression refers to the mood change that results directly from a simple partial seizure. Symptoms include anhedonia, guilt, and suicidal ideation that last for only a short period [25]. Often, these seizures progress to complex partial seizures with disruption of consciousness. Patients may experience a decline in mood for 1 to 3 days before a seizure [25]. Among 13 patients who had a seizure during a 56-day period, 6 patients had significant decline in mood the day before seizing [26]. Mood ratings improved soon after the seizure. This finding suggests that some patients may experience mood change as a prodrome to seizure activity.

Postictal depression has been noted to occur in 43% of patients who have poorly controlled epilepsy [25]. Often, these patients had interictal depression that was exacerbated following a seizure. Patients who have episodic complaints of depression that resolves rapidly should be evaluated for seizures and treated if the evaluation is positive.

Interictal depression is the most common type of depression in people who have epilepsy [25]. As mentioned previously, epileptics' presentations of depression do seem to differ from those of the general population in some important ways. Their symptoms often are chronic but somewhat milder than in classic major depression and thus may be more consistent with a diagnosis of dysthymia or interictal dysphoric disorder.

Depression has been identified as a key risk factor for lower quality of life among patients who have epilepsy. A recent analysis of quality of life among patients who have epilepsy found depression to be the second most important factor in determining health-related quality of life and estimated that it accounted for 12% of the variance in quality of life among epileptics [27]. The only variable that was more predictive was seizure frequency. Fatigue also was found to be a significant factor [27].

In spite of the high prevalence of depression in epilepsy, few studies have looked at treatment. One double-blind placebo-controlled study has been published to date. Antidepressant treatment with amitriptyline or nomifensine (an agent not commercially available in the United States) was no better than placebo at 6 weeks [28]. Only after higher-than-usual doses were used did treatment show a benefit over placebo [28]. The evidence that pharmacotherapy for depression is successful for patients who have epilepsy thus is limited, but the consensus is that treatment is beneficial. Recognizing that depression is common in epileptics may have implications for choice of antiepileptic agents. Lamotrigine, in particular, may have antidepressant efficacy and thus represent a wise choice to avoid the need for a separate antidepressant agent [29]. Psychopharmacology and its relationship to epilepsy are discussed in detail later.

A new treatment for epilepsy, vagus nerve stimulation, also has been approved for the treatment of medication-resistant depression. Although an open-label trial of vagal nerve stimulation showed response rates of 44% at 1 year and 42% at 2 years [30], a randomized, controlled trial failed to show benefit [31]. In patients who have epilepsy, however, mood improvement after placement of vagal nerve stimulation has been demonstrated in a controlled trial with a response rate of 82% [32], suggesting that it may be a viable and effective treatment for patients who have comorbid depression and epilepsy.

Suicide and Epilepsy

Epilepsy has been linked to greatly increased rates of suicide [33]. Although the rate of suicide in the general population is approximately 1.1% to 1.2%, the rate in patients who have epilepsy seems to be about 11.5% [33]. The rate of suicide attempts in patients who have epilepsy was 20.8% in a multicenter study, and the rate of current suicidal ideation was 12.2% [33]. One case-control study found that all four patients who committed suicide in a cohort of 1611 had partial complex seizures with a temporal lobe focus [34], but other studies have been inconclusive in determining whether seizure type and focus relate to suicide risk [34]. Two of the patients who committed suicide did so during a period of increased seizure activity, but the other two had relatively good control at the time of suicide; both of these completed suicides had comorbid schizophrenia [34].

ANXIETY DISORDERS

Anxiety disorders have received less attention than mood disorders in epilepsy. Patients report fear with seizures, and up to 15% report fear as part of the aura [35]. Patients who have frequent seizures actually report lower levels of anxiety about seizures than do patients who are better controlled, perhaps because of conditioning [36]. Anxiety impacts quality of life for epilepsy patients independent of depression or seizure frequency [7].

PSYCHOTIC DISORDERS

Psychosis and epilepsy have a long and intertwined history. After a period in the early twentieth century when it was thought that epilepsy and psychosis could not coexist [37], Slater and Beard [38] proposed that the disorders coexist more frequently than by chance. Since then, the prevalence of psychosis in epilepsy has been estimated to be as high as 9% [39]. Risk factors for psychosis in epilepsy seem to include bitemporal seizure focus and clustering of seizures [40], but studies differ on the relationship between age of onset of seizures and risk of psychosis [39,40].

Although the prevalence of psychosis is elevated in epileptic patients, in a subset of those who have both disorders the manifestations of the two are antagonistic or reciprocal. That is, the patients have fewer seizures when psychotic; when the epilepsy is less well controlled, the psychotic disorder remits. This pattern is widely reported in the literature under the rubric of "false normalization," a term translated from a German term meant to describe the "overnormalization" or paradoxical normalization of the electroencephalograph (EEG) in longitudinally observed epileptic patients whose EEGs appeared more normal when they were psychotic than when they were not [41]. The phenomenon occasionally occurs with other psychopathology, such as depression. The term "alternative psychosis" has been used to refer to the clinical, as opposed to EEG, phenomenon.

Patients who have interictal psychosis characteristically develop delusions and hallucinations without thought disorder or marked personality deterioration in the context of a longstanding epileptic disorder. The features of epilepsy associated with such a course have been a disputed point. Most authorities believe that temporal lobe epilepsy (TLE) is the typical substrate, but the evidence may be inconclusive [42,43]. Some researchers believe that the link is even more specific, with left-sided epilepsy and in particular the presence of "alien tissue lesions" (such as hamartomas, vascular malformations, or tumors, as against the more typical epileptic substrate of mesial temporal sclerosis) predominating in the patients who develop a schizophrenia-like psychosis. The latter claim about histopathology, which originated in the early days of surgery for TLE, has not been widely supported [43]. Some patients develop psychosis after temporal lobectomy for seizure control, as discussed later.

Cognitive testing comparing patients who have schizophrenia and patients who have epilepsy and psychosis found no differences in overall neuropsychologic profiles [44]. Biologic mechanisms proposed for the relationship between psychosis and epilepsy include the possibility that kappa opioid receptor hyperactivation by dynorphin following seizures, an endogenous method for seizure control, may cause overstimulation and psychotic experiences [45].

Postictal psychosis develops in the immediate postictal period. Postictal psychosis and interictal psychosis may have similar mechanisms involving prolonged inhibition of limbic circuit; this mechanism probably is mediated through the neurotransmitter γ-aminobutyric acid (GABA) [46]. The length of time between the development of epilepsy and the onset of psychosis has been found to be greater for postictal psychosis than for chronic interictal psychosis [47]. Postictal psychosis often follows flurries of seizures, usually after a "lucid interval" of 24 to 48 hours, and tends to recur [48,49]. Postictal psychosis is self-limited, rarely lasting more than 2 weeks even when not treated with antipsychotic agents. When compared with other patients who had epilepsy, patients who had postictal psychoses were more likely to have generalized tonic-clonic seizures and bilateral discharges on EEG monitoring than those who did not develop psychosis [49]. They also were noted to have higher rates of prior psychiatric hospitalization than epileptic patients without psychosis [49]. Patients have fewer hallucinations and delusions but report aura and odd, mystical experiences more often than those that have chronic psychotic illnesses [49].

AGGRESSION

The relationship between aggression and epilepsy is complex and not well understood. In general, two types of aggression are seen in patients who have epilepsy. Some episodes of aggression are clearly linked to seizure activity and are best understood as peri-ictal phenomenon. Other aggressive acts seem to be unrelated to the timing of seizures and may be part of the patient's underlying character structure, caused by the socioeconomic circumstances that frequently arise in epilepsy or related to the brain abnormality that underlies the epilepsy itself.

A neuroanatomic network including amygdala and other limbic structures processes affectively charged events and is believed to mediate fear-based aggression [50,51]. Alterations in this network, including seizure activity, may lead to aggression. This possibility has led to increased focus on TLE and its relation to aggression.

Patients who have TLE are not consistently found to have increased aggression [52], but a subgroup of patients with aggression and TLE was found to have significant atrophy of the amygdala [53]. This study also found that aggression in epilepsy was associated with lower IQ scores and higher rates of anxiety and depression [53], raising the possibility that treatment of psychiatric disorders may decrease episodes of aggression. A study of patients at the Maudsley Hospital showed that patients who had aggression and epilepsy were less educated and were more likely to have a personality disorder than those who had epilepsy without aggression [54]. The authors conclude that a mix of biologic and social factors contributes to the development of aggression in epilepsy.

There are numerous reports of aggression linked to epileptic activity. One multicenter study identified 14 patients who had aggression associated with epilepsy [55]. They noted that to associate the violence with epilepsy, the patients should have an established diagnosis of epilepsy, a predictable pattern of aggressive behavior, and evidence from video monitoring of an association between EEG changes and aggressive behavior [55]. These criteria for diagnosing ictal violence are difficult to meet, if only because a rare incident of severe violence is unlikely to have been recorded in the video-EEG laboratory. As a clinical rule, peri-ictal aggressive behavior is poorly organized and not purposeful. In general, the violence is directed at those in the immediate vicinity in a nonspecific fashion during a period of confusion, often when the patient is restrained. Nonetheless, some cases have been recorded of severe violence, even homicide, that can be tentatively identified as peri-ictal although not meeting the criteria of Delgado-Escueta and colleagues [56]. Three cases of postictal aggression with onset shortly after the seizure and duration of 5 to 30 minutes recently were reported from Japan [57]. When examined in aggregate with other case reports [58,59], no consistent seizure focus could be located, although frequent cases of bilateral abnormalities were noted [58].

Although aggression may not be linked consistently with a particular type of epilepsy, it clearly does occur as a consequence of seizure activity in some patients. Evaluation for seizures is particularly indicated if the violence is episodic, seems random, and is brief in duration. In patients known to have epilepsy and violence, treatment of comorbid psychiatric disorders may decrease violent acts as well as treating depression or psychosis.

PERSONALITY IN EPILEPSY

Given the high level of psychosocial disability and the chronic, sometimes life-long, course associated with epilepsy, changes in personality among those who have epilepsy would seem almost inevitable. Physicians have been interested in questions about personality in epilepsy since at least the nineteenth century, and a number of changes have been reported in patients who have TLE (Box 2). Not all studies of patients who have TLE demonstrate personality changes, and other areas of the brain, such as the frontal lobe, probably play an important role as well [60].

A detailed description of a specific personality syndrome putatively related to TLE was provided by Waxman and Geschwind [61]. They suggested that increased religiosity or "cosmic" concerns, manifest by religious conversions or intense idiosyncratic beliefs, are more common in TLE [61]. The syndrome also featured excessive writing (hypergraphia), hyposexuality, "humorless sobriety," and a tendency to be preoccupied with detail and moral righteousness [61]. This claim of an interictal personality syndrome specific to TLE, now called the Geschwind-Gastaut syndrome, has been widely discussed and disputed [22,63].

Some studies have replicated the relationship between epilepsy and personality traits. Such traits as social "viscosity" (a tendency to prolong social encounters), humorlessness, and obsessionalism have been found to be more common in patients who have left TLE or generalized seizures than in those who have right-sided foci [62]. Others have found that personality traits

---

Box 2: Personality changes reported in epilepsy [61,62]

Hyperreligiosity

Viscosity

Hypergraphia

Circumstantiality

Aggression

Anger

Increased moral concerns

Decreased sexual interest

associated with TLE, such as increased religiosity, are associated with bilateral dysfunction [64]. Other studies have failed to find an association between TLE or laterality and psychopathology [65].

Changes in sexual behavior in epilepsy have been reported repeatedly. Decreased frequency of sexual intercourse, moral repugnance toward masturbation, and a high rate (44%) of self-reporting of never having had an orgasm were found among 97 men who had epilepsy [66]. Some of the antiepileptic drugs (AEDs), including phenytoin and carbamazepine, may impede sexual function in patients who have epilepsy [67]. In addition, abnormalities of sex hormones, in particular polycystic ovary syndrome in women, have been associated with epilepsy and its treatment [68]. Social factors, including stigma, may lead to reduced sexual interest and activity. More specific biologic factors also have been postulated [69]. For example, the rise in prolactin following generalized and some partial complex seizures may play a role in sexual dysfunction in epilepsy.

Personality disorder can develop in patients who have forms of epilepsy other than TLE. A number of recent studies have investigated juvenile myoclonic epilepsy, which is a form of generalized epilepsy [70–72]. A high rate of psychiatric symptoms, and of personality disorders in particular, may reflect the frontal pathology known in this epileptic syndrome. Taken as a whole, it is likely that there is some relationship between epilepsy and personality traits, but heterogeneity of diagnostic groups (TLE in particular), difficulties with assessment, and case-report bias make exact correlation difficult.

ATTENTION AND IMPULSIVITY

Disorders of attention, including attention-deficit hyperactivity disorder (ADHD), have long been noted in both children and adults who have epilepsy. A review of the subject found an estimated prevalence of ADHD among children who had epilepsy of 14% [73]. Children who have comorbid epilepsy and ADHD have lower IQ scores than the general population and also function at a lower level than their IQ scores (when > 80) would predict [74]. Comorbid psychiatric disorders, including depression, anxiety, and oppositional defiant disorder, are common, but their frequency is similar to that seen in children who have ADHD but not epilepsy [74].

Alteration in attention may be caused by subtle changes in brain activity, particularly 3-Hz spike-and-wave discharges [73]. Treatment with AEDs has been shown to improve attention in children [75], suggesting that the disturbance in attention is related in part to seizure activity. Early onset of seizures is associated with greater impairment of attention [76], and poor control of epilepsy, particularly during sleep, also may contribute to poor attention [75]. Treatment with methylphenidate is thought to be safe in epilepsy and has been demonstrated to be effective for ADHD in adults who have epilepsy [77].

Children who have ADHD have a higher rate of abnormalities on EEG, particularly increased theta and decreased alpha waves, than controls [78]. Patients who have ADHD are two and a half times more likely to develop epilepsy than patients who do not have ADHD [79], although the increase in risk was limited to children who had the inattentive subtype of ADHD. Alterations in the noradrenergic system have been proposed as a common underlying pathway, because both children who have ADHD and rats genetically designed to be prone to epilepsy have decreased levels of norepinephrine [79].

ANTIEPILEPTIC MEDICATIONS

The majority of patients who have epilepsy are treated with AEDs to control their seizures. These medications have psychotropic effects that must be considered when evaluating patients who have epilepsy. Many of the AEDs are used in psychiatry as mood stabilizers, but other effects of the medications are less well understood. The following is a review of the psychotropic effects of commonly used AEDs (Table 1) [80–83].

Barbiturates

Barbiturates, including phenobarbital, were the standard treatment for generalized seizures before the introduction of other AEDs. They are well known to cause sedation in many patients and a syndrome of hyperactivity, irritability,

Table 1
Common antiepileptic drugs

Antiepileptic Drug	P-450 system	Psychotropic effects	Side effects
Phenytoin	Induces CYP1A2 and 3A4 Metabolized by 2C9/2C10	Possible mood stabilizer	Sedation, psychosis, encephalopathy
Carbamazepine	Induces CYP3A4 Metabolized by CYP3A4 (auto-inducer)	Antimanic agent Possible benefit for impulsive aggression	Sedation, aplastic anemia
Valproate	Inhibits CYP2C enzymes Metabolized by CYP2C19	Antimanic agent Maintenance of bipolar disorder	Sedation, weight gain
Lamotrigine	Metabolized by glucuronidation 1A4	Mood stabilizer	Rash
Topiramate	Induces CYP3A4 inhibits CYP2C enzymes	Possible mood stabilizer	Cognitive slowing, decreased verbal fluency, aggression, psychosis, depression
Levetiracetam	No extensive hepatic metabolism	No current uses	Aggression, affective disorders, psychosis

Data from Refs. [80–83].

and aggression in young and elderly patients [81]. They have been linked to worsening depression and suicidal ideation in patients who have a family history of depression [82]. Because of the availability of other options and the possibly severe psychiatric side effects of barbiturates, other agents should be used, particularly in patients who have epilepsy and a personal or family history of a mood disorder.

Phenytoin

Phenytoin is a common AED that has been in use since the 1950s. A large volume of literature suggests that it has a number of adverse effects, including sedation [81], psychosis [83], and encephalopathy [82]. It has been studied in bipolar disorder and found to be superior to placebo when used with haloperidol [84], although other studies suggest that it is comparable to placebo [85]. Because of its lack of patent protection, further studies of phenytoin are unlikely to receive industry support. Current information suggests that phenytoin may cause some degree of depression in epileptics but may be useful for patients who have comorbid bipolar disorder and epilepsy [83].

Benzodiazepines

The benzodiazepines typically are used to control acute seizures and generally are not used for long-term seizure prevention. They are used widely as anxiolytics in psychiatry but may contribute to sedation and lead to dependence. Paradoxical reactions can occur in which patients become aggressive, irritable, and hyperactive [81]. The medications must be tapered slowly when discontinued, because rapid withdrawal at times can lead to exacerbation of seizures or even coma [81]. There also have been reports of patients developing catatonia following the rapid withdrawal of high-dose benzodiazepine therapy [86].

Carbamazepine

A standard treatment for TLE, carbamazepine was discovered to have mood-stabilizing effects more than 25 years ago [87]; recently, the long-acting form was approved for the treatment of acute mania. Head-to-head comparison with lithium has been unfavorable, however [88], and its use in bipolar disorder has declined with the introduction of newer agents. It has been proposed as an effective treatment for aggression [89], particularly in patients who have a history of traumatic brain injury, but a recent meta-analysis found a lack of data supporting this claim [90]. Behavioral side effects reported in some studies include psychosis and depression [83], but the majority of studies suggest that it only rarely causes adverse behavioral effects [82]. There is limited evidence that it is an effective antidepressant [81], but it does have antimanic properties.

Valproate

Valproate is an AED used for partial and complex seizures as well as absence seizures. It also is used widely as a treatment for mania in bipolar disorder. It is believed to act through effects on the GABA system, but there is evidence that it also works by modulating sodium and calcium channels [82]. It also may play a role in the control of agitation, but one study suggests that it may be effective only in patients who have cluster B personality disorders [91]. It is not associated with common adverse behavioral side effects. Valproate has well-established antimanic properties and is a first-line agent for patients who have comorbid epilepsy and bipolar disorder.

Lamotrigine

Lamotrigine is used for partial and generalized tonic-clonic seizures and has a mechanism of action similar to that of carbamazepine [83]. It has been approved as a maintenance treatment for bipolar disorder with a particular emphasis on its role in preventing depression [82]. In patients who have epilepsy, it has been shown to be superior to valproate in improving depressive symptoms [92]. It has not been found to have significant cognitive side effects in healthy adults [93] and has performed better than carbamazepine, diazepam, and phenytoin in head-to-head comparisons of adverse cognitive effects [94]. The most concerning side effect is the development of a Stevens-Johnson-like rash. This rash occurs more frequently in children, and the medication generally is avoided in patients younger than 16 years. Among the newer AEDs, lamotrigine has the strongest evidence for being effective for mood disorders in patients with or without epilepsy.

Topiramate

Topiramate is a newer AED that has the advantage of broad-spectrum antiseizure properties and an ability to promote weight loss [95]. Numerous reports have linked it to cognitive dysfunction that includes slowing, a decline in verbal fluency, and anomia [93,94,96]. Psychiatric side effects, including irritability, aggression, and depression, have been observed in 12.6% of patients using topiramate for epilepsy [96]. It also has been linked to aggression, psychosis, and cognitive impairment in children and adolescents [97]. It has not been established as an effective treatment for bipolar disorder [98]. Given the risk of behavioral side effects, topiramate should be used with caution in epileptic patients who have comorbid psychiatric disorders.

Levetiracetam

Levetiracetam is a relatively new AED that is indicated for adjunctive treatment of partial epilepsy and generalized tonic-clonic seizures in both children and adults. It has not been approved as a stand-alone agent by the Food and Drug Administration. It is generally well tolerated, but reports of adverse psychiatric events, including mood disorders, psychosis, and aggression, have emerged [99]. These effects were more common in patients who had a history of psychiatric illness. In a study of pediatric patients who had epilepsy, 10.5% developed aggression while taking levetiracetam [100]. There is limited evidence from an open-label study of efficacy in bipolar disorder, but further study is needed [82]. Given the risks associated with levetiracetam, patients who have comorbid psychiatric illnesses should be monitored closely while taking the medication or, if possible, switched to another AED associated with lower rates of behavioral side effects.

Other New Antiepileptic Drugs

New agents, such as gabapentin, oxcarbazepine, pregabalin, tiagabine, vigabatrin, and zonisamide, have been tested in psychiatric disorders, primarily bipolar disorder, with mixed results. Gabapentin actually was found to be less effective than placebo for bipolar disorder [101] after early reports suggested efficacy. Many of these agents have been tested only in open trials. A study of oxcarbazepine, a derivative of carbamazepine, found that it improved the mood of 70% of the patients who had comorbid dysthymia [102]. Zonisamide has been linked to new-onset psychosis in case reports [82]. Overall, it is difficult to recommend any of these agents for comorbid psychiatric illness, but further study may reveal that some of them have roles to play in the treatment of patients who have epilepsy and psychiatric disorders.

Summary of Antiepileptic Drugs

Patients who have epilepsy can expect to undergo long-term AED treatment and to experience both benefits and side effects from the medication. Recently, an examination of quality of life while taking AEDs found that patients taking lamotrigine and carbamazepine had the best mood outcomes; those taking medications that modulate the GABA system (topiramate, tiagabine, vigabatrin) had the most adverse mood effects [103]. The authors concluded that medications that modulate sodium channels may have a positive effect on the limbic system that combats both epilepsy and mood disorders [103].

OTHER PSYCHOTROPICS IN EPILEPSY

Given the high rates of psychiatric disorders in epilepsy, many other psychotropics are used in epileptic patients. Many of these agents may interact with AEDs or change the seizure threshold (Table 2). Many of the newer psychotropics have proven to be relatively safe for use in epilepsy and have opened the door to safer treatment for epileptic patients. A brief review of psychotropics and their safety in epilepsy follows.

Patients who have epilepsy often require treatment with antidepressants. Before the widespread introduction of selective serotonin reuptake inhibitors (SSRIs), the estimated risk of seizures while taking antidepressants was 0.1% to 4.0% [104]. Risk is higher for patients who have a history of head trauma or cerebrovascular accident [104]. Certain medications, including clomipramine, bupropion, and maprotiline, were noted to be linked to a higher risk of seizures [104]. Bupropion was found to have a dose-dependent risk of seizure with the highest risk found at doses at or above 600 mg/d [105]. Treatment at lower doses yielded a seizure rate of 0.36%, in line with that seen with other antidepressants [105]. Maprotiline, a tetracyclic antidepressant, was found to have a seizure incidence of 0.4% in the first 6 weeks of treatment [106]. Clomipramine led to new-onset seizures in 1.66% of patients taking doses above 250 mg/d; the cumulative incidence annually for all patients taking the drug was 1.34% [104]. In what is probably the largest population-based study, treatment with other tricyclic antidepressants at normal doses led to seizures in

Table 2
Psychotropic agents and their effects on seizure threshold

Medication	Effect on seizure threshold
Bupropion	Lowers seizure threshold at high doses with immediate-release formulation; less effect at lower doses and with sustained and extended release
Chlorpromazine	Lowers seizure threshold, particularly at higher doses
Clomipramine	Lowers seizure threshold, particularly at higher doses
Clozapine	Lowers seizure threshold, particularly at higher doses
Fluoxetine	May raise seizure threshold
Haloperidol	Seems to have minimal effect
Imipramine	Safe at therapeutic doses; increased risk at high doses or in patients who have a history of epilepsy
Maprotiline	Lowers seizure threshold, particularly at higher doses
Mirtazepine	Seems to raise seizure threshold
Paroxetine	Seems to raise seizure threshold
Risperidone	Seems to have minimal effect
Sertraline	Unknown, but very rare reports of seizures even in overdose
Venlafaxine	May lower threshold in overdose

Data from Mula M, Trimble MR. Pharmacokinetic interactions between antiepileptic and antidepressant drugs. World J Biol Psychiatry 2003;4(1):21–4.

0.1% of patients [107]. Studies repeatedly noted that rates were higher for patients who had predisposing factors toward seizures, one of which, of course, is a history of epilepsy [104]. These medications should be avoided in patients who have epilepsy unless they have an established period of adequate seizure control.

The introduction of the SSRIs has led to greater use of antidepressants in general. For patients who have epilepsy, SSRIs seem to be less likely to lower the seizure threshold. Citalopram has been shown to improve depressive symptoms while having no obvious effect on seizure frequency in patients who have epilepsy [108]. Twenty-eight percent of patients had a reduction in seizure frequency of 50% or more during the 4-month trial [108]. Given the possible neurobiologic link between seizures and depression mediated by serotonin [14], this change is notable. This effect also has been noted with fluoxetine [109]. Fluoxetine and sertraline seem to be similarly safe in children and adolescents with seizures [110]. A recent review of clinical trial data concluded that the SSRIs and other newer antidepressants, other than bupropion, are anticonvulsant [111]. Given the alteration in AED levels that other SSRIs may induce, citalopram, sertraline, and escitalopram are excellent choices for patients who have comorbid epilepsy and depression.

Antipsychotic medications are known to be riskier in patients who have epilepsy. Treatment with chlorpromazine led to seizures in 1.2% of all patients and in 9% in those taking high doses [112]. The introduction of clozapine led to new treatment options for chronic mental illness, but unfortunately clozapine also was associated with a high risk of seizures. The risk of seizures was

1.3% after 6 months of treatment [113] and was estimated to be 10% after 3.8 years of treatment [114]. Rapid dose titration and high doses are associated with increased risk of seizures [114]. A prior diagnosis of a seizure disorder also contributed to the risk [113]. Valproate generally is effective for the treatment of clozapine-induced seizures [114]. The clinical trial review referred to previously found that, along with clozapine, olanzapine and quetiapine risked evoking seizures [111]. Haloperidol, a typical antipsychotic, and risperidone, an atypical antipsychotic, generally are thought to be safer in regards to the seizure threshold [115].

As mentioned previously, psychostimulants seem to be safe in children who have epilepsy and ADHD. A study of 119 children who had epilepsy or EEG abnormalities demonstrated EEG improvement and no worsening of seizures [116], and similar results have been seen in adults [77].

EPILEPSY SURGERY

Surgery for intractable TLE has become more common as techniques have improved. Patients generally have a portion of the anterior temporal lobe removed; in one series, 58% of patients experienced a remission of seizures [117]. These patients also experienced a significant improvement in quality of life when compared with those who had medical management [117]. Patients often have high rates of psychiatric comorbidity before surgery and should undergo psychiatric evaluations before surgery; unfortunately, only 20% of epilepsy surgery centers report a presurgical evaluation for every patient [118]. A presurgical evaluation should include screening for depression and psychosis as well as recommendations for treatment both before and after surgery.

Before undergoing surgery, patients have high rates of psychiatric disorders. One study found 65% of patients had an axis I diagnosis before and after surgery [119]. These diagnoses included mood disorders, anxiety disorders, and organic mood and personality disorders [118]. Patients had a transient increase in symptoms after surgery, and many patients had new onset of psychiatric disorders, but overall the group was less symptomatic 6 months after surgery [119]. There are reports of psychosis after epilepsy surgery that may be related to preoperative bilateral lesions [120,121]. One group suggested a risk of postoperative psychosis specifically associated with removal of a ganglioglioma or dysembryoplastic neuroepithelioma [122]. New symptoms of depression and anxiety arose 6 weeks after surgery in half of the patients who were psychiatrically well at the presurgical evaluation, but overall symptoms declined over a longer period [123]. In one cohort of epilepsy surgery patients, postoperative mania occurred with surprising frequency, given the general rarity of mania in epilepsy, and was associated with right-sided temporal lobectomy [124]. Mania was more likely in patients who had pre-existing abnormalities in the hemisphere contralateral to the resection. These findings emphasize that patients need to be managed actively for both existing psychiatric disorders and for new-onset symptoms in the first weeks and months following surgery. In the long run, most studies seem to point to an overall improvement for patients after surgery in regards to both seizure frequency and quality of life [125].

NONEPILEPTIC SEIZURES

Psychogenic nonepileptic seizures (PNES), sometimes referred to as "pseudo-seizures," are seizure-like behavioral events that occur in the absence of abnormal electrical discharge in the brain [126]. The reference standard of diagnosis is video-EEG monitoring [127]. Diagnosis of PNES can be complicated by comorbid epilepsy: 30% to 50% of patients who have PNES have epilepsy [128], and 20% to 60% of patients who have epilepsy have PNES [129]. A number of factors suggest PNES (Table 3).

The prevalence of PNES has been estimated at 2 to 33 per 100,000, making it a rare disorder [130]. A well-designed retrospective analysis found the incidence over 4 years to be 3.03 per 100,000 [131]. The average age of onset is between 20 and 30 years [126,132], and it is three times more common in women [126,131]. A number of psychiatric diagnoses have been associated with the development of PNES. Conversion disorder is the most common; in one series 71 of 92 consecutive admissions for PNES were found to have conversion disorder as the psychiatric diagnosis [133]. Other diagnoses included anxiety disorders, psychotic disorders, and ADHD [130]. In patients who had diagnoses other than conversion disorder, the ratio of men to women was about equal, and there was a significantly lower rate of self-reported physical or sexual abuse during childhood [130]. Patients who have pure PNES are more likely to have posttraumatic stress disorder and dissociative disorders than patients who have comorbid epilepsy [127].

The outcome of PNES is difficult to track, because patients often drop out of treatment after receiving the diagnosis. A series of 56 patients followed by telephone interview after 18 months provides a snapshot of patient outcomes [133]. Episodes resolved in 51.8% of patients, but 53.6% required rehospitalization after the initial event [133]. Depression (51.8%) and suicide attempts (19.6%) were common [133]. Patients who accepted the diagnosis were more likely to

Table 3		
Features of psychogenic nonepileptic seizures		
Factor	Epilepsy	Psychogenic nonepileptic seizures
Abnormal, asynchronous movement	Rare	Frequent
Convulsion lasting > 2 minutes	Rare	Frequent
Tongue-biting, side	Common	Rare
Early onset (< 10 years)	Common	Rare
Postictal state	Common	Rare
Physical and sexual abuse	Rare	Common

Data from Reuber M, Elger CE. Psychogenic nonepileptic seizures: review and update. Epilepsy Behav 2003;4(3):205–16; Cragar DE, Berry DTR, Fakoury TA, et al. A review of diagnostic techniques in the differential diagnosis of epileptic and nonepileptic seizures. Neuropsychol Rev 2002;12(1):31–64.

remit, but anger about the diagnosis did not predict chronicity [133]. Among patients who did not remit, none were employed 18 months later [133]. This finding suggests that patients who have PNES have high rates of severe psychiatric illness, psychosocial impairment, and chronic illness.

PNES often are linked to a history of sexual abuse. Estimates of the prevalence of a history of sexual abuse in PNES range from 27% to 77% [133–135]. Patients who have a history of chronic abuse have been found to have worse outcomes [136]. Still, no clear causative role can be proven for abuse, and alternative explanatory models have been proposed, based on skepticism about the high rates reported in the literature [137].

Treatment for PNES is aimed at assisting the patient who has comorbid psychiatric illness and improving insight into the illness. The presentation of the diagnosis is an important part of treatment [138]. Providing a positive explanation about the illness and explaining the diagnosis is recommended [138]. Offering ongoing psychiatric care is appropriate to convey to patients that they will not be abandoned. Although limited data about pharmacotherapy are available, rational treatment with SSRIs targeting depressive and anxious symptoms may be warranted [138]. Cognitive behavioral therapy has met with success in a pilot study [139], but further studies are needed. Other treatments, including supportive therapy and psychodynamic therapy, have been proposed, but almost no data have been published [140].

SUMMARY

Patients who have epilepsy face many challenges resulting from their illness and have frequent psychiatric comorbidities. Recognition of these disorders is increasing and is having a positive impact on patients' quality of life. Recent recommendations about a new classification system for psychiatric disorders related specifically to epilepsy and based on the relationship of symptoms to seizures, antiepileptic medications, and EEG changes should further research and treatment [141]. Especially insofar psychiatric syndromes specific to epilepsy can be identified, correlation of clinical phenomena with relatively well-understood pathophysiology in epilepsy will allow advances in the understanding of psychiatric illness. This progress should move the treatment of patients who have epilepsy toward a comprehensive biopsychosocial model that focuses on the whole person rather than simply on the disease process.

References

[1] Hauser WA, Annegers JF, Kurland LT. Prevalence of epilepsy in Rochester, Minnesota: 1940-1980. Epilepsia 1991;32(4):429–45.

[2] Placencia M, Sander JWAS, Roman M, et al. The characteristics of epilepsy in a largely untreated population in rural Ecuador. J Neurol Neurosurg Psychiatry 1994;57(3):320–5.

[3] Forsgren L, Nystrom L. An incident case-referent study of epileptic seizures in adults. Epilepsy Res 1990;6(1):66–81.

[4] McAfee AT, Chilcott KE, Johannes CB, et al. The incidence of first provoked and unprovoked seizure in pediatric patients with and without psychiatric diagnoses. Epilepsia 2007;48(6):1075–82.

[5] Zeber JE, Copeland LA, Amuan M, et al. The role of comorbid psychiatric conditions in health status in epilepsy. Epilepsy Behav 2007;10(4):539–46.

[6] Hermann BP, Jones JE. Intractable epilepsy and patterns of psychiatric comorbidity. Adv Neurol 2006;97:367–74.

[7] Johnson EK, Jones JE, Seidenberg M, et al. The relative impact of anxiety, depression, and clinical seizure features on health-related quality of life in epilepsy. Epilepsia 2004;45(5): 544–50.

[8] Kessler RC, Berglund P, Demler O, et al. The epidemiology of major depressive disorder: results from the National Comorbidity Study Replication (NCS-R). JAMA 2003;289(23): 3095–105.

[9] Kobau R, Gilliam F, Thurman DJ. Prevalence of self-reported epilepsy or seizure disorder and its associations with self-reported depression and anxiety: results from the 2004 Heathstyles Survey. Epilepsia 2006;47(11):1915–21.

[10] Ettinger A, Reed M, Cramer J. Depression and comorbidity in community-based patients with epilepsy or asthma. Neurology 2004;63(6):1008–14.

[11] Hesdorffer DC, Hauser WA, Annegers JF, et al. Major depression is a risk factor for seizures in older adults. Ann Neurol 2000;47(2):246–9.

[12] Hesdorffer DC, Hauser WA, Olafsson E, et al. Depression and suicidae attempt as risk factors for incident unprovoked seizures. Ann Neurol 2006;59(1):35–41.

[13] Nilsson FM, Kessing LV, Bolwig TG. On the increased risk of developing late-onset epilepsy for patients with major affective disorder. J Affect Disord 2003;76(1–3):39–48.

[14] Jobe PC, Dailey JW, Wernicke JF. A noradrenergic and serotonergic hypothesis of the linkage between epilepsy and affective disorders. Crit Rev Neurobiol 1999;13(4): 317–56.

[15] Briellmann RS, Hopwood MJ, Jackson GD. Major depression in temporal lobe epilepsy with hippocampal sclerosis: clinical and imaging correlates. J Neurol Neurosurg Psychiatry 2007 Jan 26; [Epub ahead of print].

[16] Bromfield EB, Altshuler L, Leideran DB, et al. Cerebral metabolism and depression in patients with complex partial seizures. Arch Neurol 1992;49(6):617–23.

[17] Grabowska-Grzyb A, Jedrzejczak J, Naganska E, et al. Risk factors for depression in patients with epilepsy. Epilepsy Behav 2006;8(2):411–7.

[18] Turner K, Piazzini A, Franza A, et al. Postpartum depression in women with epilepsy versus women without epilepsy. Epilepsy Behav 2006;9(2):293–7.

[19] Mendez MF, Doss RC, Taylor JL, et al. Depression in epilepsy: relationship to seizures and anticonvulsant therapy. J Nerv Ment Dis 1993;181(7):444–7.

[20] Blumer D, Montouris G, Davies K. The interictal dysphoric disorder: recognition, pathogenesis, and treatment of the major psychiatric disorder of epilepsy. Epilepsy Behav 2004;5(6):836–40.

[21] Kanner AM, Kozak AM, Frey M. The use of sertraline in patients with epilepsy: is it safe? Epilepsy Behav 2000;1(2):100–5.

[22] Swinkels WA, Kuyk J, van Dyck R, et al. Psychiatric comorbidity in epilepsy. Epilepsy Behav 2005;7(1):37–50.

[23] Schmitz B. Depression and mania in patients with epilepsy. Epilepsia 2005;46(Suppl 4): 45–9.

[24] Gilliam FG, Barry JJ, Hermann BP, et al. Rapid detection of major depression in epilepsy: a multicentre study. Lancet Neurol 2006;5(5):399–405.

[25] Kanner AM. Depression in epilepsy: prevalence, clinical semiology, pathogenic mechanisms, and treatment. Biol Psychiatry 2003;54(3):388–98.

[26] Blanchet P, Frommer GP. Mood change preceding epileptic seizures. J Nerv Ment Dis 1986;174(8):471–6.

[27] Senol V, Soyuer F, Arman F, et al. Influence of fatigue, depression, and demographic, socioeconomic, and clinical variable on quality of life of patients with epilepsy. Epilepsy Behav 2007;10(1):96–104.

[28] Robertson MM, Trimble MR. The treatment of depression in patients with epilepsy: a double-blind trial. J Affect Disord 1985;9(2):127–36.

[29] Fakhoury TA, Barry JJ, Mitchell Miller J, et al. Lamotrigine in patients with epilepsy and comorbid depressive symptoms. Epilepsy Behav 2007;10(1):155–62.

[30] Nahas Z, Marangell LB, Husain MM, et al. Two-year outcome of vagus nerve stimulation (VNS) for treatment of major depressive episodes. J Clin Psychiatry 2005;66(9):1097–104.

[31] Rush AJ, Marangell LB, Sackeim HA, et al. Vagus nerve stimulation for treatment-resistant depression: a randomized, controlled acute phase trial. Biol Psychiatry 2005;58(5):347–54.

[32] Elger G, Hoppe C, Falkai P, et al. Vagus nerve stimulation is associated with mood improvements in epilepsy patients. Epilepsy Res 2000;42(2–3):203–10.

[33] Jones JA, Hermann BP, Barry JJ, et al. Rates and risk factors for suicide, suicidal ideation, and suicide attempts in chronic epilepsy. Epilepsy Behav 2003;4(Suppl 3):S31–8.

[34] Mendez MF, Doss RC. Ictal and psychiatric aspects of suicide in epileptic patients. Int J Psychiatry Med 1992;22(3):213–37.

[35] Torta R, Keller R. Behavioral, psychotic, and anxiety disorders in epilepsy: etiology, clinical features, and therapeutic implications. Epilepsia 1999;40(Suppl 10):S2–20.

[36] Goldstein MA, Harden CL, Ravdin LD, et al. Does anxiety in epilepsy patients decrease with increasing seizure frequency? Epilepsia 1999;40(Suppl 7):S60–1.

[37] Krishnamoorthy ES, Reghu R. The psychoses of epilepsy. In: Ettinger AB, Kanner AM, editors. Psychiatric issues in epilepsy: a practical guide to diagnosis and treatment. 2nd edition. Philadelphia: Lippincott Williams & Wilkins; 2007. p. 264–71.

[38] Slater E, Beard AW. The schizophrenia-like psychoses of epilepsy I. Psychiatric aspects. Br J Psychiatry 1963;109:95–150.

[39] Mendez MF, Grau R, Doss RC, et al. Schizophrenia in epilepsy: seizure and psychosis variables. Neurology 1993;43(6):1073–7.

[40] Umbricht D, Degreef G, Barr WB, et al. Postictal and chronic psychoses in patients with temporal lobe epilepsy. Am J Psychiatry 1995;152(2):224–31.

[41] Krishnamoorthy ES, Trimble MR. Forced normalization: clinical and therapeutic relevance. Epilepsia 1999;40(Suppl 10):S57–64.

[42] Trimble MR. The psychoses of epilepsy. New York: Raven Press; 1991.

[43] Kanemoto K, Tsuji T, Kawasaki J. Reexamination of interictal psychoses based on DSM IV psychosis classification and international epilepsy classification. Epilepsia 2001;42(1):98–103.

[44] Nathaniel-James DA, Brown RG, Maier M, et al. Cognitive abnormalities in schizophrenia and schizophrenia-like psychosis of epilepsy. J Neuropsychiatry Clin Neurosci 2004;16(4):472–9.

[45] Bortolato M, Solbrig MV. The price of seizure control: dynorphins in interictal and postictal psychosis. Psychiatry Res 2007;151(1–2):139–43.

[46] Sachdev PS. Alternating and postictal psychoses: review and a unifying hypothesis. Schizophr Bull 2007;33(4):1029–37.

[47] Kanemoto K, Kawasaki J, Kawai I. Postictal psychosis: a comparison with acute interictal and chronic psychoses. Epilepsia 1996;37(6):551–6.

[48] Logsdail SJ, Toone BK. Post-ictal psychoses. A clinical and phenomenological description. Br J Psychiatry 1988;152:246–52.

[49] Devinsky O, Abramson H, Alper K, et al. Postictal psychosis: a case control series of 20 patients and 150 controls. Epilepsy Res 1995;20(3):247–53.

[50] Charney DS, Deutch A. A functional neuroanatomy of anxiety and fear: implications for the pathophysiology and treatment of anxiety disorders. Crit Rev Neurobiol 1996;10(3–4):419–46.

[51] Gallagher M, Chiba AA. The amygdala and emotion. Curr Opin Neurobiol 1996;6(2):221–7.

[52] Kligman D, Goldberg DA. Temporal lobe epilepsy and aggression. J Nerv Ment Dis 1975;160(5):324–41.

[53] Tebartz van Elst L, Woermann FG, Lemieux L, et al. Affective aggression in patients with temporal lobe epilepsy: a quantitative MRI study of the amygdala. Brain 2000;123(Pt 2): 234–43.

[54] Herzberg JL, Fenwick PBC. The aetiology of aggression in temporal-lobe epilepsy. Br J Psychiatry 1988;153:50–5.

[55] Delgado-Escueta AV, Mattson RH, King L, et al. Special report. The nature of aggression during epileptic seizures. N Engl J Med 1981;305(12):711–6.

[56] Fenwick P. The nature and management of aggression in epilepsy. J Neuropsychiatry Clin Neurosci 1989;1(4):418–25.

[57] Ito M, Okazaki M, Takahashi S, et al. Subacute postictal aggression in patients with epilepsy. Epilepsy Behav 2007;10(4):611–4.

[58] Gerard ME, Spitz MC, Towbin JA, et al. Subacute postictal aggression. Neurology 1998;50(2):384–8.

[59] Yankovsky AE, Veilleux M, Dubeau F, et al. Post-ictal rage and aggression: a video-EEG study. Epileptic Disord 2005;7(2):143–7.

[60] Devinsky O, Vasquez B. Behavioral changes associated with epilepsy. Neurol Clin 1993;11(1):127–49.

[61] Waxman SG, Geschwind N. The interictal behavior syndrome of temporal lobe epilepsy. Arch Gen Psychiatry 1975;32(12):1580–6.

[62] Brandt J, Seidman LJ, Kohl D. Personality characteristics of epileptic patients: a controlled study of generalized and temporal lobe cases. J Clin Exp Neuropsychol 1985;7(1): 25–38.

[63] Bear D, Hermann B, Fogel B. Interictal behavior syndrome in temporal lobe epilepsy: the views of three experts. J Neuropsychiatry Clin Neurosci 1989;1(3):308–18.

[64] Trimble M, Freeman A. An investigation of religiosity and the Gastaut-Geschwind syndrome in patients with temporal lobe epilepsy. Epilepsy Behav 2006;9(3):407–14.

[65] Swinkels WA, van Emde Boas W, Kuyk J, et al. Interictal depression, anxiety, personality traits, and psychological dissociation in patients with temporal lobe epilepsy (TLE) and extra-TLE. Epilepsia 2006;47(12):2092–103.

[66] Fenwick PBC, Toone BK, Wheller MJ, et al. Sexual behaviors in a centre for epilepsy. Acta Neurol Scand 1985;71(6):428–35.

[67] Herzog AG, Drislane FW, Schomer DL, et al. Differential effects of antiepileptic drugs on sexual function and hormones in men with epilepsy. Neurology 2005;65(7):1016–20.

[68] Herzog AG, Fowler KM. Sexual hormones and epilepsy: threat and opportunities. Curr Opin Neurol 2005;18(2):167–72.

[69] Herzog AG. A relationship between particular reproductive endocrine disorders and the laterality of epileptiform discharges in women with epilepsy. Neurology 1993;43(10): 1907–10.

[70] de Araujo Filho GM, Pascalicchio TF, Sousa Pda S, et al. Psychiatric disorders in juvenile myoclonic epilepsy: a controlled study of 100 patients. Epilepsy Behav 2007;10(3): 437–41.

[71] Plattner B, Pahs G, Kindler J, et al. Juvenile myoclonic epilepsy: a benign disorder? Personality traits and psychiatric symptoms. Epilepsy Behav 2007;10(4):560–4.

[72] Trinka E, Kienpointner G, Unterberger I, et al. Psychiatric comorbidity in juvenile myoclonic epilepsy. Epilepsia 2006;47(12):2086–91.

[73] Schubert R. Attention deficit disorder and epilepsy. Pediatr Neurol 2005;32(1):1–10.

[74] Gonzalez-Heydrich J, Dodds A, Whitney J, et al. Psychiatric disorders and behavioral characteristics of pediatric patients with both epilepsy and attention-deficit hyperactivity disorder. Epilepsy Behav 2007;10(3):384–8.

[75] Binnie CD. Significance and management of transitory cognitive impairment due to subclinical EEG discharges in children. Brain Dev 1993;15(1):23–30.

[76] Sanchez-Carpintero R, Neville BGR. Attentional ability in children with epilepsy. Epilepsia 2003;44(10):1340–9.

[77] Van der Feltz-Cornelis CM, Aldenkamp AP. Effectiveness and safety of methylphenidate in adult attention deficit hyperactivity disorder in patients with epilepsy: an open treatment trial. Epilepsy Behav 2006;8(3):659–62.

[78] Becker K, Holtmann M. Role of electroencephalography in attention-deficit hyperactivity disorder. Expert Rev Neurother 2006;6(5):731–9.

[79] Hesdorffer DC, Ludvigsson P, Olafsson E, et al. ADHD as a risk factor for incident unprovoked seizures and epilepsy in children. Arch Gen Psychiatry 2004;61(7):731–6.

[80] Mula M, Trimble MR. Pharmacokinetic interactions between antiepileptic and antidepressant drugs. World J Biol Psychiatry 2003;4(1):21–4.

[81] Rivinus TM. Psychiatric effects of the anticonvulsant regimens. J Clin Psychopharmacol 1982;2(3):165–92.

[82] Ettinger AB. Psychotropic effects of antiepileptic drugs. Neurology 2006;67(11): 1916–25.

[83] Reijs R, Aldenkamp AP, De Krom M. Mood effects of antiepileptic drugs. Epilepsy Behav 2004;5(Suppl 1):S66–76.

[84] Bersudsky Y. Phenytoin: an anti-bipolar anticonvulsant? Int J Neuropsychopharmacol 2006;9(4):429–84.

[85] Mishory A, Yaroslavsky Y, Bersudsky Y, et al. Phenytoin as an antimanic anticonvulsant: a controlled study. Am J Psychiatry 2000;157(3):463–5.

[86] Hauser P, Devinsky O, De Bellis M, et al. Benzodiazepine withdrawal delirium with catatonic features. Occurrence in patients with partial seizure disorders. Arch Neurol 1989;46(6):696–9.

[87] Ballenger JC, Post RM. Carbamazepine in manic-depressive illness: a new treatment. Am J Psychiatry 1980;137(7):782–90.

[88] Hartong EG, Moleman P, Hoogduin CA, et al. Prophylactic efficacy of lithium versus carbamazepine in treatment-naïve bipolar patients. J Clin Psychiatry 2003;64(2):144–51.

[89] Stone JL, McDaniel KD, Hughes JR, et al. Episodic dyscontrol disorder and paroxysmal EEG abnormalities: successful treatment with carbamazepine. Biol Psychiatry 1986;21(2): 208–12.

[90] Fleminger S, Greenwood RJ, Oliver DL. Pharmacological management for agitation and aggression in people with acquired brain injury. Cochrane Database Syst Rev 2006;4:CD003299.

[91] Hollander E, Tracy KA, Swann AC, et al. Divalproex in the treatment of impulsive aggression: efficacy in cluster B personality disorders. Neuropsychopharmacology 2003;28(6): 1186–97.

[92] Edwards KR, Sackellares JC, Vuong A, et al. Lamotrigine monotherapy improves depressive symptoms in epilepsy: a double-blind comparison with valproate. Epilepsy Behav 2001;2(1):28–36.

[93] Martin R, Kuzniecky R, Ho S, et al. Cognitive effects of topiramate, gabapentin, and lamotrigine in healthy young adults. Neurology 1999;52(2):321–7.

[94] Drane DL, Meador KJ. Cognitive and behavioral effects of antiepileptic drugs. Epilepsy Behav 2002;3(5S):S49–53.

[95] Li Z, Maglione M, Tu W, et al. Meta-analysis: pharmacologic treatment of obesity. Ann Intern Med 2005;142(7):532–46.

[96] Kanner AM, Wuu J, Faught E, et al. A past psychiatric history may be a risk factor for topiramate-related psychiatric and cognitive adverse events. Epilepsy Behav 2003;4(5): 548–52.

[97] Reith D, Burke C, Appleton DB, et al. Tolerability of topiramate in children and adolescents. J Paediatr Child Health 2003;39(6):416–9.

[98] Vasudev K, Macritchie K, Geddes J, et al. Topiramate for acute affective episodes in bipolar disorder. Cochrane Database Syst Rev 2006;1:CD003384.

[99] Mula M, Trimble MR, Yuen A, et al. Psychiatric adverse events during levetiracetam therapy. Neurology 2003;61(5):704–6.

[100] Opp J, Tuxhorn I, May T, et al. Levetiracetam in children with refractory epilepsy: a multicenter open label study in Germany. Seizure 2005;14(7):476–84.

[101] Pande AC, Crockatt JG, Janney CA, et al. Gabapentin in bipolar disorder: a placebo-controlled trial of adjunctive therapy. Gabapentin Bipolar Disorder Study Group. Bipolar Disord 2000;2(3 Pt 2):249–55.

[102] Mazza M, Della Marca G, Di Nicola M, et al. Oxcarbazepine improves mood in patients with epilepsy. Epilepsy Behav 2007;10(3):397–401.

[103] Selai C, Bannister D, Trimble M. Antiepileptic drugs and the regulation of mood and quality of life (QOL): the evidence from epilepsy. Epilepsia 2005;46(Suppl 4):50–7.

[104] Rosenstein DL, Nelson JC, Jacobs SC. Seizures associated with antidepressants: a review. J Clin Psychiatry 1993;54(8):289–99.

[105] Johnston JA, Lineberry CG, Ascher JA, et al. A 102-center prospective study of seizure in association with bupropion. J Clin Psychiatry 1991;52(11):450–6.

[106] Dessain EC, Schatzberg AF, Woods BT, et al. Maprotiline treatment in depression: a perspective on seizures. Arch Gen Psychiatry 1986;43(1):86–90.

[107] Jick H, Dinan BJ, Hunter JR, et al. Tricyclic antidepressants and convulsions. J Clin Psychopharmacol 1983;3(3):182–5.

[108] Specchio LM, Iudice A, Spechio N, et al. Citalopram as treatment of depression in patients with epilepsy. Clin Neuropharmacol 2004;27(3):133–6.

[109] Favale E, Rubino V, Mainardi P, et al. Anticonvulsant effect of fluoxetine in humans. Neurology 1995;45(10):1926–7.

[110] Thome-Souza MS, Kuczynski E, Valente KD. Sertraline and fluoxetine: safe treatments for children and adolescents with epilepsy and depression. Epilepsy Behav 2007;10(3):417–25.

[111] Alper K, Schwartz KA, Kolts RL, et al. Seizure incidence in psychopharmacological clinical trials: an analysis of Food and Drug Administration (FDA) summary basis of approval reports. Biol Psychiatry 2007;62(4):345–54.

[112] Logothetis J. Spontaneous epileptic seizures and electroencephalographic changes in the course of phenothiazines therapy. Neurology 1967;17(9):869–77.

[113] Pacia SV, Devinsky O. Clozapine-related seizures: experience with 5,629 patients. Neurology 1994;44(12):2247–9.

[114] Toth P, Franeknburg FR. Clozapine and seizures: a review. Can J Psychiatry 1994;39(4):236–8.

[115] Pisani F, Oteri G, Costa C, et al. Effects of psychotropic drugs on seizure threshold. Drug Saf 2002;25(2):91–110.

[116] Gucuyener K, Erdemoglu AK, Senol S, et al. Use of methylphenidate for attention-deficit hyperactivity disorder in patients with epilepsy or electroencephalographic abnormalities. J Child Neurol 2003;18(2):109–12.

[117] Wiebe S, Blume WT, Girvin JP, et al. A randomized, controlled trial of surgery for temporal-lobe epilepsy. N Engl J Med 2001;345(5):311–8.

[118] Balabanov AJ, Kanner AM. Psychiatric aspects of epilepsy surgery. In: Ettinger AB, Kanner AM, editors. Psychiatric issues in epilepsy: a practical guide to diagnosis and treatment. 2nd edition. Philadelphia: Lippincott Williams & Wilkens; 2006. p. 405–19.

[119] Glosser G, Zwil AS, Glosser DS, et al. Psychiatric aspects of temporal lobe epilepsy before and after anterior temporal lobectomy. J Neurol Neurosurg Psychiatry 2000;68(1):53–8.

[120] Shaw P, Mellers J, Henderson M, et al. Schizophrenia-like psychosis arising de novo following a temporal lobectomy: timing and risk factors. J Neurol Neurosurg Psychiatry 2004;75(7):1003–8.

[121] Christodoulou C, Koutroumanisis M, Hennessy MJ, et al. Postictal psychosis after temporal lobectomy. Neurology 2002;59(9):1432–5.

[122] Andermann LF, Savard G, Meencke HJ, et al. Psychosis after resection of ganglioglioma or DNET: evidence for an association. Epilepsia 1999;40(1):83–7.

[123] Ring HA, Moriarty J, Trimble MR. A prospective study of the early postsurgical psychiatric associations of epilepsy surgery. J Neurol Neurosurg Psychiatry 1998;64(5):601–4.

[124] Carran MA, Kohler CG, O'Connor MJ, et al. Mania following temporal lobectomy. Neurology 2003;61(6):770–4.

[125] Devinsky O, Barr WB, Vickery BG, et al. Changes in depression and anxiety after resective surgery for epilepsy. Neurology 2005;65(11):1744–9.

[126] Reuber M, Elger CE. Psychogenic nonepileptic seizures: review and update. Epilepsy Behav 2003;4(3):205–16.

[127] Cragar DE, Berry DTR, Fakoury TA, et al. A review of diagnostic techniques in the differential diagnosis of epileptic and nonepileptic seizures. Neuropsychol Rev 2002;12(1): 31–64.

[128] Reuber M, Fernandez G, Helmstaeder C, et al. Evidence of brain abnormality in patients with psychogenic nonepileptic seizures. Epilepsy Behav 2002;3(3):249–54.

[129] D'Alessio L, Giagante B, Oddo S, et al. Psychiatric disorders in patients with psychogenic non-epileptic seizures, with and without comorbid epilepsy. Seizure 2006;15(5):333–9.

[130] Benbadis SR, Allen HW. An estimate of the prevalence of psychogenic non-epileptic seizures. Seizure 2000;9(4):280–1.

[131] Szaflarski JP, Ficker DM, Cahill WT, et al. Four-year incidence of psychogenic nonepileptic seizures in adults in Hamilton County, OH. Neurology 2000;55(10):1561–3.

[132] Ettinger AB, Devisnky O, Weisbrot DM, et al. A comprehensive profile of clinical, psychiatric, and psychosocial characteristics of patients with psychogenic nonepileptic seizures. Epilepsia 1999;40(8):1292–8.

[133] Alper K, Devinsky O, Perrine K, et al. Psychiatric classification of nonconversion nonepileptic seizures. Arch Neurol 1995;52(2):199–201.

[134] Betts T, Boden S. Diagnosis, management and prognosis of a group of 128 patients with non-epileptic attack disorder. Part II. Previous childhood sexual abuse in the aetiology of these disorders. Seizure 1992;1(1):27–32.

[135] Bowman ES. Etiology and clinical course of pseudoseizures: relationship to trauma, depression, and dissociation. Psychosomatics 1993;34(4):333–42.

[136] Kanner AM, Parra J, Frey M, et al. Psychiatric and neurologic predictors of psychogenic pseudoseizure outcome. Neurology 1999;53(5):933–8.

[137] Sharpe D, Faye C. Non-epileptic seizures and child sexual abuse: a critical review of the literature. Clin Psychol Rev 2006;26(8):1020–40.

[138] LaFrance WC Jr, Devinsky O. Treatment of nonepileptic seizures. Epilepsy Behav 2002;3(5 Suppl):S19–23.

[139] Goldstein LH, Deale AC, Mitchell-O'Mallet SJ, et al. An evaluation of cognitive behavioral therapy as a treatment for dissociative seizures. Cogn Behav Neurol 2004;17(1):41–9.

[140] LaFrance WC Jr, Barry JJ. Update on treatments of psychological nonepileptic seizures. Epilepsy Behav 2005;7(3):364–74.

[141] Krishnamoorthy ES, Trimble MR, Blumer D. The classification of neuropsychiatric disorders in epilepsy: a proposal by the ILAE commission on psychobiology of epilepsy. Epilepsy Behav 2007;10(3):349–53.

Psychiatr Clin N Am 30 (2007) 803–817

PSYCHIATRIC CLINICS
OF NORTH AMERICA

Psychiatric Issues in Multiple Sclerosis

Lydia A. Chwastiak, MD, MPH[a],*, Dawn M. Ehde, PhD[b,c]

[a]Departments of Psychiatry and Medicine, Yale University School of Medicine, Yale New Haven Psychiatric Hospital, 184 Liberty Street; LV-119, New Haven, CT 06519, USA
[b]Department of Rehabilitation Medicine, University of Washington School of Medicine, Harborview Medical Center, Box 359740, 325 9th Avenue, Seattle, WA 98104-2499, USA
[c]University of Washington Multiple Sclerosis Rehabilitation Research and Training Center, University of Washington Medical Center, SS812, Box 356157, 1959 NE Pacific Street, Seattle, WA 98195, USA

OVERVIEW

Multiple sclerosis (MS) is the most common chronic disabling disease of the central nervous system in young adults, affecting 1 in 1000 people in Western countries [1]. MS is a demyelinating disease of the central nervous system; a diagnosis of MS requires the occurrence of at least two neurologic events consistent with demyelination in the central nervous system that are separated temporally and anatomically. Early onset (typically between 20 and 40 years of age) and long duration of disease result in tremendous individual, family, and societal costs as well as reductions in quality of life and work productivity [2]. MS has a variable and unpredictable course, with symptoms that can include weakness, visual loss, bowel and bladder incontinence, fatigue, cognitive impairment, and mood symptoms. Persons who have MS seem to have a higher prevalence of a number of psychiatric symptoms and disorders (Table 1) [3–6]. Depression and anxiety, in particular, have been associated with decreased adherence to treatment [7], functional status [8], and quality of life [9]. This article seeks to summarize the existing literature on the epidemiology, impact, and treatment of psychiatric disorders among persons who have MS and to identify the areas in which further research is needed.

IMPACT OF PSYCHIATRIC DISORDERS ON MULTIPLE SCLEROSIS

The most compelling reason to investigate psychiatric disorders among persons who have MS is that reported rates of completed suicide in MS populations are high [10], and psychiatric disorders seem to be the major risk factor for suicidality [11]. Death certificate–based reviews indicate that suicide may be the cause of death as many as 15% of MS clinic patients [12]. In retrospective analyses of completed suicides in MS populations, depression has been the most

*Corresponding author. E-mail address: lydia.chwastiak@yale.edu (L.A. Chwastiak).

0193-953X/07/$ – see front matter
doi:10.1016/j.psc.2007.07.003
© 2007 Elsevier Inc. All rights reserved.
psych.theclinics.com

Table 1
Prevalence of psychiatric disorders among persons who have MS compared with the general population

Disorder	Prevalence in multiple sclerosis (%)	Prevalence in general population (%)
Major depressive disorder, 12-month	15.7 [37]	7.4 [37]
Major depressive disorder, lifetime	22.8 [44]	16.2 [3]
Any anxiety disorder, lifetime	36 [14,66]	25 [67]
Generalized anxiety disorder	18.6 [14,66]	3.0 [4]
Bipolar disorder, lifetime	0.3 [76]	0.2 [5]
Alcohol abuse, lifetime	13.6 [81]	7.4 [6]
Substance misuse, past month	18.7 [82]	11.1 [6]

important risk factor for suicide [13]. Anxiety disorders also seem to be linked to suicidal intent and self-harm attempts [14]. Social isolation, a history of previous suicide attempts, and recent functional deterioration also seem to be important determinants of suicidal intent [15]; but the level of neurologic disability, per se, does not seem to be a risk factor for suicide. This epidemiologic research led an expert consensus panel to conclude that the single most useful step that can be taken with regard to the primary prevention of suicide in MS is better identification and treatment of depressive disorders [16].

Psychiatric disorders seem to have profound effects on wide-ranging aspects of the lives of persons who have MS. Depression has been the most-studied psychiatric disorder among persons who have MS; only a limited number of rigorous studies of the prevalence and impact of anxiety disorders, substance use disorders, or serious mental illness such as bipolar disorder or schizophrenia have been reported. Depressed patients who have MS report subjective cognitive difficulties, including memory complaints [17], and in some studies perform more poorly on objective neuropsychologic measures than nondepressed patients who have MS [18]. Quality of life is significantly lower among depressed MS patients than among nondepressed control MS patients, even when controlling for factors such as level of neurologic disability and fatigue [9]. Depression adversely affects functional status (eg, increasing the time lost from work) among patients who have MS [19]. Depressed MS patients experience disruption of their social support and family systems beyond the level that can be attributed to neurologic disease factors alone. There also is evidence that depression decreases adherence to treatment regimens for MS, and that adherence improves with treatment of depression [7]. Finally, a recent meta-analysis demonstrates a consistent association between stressful life events and subsequent MS exacerbation [20]. There is, however, no definitive evidence that major depressive disorder or other psychiatric disorders affect the neurobiologic course of MS.

PSYCHIATRIC EFFECTS OF TREATMENT OF MULTIPLE SCLEROSIS

Pharmacologic treatments for MS include corticosteroids, beta interferon (IFNβ), glatiramer acetate, and immunosuppressants. Corticosteroids, which are used in high doses for short courses to treat acute exacerbations, have been associated with a variety of neuropsychiatric side effects, including increased energy, decreased sleep, and significant mood symptoms such as mood lability, euphoria, and depressed mood [21,22]. Epidemiologic studies suggest an incidence of neuropsychiatric side effects from corticosteroid treatment of 5% to 8% [22,23]. It is difficult to predict which patients are at highest risk for the emergence of neuropsychiatric symptoms during corticosteroid treatment. There is no clear evidence that a previous psychiatric history increases the risk of adverse neuropsychiatric events from steroid treatment [24], and overall there is little data to help identify individuals who are at increased risk. The potential risks of multiple courses of steroid treatment have not been explored.

The majority (75%) of cases of neuropsychiatric side effects from corticosteroids fit an affective profile of mania and/or depression. Mania occurs more frequently than depression. Psychotic symptoms (in particular, hallucinations) are present in up to half of these cases. Fewer than 25% of cases of neuropsychiatric side effects have symptoms consistent with delirium. Psychotic symptoms typically last about a week, but affective symptoms often last for longer periods. Although no large studies of neuropsychiatric side effects of corticosteroids have been conducted specifically among patients who have MS, a study of a short course (14 days) of corticosteroid treatment in asthma patients demonstrated that mild mood changes occurred early (3–7 days) in the treatment and returned to baseline 10 days after discontinuation of prednisone [25]. Depressive symptoms can occur after the initial administration of corticosteroids, with long-term use, or with discontinuation of the steroid dosing. Cognitive deficits have been reported in association with short-term steroid treatment [26]. Treatment of neuropsychiatric side effects involves tapering of the corticosteroid dose and administration of antidepressant or antipsychotic medications for symptom relief. Across studies, the outcome is complete recovery in more than 90% of cases [27].

Currently approved disease-modifying therapies for MS include glatiramer acetate and IFNβ [28]. Glatiramer acetate has not been associated with neuropsychiatric side effects [16]. Two types of IFNβ have been approved for the treatment of MS. IFNβ-1a (Avonex, Rebif) is administered through an intramuscular injection, given weekly or monthly. IFNβ-1b (Betaseron) is administered by subcutaneous injection every other day. The side effects of both IFNβ-1a and -1b include flulike symptoms (fever and myalgias), elevations in liver function tests, and anemia. The data regarding the risk of mood symptoms related to IFN use are conflicting. Several clinical trials have reported an increase in depression in patients during the first 2 to 6 months of treatment with both IFNβ-1b [29] and IFNβ-1a [30], but these increases in depressive symptoms seem to be related more to pretreatment levels of depression than to the administration of IFN [31]. Two randomized controlled trials, however, have found that depression is not an effect of treatment with IFNβ-1a. In the SPECTRIMS trial of Rebif in secondary progressive MS, depression ratings were no different in the IFN group than in the placebo group [32]. A second study found no change on Beck Depression Inventory scores in a cohort of patients who had MS before and 12 months after initiation of IFNβ-1a [33]. The results of these studies show no clear evidence that the administration of IFN to patients who have MS increases the risk for depressive disorders [34]. Nonetheless, given the high prevalence of depression among persons who have MS, expert panels have recommended that patients should be educated about depression and complete a measure of depression severity at regular intervals during the course of IFN treatment [35].

There have been no reports to date of psychiatric side effects associated with two newer pharmacotherapies for MS. Mitoxantrone (Novantrone), an immunosuppressant, is approved for treatment of secondary progressive, progressive-relapsing, and worsening relapsing-remitting MS. Natalizumab (Tysabri) is a monoclonal antibody against integrin-α4 that was approved by the Food and Drug Administration in 2006 for treatment of patients who have relapsing forms of MS and who have not responded to or are unable to tolerate the other treatments of MS. Because natalizumab increases the risk of progressive multifocal leukoencephalopathy, this medication is available only through a special, restricted distribution program and is not used widely.

MAJOR DEPRESSIVE DISORDER
Epidemiology and Clinical Correlates of Depression
Depression may be more common in MS than in other chronic neurologic conditions [36]. The 12-month prevalence of major depressive disorder (MDD) among persons who have MS is 15.7%, nearly double the prevalence of MDD in persons who do not have MS (7.4%) [37]. Reports of the lifetime risk for MDD in MS populations have ranged from 27% to 54% [36–38]. The prevalence of clinically significant depressive symptoms is much higher [39] than the prevalence of MDD, but few studies have evaluated other depressive disorders such as dysthymia [40].

The depressive syndromes associated with MS occur throughout the natural history of the disease, including in patients who have very mild forms of MS [41]. Some studies have found associations between depression and severity of MS as reflected by degree of disability [42], but other studies have not replicated these findings [37,43]. The association of depression with the duration of MS illness also is unclear, with most studies finding no correlation [42,43], but others reporting a greater risk of depression in the first year after diagnosis [39] and in patients younger than 35 years [44]. Most studies have not found a correlation between depression and female gender among persons who have MS [39,42,43].

Neurobiology of Depression in Multiple Sclerosis

Several lines of evidence suggest that neurobiologic risk factors specifically associated with MS contribute to the increased incidence of depressive disorders among MS patients. There is, however, no clear consensus about what the neurobiologic differences between depressed MS patients and nondepressed MS patients might be. Although some comparative studies using MRI have found no differences in lesion distribution between depressed and nondepressed MS patients [42], other studies have suggested an increase in lesions in specific brain areas among depressed MS patients, including the right temporal lobe [45], the left hemisphere supra-sylvian region [46], and the superior frontal or parietal regions [47].

Similarly, little is known about the specific nature of the interactions between the neuroimmunology of MS and depressive disorders. Regulation of hypothalamic feedback is abnormal in many MS patients, with 50% of MS patients demonstrating a failure of suppression on the dexamethasone suppression test. This lack of regulation is similar to the pattern seen in many patients who have major depressive episodes [48]. Failure to respond to dexamethasone challenge also has been associated with the presence of gadolinium-enhancing lesions on MRI in MS patients, suggesting that some of the depressive symptomatology in MS could be related to disease activity [49].

Treatment of Depression in Multiple Sclerosis

Depression in MS patients seems to be underdetected and undertreated by neurologists, consistent with studies of primary care samples [50]. In a study of 260 outpatients who had MS treated by 35 neurologists in a large health maintenance organization, 26% of patients met criteria for MDD. Among these patients, 66% received no antidepressant medication, and 4.7% received subthreshold doses from their neurologist [51]. Despite the development of reliable, user-friendly screening tools to detect depression in MS patients [52] and the recommendation by expert consensus panels for routine screening for MDD in MS clinics, screening has not been widely adopted.

Treatment for depression in persons who have MS should be individualized and involve psychotherapy, psychopharmacology, or a combination [16]. A meta-analysis published in 1999 found that both psychotherapy and pharmacotherapy are effective for decreasing depressive symptoms in persons who have MS; but only five studies were of sufficient methodologic rigor (randomized clinical trials using an objective measure of depressive symptoms) to be included in the meta-analysis [53].

Pharmacotherapy

Although antidepressant use is common among persons who have MS [54], the literature on the effectiveness of antidepressants in MS is small and largely anecdotal. Only two randomized trials of pharmacotherapy for depression have been published to date, neither of which used a placebo control. A small trial (N = 28) found desipramine to be effective relative to a case-management control [55]. The second trial evaluated the efficacy of sertraline (n = 21) relative to two psychologic treatments: individual cognitive behavior therapy (CBT; n = 20) and supportive-expressive group therapy (SET; n = 22). In this study, 24% of those in the sertraline group had a treatment response, compared with 50% in the CBT group and 14% in the SET group. Attrition was greatest for the sertraline group, with 29% dropping out before completing the study [56].

Several conclusions can be drawn from the available literature on pharmacotherapy for depression in MS. First, antidepressants reduce the severity of depressive symptoms in persons who have MS and should be considered for treating MDD in this patient population. Although depressive symptoms may be responsive to pharmacotherapy, not all MS patients who use them experience full remission of these symptoms. Research on methods for identifying MS patients or symptoms that are particularly responsive to antidepressant medications would improve the treatment of MDD in patients who have MS. Given the clinical characteristics of MS, side effects of antidepressants may be particularly bothersome in this population and lead to higher rates of nonadherence and premature treatment termination in clinical practice than in clinical trials. The small sample sizes in the existing studies suggest that it is difficult to enroll large numbers of participants into pharmacotherapy clinical trials in this disease group. Future research evaluating antidepressants should consider multicenter trials.

Psychotherapy

Several randomized, controlled trials have demonstrated the effectiveness of CBT for treatment of major depressive disorder among persons who have MS [56,57]. In these studies, response rates to CBT have approached 50%, equal to or higher than response rates to antidepressant medications or to other psychotherapy modalities [56]. Moreover, in these trials the attrition for the CBT intervention typically is very low (5%). Recent studies also have shown that CBT delivered by telephone is an effective form of psychotherapy for depression in MS relative to usual care [57] and relative to a telephone-delivered SET-focused therapy [58]. Attrition also was low for the telephone-delivered interventions, and in one study, adherence to MS disease–modifying medications was significantly better at follow-up among those who participated in the telephone CBT [58]. Telephone-delivered CBT shows considerable promise as a viable and potentially cost-effective treatment for MDD that may overcome many of the common barriers to face-to-face treatment such as fatigue, stigma, and logistic issues (lack of access to treatment, transportation, child care, or financial limitations). Unfortunately, at this time, most health insurance carriers usually do not cover psychotherapy delivered by telephone. Interpersonal therapy or behavioral activation has not been evaluated empirically as treatment for depression in the MS literature. The Goldman Consensus Group has recommended that psychotherapy, particularly CBT, be offered as a treatment option for persons who have MS and depression [16]. Because skills learned through CBT produce improvements beyond the nonspecific effects of supportive treatment [56], standard CBT for depression may be considered the treatment of choice.

Exercise

Although physical exercise has not been studied formally as a treatment for MDD in MS, it has widespread beneficial effects among persons who have MS, including improvements in mood, pain, fatigue, quality of life, sexual functioning, recreation, and psychosocial functioning [59]. The effect of exercise on MDD has been studied in healthy adults, persons who have psychiatric conditions, and older adults [60]. Across studies, exercise seems to be more beneficial than no treatment, and in some studies it has been as effective as antidepressant medication and psychotherapy for mild-to-moderate depression [61]. In depression, exercise also has been associated with lower rates of relapse than pharmacotherapy [60,62]. Moderate exercise (walking 20 minutes a day at 60% maximum heart rate) has been more effective than vigorous exercise and is associated with fewer drop-outs [63].

ANXIETY DISORDERS IN MULTIPLE SCLEROSIS

In contrast to the extensive literature on depression in patients who have MS, less attention has been paid to anxiety disorders. Several studies using self-report scales of anxiety symptoms have found a point prevalence of clinically significant anxiety ranging from 25% to 41% [42,64,65]. Only two studies have used structured clinical interviews to evaluate formal diagnoses of anxiety disorders, and both of these found lifetime prevalence rates of 36% [14,66], which is much higher than the 25% lifetime rate of anxiety disorders in the general population reported in the National Comorbidity Survey [67]. Generalized anxiety disorder seems to be the most common anxiety disorder among persons who have MS, with 18.6% of patients meeting criteria for this disorder [14,66]. Panic disorder and obsessive compulsive disorder also may be much more common among patients who have MS than among the general population. MS patients who had anxiety disorders were more likely to be female and to have a lifetime diagnosis of MDD or alcohol abuse. They also were more likely to report greater social stress, less social support, and to have contemplated suicide. In one of the studies, only 34% of those who had an anxiety disorder had previously been given a documented psychiatric diagnosis, and none had been given a diagnosis of an anxiety disorder. More than half of the patients were not receiving any treatment [14]. There have been no studies specifically evaluating posttraumatic stress disorder among persons who have MS.

SERIOUS MENTAL ILLNESS IN MULTIPLE SCLEROSIS

Numerous case reports have documented an association between bipolar disorder and MS [68–71]. Bipolar symptoms may precede other neurologic signs of MS, and there have been reports of MS presenting as frank mania [70,71]. Affective lability, in particular, may occur in tandem with an MS exacerbation. Some researchers have hypothesized that the comorbidity of bipolar disorder may be related to the location of the MS lesions [69]. Several clinical studies have identified elevated rates of MS among patients who have bipolar disorder [72,73]. Other small clinical studies have identified elevated rates of bipolar disorder among MS patients [40,74], with some reporting bipolar disorder in more than 10% of MS patients [40]. The few epidemiologic studies that have been conducted have documented the comorbidity of MS and bipolar disorder at more than twice the expected rate based on the prevalence of each disorder in the population [74,75]. In a recent study of more than 650 outpatients who had MS, the prevalence of bipolar disorder was 0.3%, significantly greater than the prevalence of 0.2% in the general population [76]. These epidemiologic studies have been limited by either small sample sizes or the method of diagnosing bipolar disorder. To date, there have been no large, population-based epidemiologic studies of the prevalence of bipolar disorder among persons who have MS. Finally, there have been no epidemiologic studies of the relationship between multiple sclerosis and schizophrenia spectrum disorders.

SUBSTANCE USE DISORDERS IN MULTIPLE SCLEROSIS

Alcohol and illicit drug use may be more problematic in people who have MS than in the general population, potentially causing further neurologic damage to an already compromised central nervous system or leading to dangerous interactions with prescription medications. Heavy alcohol use can magnify the subtle cognitive impairment associated with MS [77] and has been shown to cause persistent cognitive impairment, even in persons who do not meet the criteria for alcohol abuse or dependence [78] Moreover, alcohol tolerance may diminish as MS progresses, resulting in more impaired balance and coordination [77]. Substance abuse is associated with a poorer psychologic adjustment in people who have disabilities [79] and with suicidal intent in persons who have MS [13]. Substance abuse may exacerbate depression symptoms and complicate treatment of comorbid depression [80].

Alcohol Use Disorders

Several studies have shown higher rates of "problem drinking" among MS patients (when compared with the general population) [44,81,82]. In a detailed study of alcohol consumption patterns of 140 MS clinic patients, no subjects met criteria for alcohol dependence, but 13.6% had a lifetime prevalence of alcohol abuse by structured psychiatric interview (SCID-IV) [83]. An additional 5% of subjects met the national guidelines criteria for "problem drinking" [84]. In a large community-based sample, 14% of subjects screened positive for possible alcohol abuse within the previous month, using the alcohol screen from the Patient Health Questionnaire [85]. In this study, alcohol misuse was significantly and independently correlated with severity of depression symptoms [82]. Because rates of alcohol problems are comparable to those in primary medical care settings, MS clinicians should consider routine screening for alcohol misuse as is recommended in primary care [86]. As with depression, brief screening measures, such as the CAGE [87] or the Patient Health Questionnaire alcohol screen [85], are relatively easy to integrate into routine clinical practice. Physician advice to stop or cut down on alcohol use is an effective means of reducing problem drinking, particularly for those patients who have less severe alcohol problems [88].

Substance Use Disorders

The only published study reporting substance abuse rates among persons who have MS was a community survey in which drug abuse was evaluated by a single question from the 1992 National Household Survey on Drug Abuse [89]. In this study, 18.7% of subjects reported either drug misuse or possible alcohol abuse within the past month. Significantly higher rates of alcohol and/or drug misuse were found among MS patients who were younger, still employed, and had less severe MS [82].

Cannabis

Cannabinoids have been purported to alleviate a variety of MS-related symptoms including spasticity, pain, tremor, and bladder dysfunction [90], but clinical trials of cannabinoids in MS have not demonstrated beneficial effects consistently. A large randomized, controlled trial (N = 660) compared the effects of oral cannabis extracts with pure oral tetrahydrocannabinol and placebo on spasticity. The study found no differences with respect to spasticity but did note significant subjective improvements in pain and sleep [91]. Even though cannabis remains illegal, and there is limited evidence for its clinical efficacy in relieving MS symptoms, almost a third of MS patients have used cannabis in an attempt to alleviate symptoms [92], with rates of current medicinal cannabis use of 14% to 18% [92,93]. In a large (N = 337) survey of MS clinic patients at three hospital-based clinics, 43% reported using cannabis at least once in their lifetime, with first cannabis use being split evenly between before and after MS diagnosis. Ninety percent of the subjects who started using cannabis after MS diagnosis reported that they started using it because of MS symptoms, most commonly for pain and spasms. The majority of patients using it for these symptoms reported benefit. Seventy-one percent of individuals who had never used cannabis stated that they would try the drug if it were legal or available by prescription [92].

PSEUDOBULBAR AFFECT

In addition to mood disorders, MS patients also may experience disorders of affect, typically an expression of affect that is not representative of the underlying emotion [94]. Some MS patients may laugh or cry out of proportion to or in the absence of the expected feeling, a phenomenon that has been referred to as "pathological laughing and crying," or pseudobulbar affect (PBA). PBA has been recognized in association with MS for many years, but even today its causes are not well understood. PBA traditionally has been considered to be a disconnection syndrome resulting in the loss of brainstem inhibition of a putative center for laughing and crying. PBA occurs in approximately 10% of patients who have MS [94]. In general, patients who have MS with PBA have greater physical disability and are more likely to be in the chronic progressive stage of the disease (compared with MS patients not exhibiting PBA). Evidence suggests that PBA can be modulated through pharmacologic intervention. Most commonly, patients who have MS are treated with tricyclic antidepressants [95] or selective serotonin reuptake inhibitors [96]. There is evidence that other medications, such as levodopa or dextromethorphan/ quinidine also may be beneficial [97,98], but these medications are not commonly used for this indication.

RESILIENCE AND POSTTRAUMATIC GROWTH

Although psychiatric conditions are highly prevalent among individuals living with MS, many persons who have MS do not exhibit clinically significant levels of depression, anxiety, or other serious mental illness. The ability to maintain psychologic well being and functioning in the face of adversity such as loss, trauma, and serious medical illness often is referred to as "resilience" [99]. Being resilient does not mean that the individual never experiences any negative emotions, thoughts, or actions in response to adversity or loss. Such experiences are common and may, in fact, be part of the resilience process, but in resilient individuals they typically are transient, occur with positive emotions, and do not interfere significantly with functioning [99]. "Posttraumatic growth" has been defined as positive psychologic changes resulting from or in response to a challenging circumstance such as a traumatic event or loss [100]. It is thought to involve more than resilience, namely, growth and improved functioning be- yond a return to a pre-event level of psychologic functioning. Posttraumatic growth can be manifested in a variety of ways, including an increased appreci- ation for life, feeling increased personal strength, experiencing improved inter- personal relationships, changing life priorities, gaining positive spiritual changes, or finding new meaning and purpose in life. Future research should be con- ducted using theoretically driven models of psychosocial functioning that take into account not only what goes "wrong" after the onset of MS, but perhaps more importantly, on what goes "right," and the risk and protective factors pre- dicting both. Such research may lead to greater recognition of and interventions for promoting psychologic well being after the onset of MS.

SUMMARY

MDD and anxiety disorders are highly prevalent among persons who have MS and have been associated with decreased adherence to MS treatment and poorer functional status and quality of life. Effective treatment is available for MDD, but this disorder continues to be underdetected and undertreated by MS providers. Treatment with pharmacotherapy is particularly challenging in this patient population, given the somatic symptom overlap between MS and depression and the increased burden of side effects. Larger randomized, controlled trials are needed to elucidate further the effectiveness of pharmaco- therapy and to identify subgroups of patients who would benefit from this type of treatment for depression. There have been few rigorous studies of the prevalence and impact of anxiety disorders, substance use disorders, or serious mental illness such as bipolar disorder or schizophrenia, in MS samples.

References

[1] Hogancamp WE, Rodriguez M, Weinshenker BG. The epidemiology of multiple sclerosis. Mayo Clin Proc 1997;72:871–8.

[2] Grima DT, Torrance GW, Francis G, et al. Cost and health related quality of life consequences of multiple sclerosis. Mult Scler 2000;6:91–8.

[3] Kessler RC, Berglund P, Demler O, et al. The survey replication epidemiology of major depressive disorder results from the National Comorbidity Survey Replication. JAMA 2003;289:3095–105.

[4] Kessler RC, Keller MB, Wittchen HU. The epidemiology of generalized anxiety disorder. Psychiatr Clin North Am 2001;24(1):19–39.

[5] Perala J, Suvisaari J, Saarni SI, et al. Lifetime prevalence of psychotic and bipolar I disorders in a general population. Arch Gen Psychiatry 2007;64(1):19–28.

[6] Results from the 2001 National Household Survey on Drug Abuse, volume I. Summary of national findings. Rockville (MD): US Department of Health and Human Services. Substance Abuse and Mental Health Services Administration; 2002.

[7] Mohr DC, Goodkin DE, Likosky W, et al. Treatment of depression improves adherence to interferon beta-1b therapy for multiple sclerosis. Arch Neurol 1997;54:531–3.

[8] Tsivgoulis G, Triantafyllou N, Papageorgiou C, et al. Associations of the Expanded Disability Status Scale with anxiety and depression in multiple sclerosis outpatients. Acta Neruol Scand 2007;115:67–72.

[9] Amato MP, Ponziani G, Rossi F, et al. Quality of life in multiple sclerosis: the impact of depression, fatigue and disability. Mult Scler 2001;7:340–4.

[10] Stenager EN, Stenager E, Koch-Henrikksen N, et al. Suicide and multiple sclerosis: an epidemiological investigation. J Neurol Neurosurg Psychiatry 1992;55:542–5.

[11] Stenager EN, Koch-Henrikksen N, Stenager E. Risk factors for suicide in multiple sclerosis. Psychother Psychosom 1996;65:86–90.

[12] Sadovnick AD, Eisen K, Ebers GC, et al. Cause of death in patients attending multiple sclerosis clinics. Neurology 1991;41:1193–6.

[13] Feinstein A. Multiple sclerosis, depression and suicide. BMJ 1997;315:691–2.

[14] Korostil M, Feinstein A. Anxiety disorders and their clinical correlates in multiple sclerosis patients. Mult Scler 2007;13:67–72.

[15] Feinstein A. An examination of suicidal intent in patients with multiple sclerosis. Neurology 2002;59:674–8.

[16] Goldman Consensus Group. The Goldman consensus statement on depression in multiple sclerosis. Mult Scler 2005;11:328–37.

[17] Julian L, Merluzzi NM, Mohr DC. The relationship among depression, subjective cognitive impairment, and neuropsychological performance in MS. Mult Scler 2007;13:81–6.

[18] Gilchrist AC, Creed FH. Depression, cognitive impairment and social stress in multiple sclerosis. J Psychosom Res 1994;38:193–201.

[19] Smith MM, Arnett PA. Factors related to employment status changes in individuals with multiple sclerosis. Mult Scler 2005;11:602–9.

[20] Mohr DC, Hart SL, Julian L, et al. Association between stressful life events and exacerbation in multiple sclerosis: a meta-analysis. BMJ 2004;328:731–5.

[21] Minden SL, Orav J, Schildkraut JJ. Hypomanic reactions to ACTH and prednisone treatment for multiple sclerosis. Neurology 1988;38:1631–4.

[22] Kershner P, Wang-Cheng R. Psychiatric side effects of steroid therapy. Psychosomatics 1989;30:135–9.

[23] Lewis DA, Smith RE. Steroid-induced psychiatric syndromes. A report of 14 cases and a review of the literature. J Affect Disord 1983;5:319–32.

[24] Patten SB, Neutel CI. Corticosteroid-induced adverse psychiatric effects: incidence, diagnosis and management. Drug Saf 2000;22:111–22.

[25] Brown ES, Suppes T, Khan DA, et al. Mood changes during prednisone bursts in outpatients with asthma. J Clin Psychopharmacol 2002;22:55–61.

[26] Naber D, Sand P, Heigi B. Psychopathological and neuropsychological effects of 8-days corticosteroid treatment: a prospective study. Psychoneuroendocrinology 1996;21: 25–31.

[27] Sirois F. Steroid psychosis: a review. Gen Hosp Psychiatry 2003;25:27–33.

[28] Polman CH, Thompson AJ, Murray TJ, McDonald WI, editors. Multiple sclerosis: the guide to treatment and management. 5th edition. New York: Demos Publishing; 2001. p. 7–43.

[29] Neilley LK, Goodin DS, Goodkin DE, et al. Side effect profile of interferon beta-1b in MS: results of an open label trial. Neurology 1996;46:552–4.

[30] Mohr DC, Likosky W, Dwyer P, et al. Course of depression during initiation of interferon beta-1a treatment for multiple sclerosis. Arch Neurol 1999;56:1263–5.

[31] Feinstein A, O'Connor P, Feinstein K. Multiple sclerosis, interferon beta 1b and depression. J Neurol 2002;24:815–20.

[32] Patten SB, Metz LM. SPECTRIMS Study Group. Interferon beta 1a and depression in secondary progressive MS: data from the SPECTRIMS trial. Neurology 2002;59:744–6.

[33] Zephir H, DeSeze J, Stojkovic T, et al. Multiple sclerosis and depression: influence of interferon beta therapy. Mult Scler 2003;9:284–8.

[34] Feinstein A. Multiple sclerosis, disease modifying treatment and depression: a critical methodological review. Mult Scler 2000;6:343–8.

[35] Lublin FD, Whitaker JN, Eidelman BH, et al. Management of patients receiving interferon beta-1b for multiple sclerosis: report of a consensus conference. Neurology 1996;46: 12–8.

[36] Schubert DS, Foliart RH. Increased depression in multiple sclerosis patients: a meta-analysis. Psychosomatics 1993;34:124–30.

[37] Patten SB, Beck CA, Williams JV, et al. Major depression in multiple sclerosis: a population-based perspective. Neurology 2003;61:1524–7.

[38] Minden SL, Orav J, Reich P. Depression in multiple sclerosis. Gen Hosp Psychiatry 1987;9: 426–34.

[39] Chwastiak L, Ehde DM, Gibbons, et al. Depressive symptoms and severity of illness in multiple sclerosis: epidemiologic study of a large community sample. Am J Psychiatry 2002; 159:1862–8.

[40] Minden SL. Mood disorders in multiple sclerosis: diagnosis and treatment. J Neurovirol 2000;6(Suppl 2):S160–7.

[41] Sullivan MJ, Weinshenker B, Mikail S, et al. Depression before and after diagnosis of multiple sclerosis. Mult Scler 1995;1:104–8.

[42] Zorzon M, de Masi R, Nasuelli D, et al. Depression and anxiety in multiple sclerosis. A clinical and MRI study in 95 subjects. J Neurol 2001;248:416–21.

[43] Moller A, Wiedemann G, Rohde U, et al. Correlates of cognitive impairment and depressive mood disorder in multiple sclerosis. Acta Psychiatr Scand 1994;89:117–21.

[44] Patten SB, Metz LM, Reimer MA. Biopsychosocial correlates of lifetime major depression in a multiple sclerosis population. Mult Scler 2000;6:115–20.

[45] Berg D, Supprian T, Thomas J, et al. Lesion pattern in patients with multiple sclerosis and depression. Mult Scler 2000;6:156–62.

[46] Pujol J, Bello J, Deus J, et al. Lesions in the left arcuate fasciculus region and depressive symptoms in multiple sclerosis. Neurology 1997;49:1105–10.

[47] Bakshi R, Czarnecki D, Shaikh ZA, et al. Brain MRI lesions and atrophy are related to depression in multiple sclerosis. Neuroreport 2000;11:1153–8.

[48] Reder AT, Makowiec RL, Lowy MT. Adrenal size is increased in multiple sclerosis. Arch Neurol 1994;51:151–4.

[49] Fassbender K, Schmidt R, Mossner R, et al. Mood disorders and dysfunction of the hypothalamic-pituitary-adrenal axis in multiple sclerosis. Arch Neurol 1998;55:66–72.

[50] Katon WJ, Unutzer J, Simon G, et al. Treatment of depression in primary care: where we are, where we can go. Med Care 2004;42:1153–7.

[51] Mohr DC, Hart SL, Fonareva I, et al. Treatment of depression for patients with multiple sclerosis in neurology clinics. Mult Scler 2006;12:204–8.

[52] Mohr DC, Hart SL, Julian L, et al. Screening for depression among patients with multiple sclerosis: two questions may be enough. Mult Scler 2007;13:215–9.

[53] Mohr DC, Goodkin DE. Treatment of depression in multiple sclerosis: review and meta-analysis. Clinical Psychology: Science and Practice 1999;6:1–9.

[54] Cetin K, Johnson KL, Ehde DM, et al. Antidepressant use in multiple sclerosis: epidemiologic study of a large community sample. Mult Scler 2007 Jul 10; [Epub ahead of print].

[55] Schiffer RB, Wineman NM. Antidepressant pharmacotherapy of depression associated with multiple sclerosis. Am J Psychiatry 1990;147:1493–7.

[56] Mohr DC, Boudewyn AC, Goodkin DE, et al. Comparative outcomes for individual cognitive-behavioral therapy, supportive-expressive group psychotherapy and sertraline for the treatment of depression in multiple sclerosis. J Consult Clin Psychology 2001;69:942–9.

[57] Mohr DC, Likosky W, Bertagnolli A, et al. Telephone-administered cognitive-behavioral therapy for the treatment of depressive symptoms in multiple sclerosis. J Consult Clin Psychol 2000;68:356–61.

[58] Mohr DC, Hart SL, Julian L, et al. Telephone-administered psychotherapy for depression. Arch Gen Psychiatry 2005;62:1007–14.

[59] Petajan JH, Gappmaier E, White AT, et al. Impact of aerobic training on fitness and quality of life in multiple sclerosis. Ann Neurol 1996;39:432–3.

[60] Blumenthal JA, Babyak MA, Moore KA, et al. Effects of exercise training on older patients with major depression. Arch Intern Med 1999;159:2349–56.

[61] Martinsen EW. Physical activity and depression: clinical experience. Acta Psychiatr Scand Suppl 1994;377:23–7.

[62] Babyak M, Blumenthal JA, Herman S, et al. Exercise treatment for major depression: maintenance of therapeutic benefit at 10 months. Psychosom Med 2000;62:633–8.

[63] Brown WJ, Ford JH, Burton NW, et al. Prospective study of physical activity and depressive symptoms in middle-aged women. Am J Prev Med 2005;29:265–72.

[64] Janssens AC, van Doorn PA, de Boer JB, et al. Anxiety and depression influence the relation between disability status and quality of life in multiple sclerosis. Mult Scler 2003;9:397–403.

[65] Feinstein A, O'Connor P, Gray T, et al. The effects of anxiety and psychiatric morbidity in patients with multiple sclerosis. Mult Scler 1999;5:323–6.

[66] Galeazzi GM, Ferrari S, Giaroli G, et al. Psychiatric disorders and depression in multiple sclerosis outpatients: impact of disability and interferon beta therapy. Neurol Sci 2005;26:255–62.

[67] Kessler RC, McGonagle KA, Zhao S, et al. Lifetime and 12-month prevalence of DSM-III-R psychiatric disorders in the United States. Results from the National Comorbidity Survey. Arch Gen Psychiatry 1994;51:8–19.

[68] Kellner CH, Davenport Y, Post RM, et al. Rapid cycling bipolar disorder and multiple sclerosis. Am J Psychiatry 1984;141:112–3.

[69] Salmaggi A, Eoli M, La Mantia L, et al. Parallel fluctuations of psychiatric and neurological symptoms in a patient with multiple sclerosis and bipolar affective disorder. Ital J Neurol Sci 1995;16:551–3.

[70] Kwentus JA, Hart RP, Calabrese V, et al. Mania as a symptom of multiple sclerosis. Psychosomatics 1986;27:729–31.

[71] Heila H, Turpeinen P, Erkinjuntti T. Case study: mania associated with multiple sclerosis. J Am Acad Child Adolesc Psychiatry 1995;34:1591–5.

[72] Krishnan KRR. Psychiatric and medical comorbidities of bipolar disorder. Psychosom Med 2005;67:1–8.

[73] Pine DS, Douglas CJ, Charles E, et al. Patients with multiple sclerosis presenting to psychiatric hospitals. J Clin Psychiatry 1995;56:297–306.

[74] Fisk JD, Morehouse SA, Brown MG, et al. Hospital-based psychiatric service utilization and morbidity in multiple sclerosis. Can J Neurol Sci 1998;25:230–5.

[75] Schiffer RB, Wineman M, Weitkamp LR. Association between bipolar affective disorder and multiple sclerosis. Am J Psychiatry 1986;143:94–5.

[76] Edwards LJ, Constantinescu CS. A prospective study of conditions associated with multiple sclerosis in a cohort of 658 consecutive outpatients attending a multiple sclerosis clinic. Mult Scler 2004;10:575–81.

[77] Lechtenberg R. Multiple sclerosis fact book. 2nd edition. Philadelphia: FA Davis; 1995.

[78] Parsons O, Nixon S. Cognitive functioning in sober social drinkers: a review of the research since 1986. J Stud Alcohol 1998;59:180–90.

[79] Moore D, Li L. Prevalence and risk factors of illicit drug use by people with disabilities. Am J Addict 1998;7:93–102.

[80] Sullivan LE, Fiellin DA, O'Connor PG. The prevalence and impact of alcohol problems in major depression: a systematic review. Am J Med 2005;118:330–41.

[81] Quesnel S, Feinstein A. Multiple sclerosis and alcohol: a study of problem drinking. Mult Scler 2004;10:197–201.

[82] Bombardier CH, Blake KD, Ehde DM, et al. Alcohol and drug abuse among persons with multiple sclerosis. Mult Scler 2004;10:35–40.

[83] First MB, Spitzer RL, Gibbon M, et al. Structured clinical interview for axis I DSM-IV disorders—patient edition. SCID-/p, Version 2.0. New York: New York State Psychiatric Institute; 1994.

[84] Bondy SJ, Rehm J, Ashley MJ, et al. Low-risk drinking guidelines: the scientific evidence. Can J Pub Health 1999;90:264–70.

[85] Spitzer RL, Williams JB, Kroenke K, et al. Utility of a new procedure for diagnosing mental disorders in primary care. The PRIME-MD 1000 study. JAMA 1994;272:1749–56.

[86] Institute of Medicine. Broadening the base of treatment for alcohol problems. Washington, DC: National Academy Press; 1990.

[87] Mayfield D, McLeod G, Hall P. The CAGE questionnaire: validation of a new alcoholism screening instrument. Am J Psychiatry 1974;131:1121–3.

[88] Fleming M, Barry K, Manwell L, et al. Brief physician advice for problem alcohol drinkers. J Am Med Assoc 1997;277:1039–45.

[89] Choy W, Gerstein DR, Ghadialy R, et al. National household survey on drug abuse: main findings, 1992. Rockville (MD): Substance Abuse and Mental health Services Administration; 1995.

[90] Goodin D. Marijuana and multiple sclerosis. Lancet Neurol 2004;3:79–80.

[91] Zajicek J, Fox P, Sanders H, et al. Cannabinoids for treatment of spasticity and other symptoms related to multiple sclerosis (CAMS study): multicentre randomised placebo-controlled trial. Lancet 2003;362:1517–26.

[92] Chong MS, Wolff K, Wise K, et al. Cannabis use in patients with multiple sclerosis. Mult Scler 2006;12:646–51.

[93] Clark AJ, Ware MA, Yazer E, et al. Patterns of cannabis use among patients with multiple sclerosis. Neurology 2004;62:2098–100.

[94] Feinstein A, Feinstein K, Gray T, et al. Prevalence and neurobehavioral correlates of pathological laughing and crying in multiple sclerosis. Arch Neurol 1997;54:1116–21.

[95] Schiffer RB, Herndon RM, Rudick RA. Treatment of pathologic laughing and weeping with amitriptyline. N Engl J Med 1985;312:1480–2.

[96] Seliger GM, Hornstein A. Serotonin, fluoxetine, and pseudobulbar affect. Neurology 1989;39(10):1400.

[97] Udaka F, Yamao S, Nagata H, et al. Pathologic laughing and crying treated with levodopa. Arch Neurol 1984;41:1095–6.
[98] Panitch HS, Thisted RA, Smith RA, et al. Randomized controlled trial of dextromethorphan/quinidine for pseudobulbar affect in multiple sclerosis. Ann Neurol 2006;59(5):780–7.
[99] Bonanno GA. Loss, trauma, and human resilience: have we underestimated the human capacity to thrive after extremely aversive events? Am Psychol 2004;59:20–8.
[100] Tedeschi RG, Calhoun LG. The Posttraumatic Growth Inventory: measuring the positive legacy of trauma. J Trauma Stress 1996;9:455–71.

Psychiatr Clin N Am 30 (2007) 819–835

PSYCHIATRIC CLINICS
OF NORTH AMERICA

Late Consequences of Chronic Pediatric Illness

Susan Turkel, MD[a], Maryland Pao, MD[b],*

[a]Childrens Hospital Los Angeles, University of Southern California Keck School of Medicine, 4650 Sunset Blvd #82, Los Angeles, CA 90027, USA
[b]Office of the Clinical Director, National Institute of Mental Health, National Institutes of Health, Building 10, Room 6-5340, 10 Center Drive, Bethesda, MD 20892, USA

With the advent of new treatments for chronic pediatric disorders such as cystic fibrosis (CF), juvenile rheumatoid arthritis, and congenital heart disease, more children and adolescents are surviving into adulthood than ever before. Seventy years ago, individuals who had CF survived an average of 5 years; currently the life expectancy for CF is more than 30 years [1]. Increased survival has brought new morbidities [2] and may affect psychosocial outcomes of adult life [3]. The prevalence of children suffering from a chronic illness varies widely, but the overall rate is 10% to 20% [4]. Children who have chronic illnesses are more likely to have emotional, behavioral, and psychiatric symptoms than healthy children [5] and may be psychologically affected or traumatized by medical treatments [6]. On the other hand, resilience is common [7], and chronically ill children do not inevitably develop psychiatric difficulties. This article is aimed at helping psychiatric consultants understand how medical, developmental, and psychosocial needs are altered in adults who have grown up with chronic pediatric illnesses. Three childhood conditions, congenital heart disease, CF, and rheumatologic disorders, are discussed in detail. These conditions are used as models to illustrate the impact of congenital malformations, genetic disorders, and typically adult disorders occurring in the pediatric age group.

EVALUATING CHRONICALLY ILL CHILDREN AND ADOLESCENTS

Three aspects of psychiatric consultation in the medically and surgically ill that are specific to working with youth are (1) an awareness of the cognitive and emotional developmental levels of the patient, (2) the essential role of the family, and

This research was supported in part by the National Institute of Mental Health. Dr. Pao's views are her own and do not necessarily reflect the opinions of the United States government.

*Corresponding author. E-mail address: paom@mail.nih.gov (M. Pao).

(3) a focus on facilitating coping and adjustment to illness to follow an optimal developmental trajectory, rather than a focus on psychopathology. Clinicians must be familiar with normal physical, motor, language, cognitive, sexual, and emotional development in chronically ill children to distinguish normal responses to stress from unhealthy ones [8]. Understanding a child's cognitive ability to process information is essential when communicating about his/her disease. Clinicians cannot assume that chronologic age is equivalent to mental age. Children who have medical illness may not develop at the same rate as healthy children because of delayed neurocognitive development, disruptions in education, and limited social experiences in addition to the influences of the medical condition and treatment on intellectual and somatic growth and maturation [9].

The hospital or clinic environment is often distressing or even traumatic for the chronically ill child. Injections, procedures, and surgeries are highly stressful experiences for children. Pain from medical conditions and treatments can provoke anxiety and affect later pain sensitivities and neurologic development [10]. Posttraumatic stress disorder is a risk with traumatic injury or intense hospital experiences such as transplantations. Identifying and easing potentially traumatic situations may decrease the child's stress and improve medical outcomes [11]. Clinicians should inquire into a patient's childhood medical disorders and treatments because these early experiences surely influence the patient's trust and use of the medical system as they develop into adults.

IMPAIRED GROWTH AND DEVELOPMENT AND IMPACT OF CHRONIC STEROID USE

Physical growth is a dynamic process that starts at conception and ends after full pubertal development [12]. Chronic illness may lead to growth retardation, either because of the illness itself or because of treatments required for it. Short stature commonly is perceived to be associated with social and psychologic disadvantage [13]. Parents often attribute behavioral disorders, anxiety, depression, social, and attentional problems to short stature and are concerned that their children are subjected to height-related stressors of being teased or infantilized [13]. It is difficult, however, to determine if problems in psychosocial functioning are caused by the underlying illness, treatment, or resultant effects such as impaired growth.

Long-term administration of systemic corticosteroids (eg, dexamethasone, prednisone) is a major cause of impaired growth but often is required for children and adolescents who have a range of chronic inflammatory, autoimmune, and neoplastic diseases. These agents also are often used to treat inflammatory bowel disease (IBD), asthma, CF, bone marrow and solid-organ transplants, nephrotic syndrome and other causes of renal failure, systemic lupus erythematosus (SLE), and juvenile arthritis. Children and adolescents who have these conditions are at high risk for growth failure, both from their underlying disease and from glucocorticoid therapy.

Multiple mechanisms play a role in the impact of glucocorticoids on bone development and growth. In the short term, bone loss and deterioration depend on the type and dose of glucocorticoid and occur most prominently in the first 6 months of treatment. Treatments directed at preventing bone loss during this period are more effective than attempts to compensate for lost growth later on [14]. Glucocorticoids have direct effects on the growth plate and disrupt growth plate vasculature. They have a suppressive effect on osteoblastogenesis and promote apoptosis of osteoblasts and osteocytes. This process may lead to decreased bone formation and osteonecrosis or to avascular necrosis of bone. Glucocorticoids may promote calcium loss through the kidneys and gastrointestinal tract, increasing bone remodeling and osteoclastic activity caused by secondary hyperparathyroidism. High-dose glucocorticoid therapy can attenuate physiologic growth hormone secretion and increase somatostatin tone and may also impair attainment of peak bone mass and delay growth through direct effects on gonadotropin and sex steroids [15].

Growth retardation has been reported in children who have chronic IBD, including ulcerative colitis, and especially in those who have Crohn's disease [16]. Typically children who have IBD grow more slowly before diagnosis and when disease is active. Growth retardation has been reported in 15% to 40% of children who have IBD [17]. Decreased height velocity may be the earliest indicator preceding the diagnosis of Crohn's disease. Chronic low nutrition generally is considered an important reason for growth impairment. Treating IBD may restore growth velocity, but ultimately the prolonged use of glucocorticoids may itself lead to growth retardation. Eventual height usually is normal in ulcerative colitis and is nearly normal in Crohn's disease, and delayed puberty may compensate for the period of poor growth earlier in life [16]. The incidence of osteoporosis, glaucoma, and cataracts also is higher in pediatric patients who have IBD treated with glucocorticoids than in adult patients [18]. Steroid-sparing agents such as 6-mercaptopurine may prevent growth retardation associated with chronic steroid use [17]. Mercaptopurine and its prodrug, azathioprine, are effective in maintaining remission in children who have Crohn's disease and may improve growth velocity and final adult height by controlling the disorder and sparing the child long-term glucocorticoid treatment [19].

Children who have chronic renal disease also may have growth retardation and often require glucocorticoid treatment to control their disease. Prednisone is associated with impairment of growth and body height in a dose-dependent fashion [20]. Children who have severe steroid-dependent nephrotic syndrome are at risk of permanent growth retardation caused by prolonged courses of steroid treatment [21]. Suboptimal final height and marked weight gain are common after renal transplantation and may result in significant obesity. After transplantation some children show improved growth, but height remains suboptimal, and steroids needed to maintain the transplant contribute to obesity [22]. Management of growth retardation before transplantation and further reduction in the steroid dose after transplantation may increase final height of children who have chronic renal failure [23].

In children who have severe rheumatic disorders, treatment with glucocorticoids is frequently needed and is associated with growth retardation and osteopenia [24]. Growth hormone treatment may improve growth and lean body mass, but these benefits disappear when growth hormone therapy is stopped. Long-term growth hormone treatment is necessary to maintain a potential positive effect on bone density and metabolism [25]. Children who have mild or moderate juvenile idiopathic arthritis (JIA) and lower medication requirements respond better to growth hormone therapy than those who have active disease [26]. Using growth hormone earlier may prevent growth deterioration and metabolic complications induced by chronic inflammation and prolonged steroid therapy [27]. Chronic inflammation and prednisone therapy may affect growth adversely, and final height may depend closely both on the severity of growth retardation during the active phase of the disease and on linear growth after remission [28]. After remission of active disease and discontinuation of prednisone treatment, 70% of children show catch-up growth, but 30% show persistent loss of height [29]. This observation has led to the recommendation that early initiation of growth hormone therapy may prevent growth deterioration and other metabolic complications induced by chronic inflammation and long-term steroid therapy [29]. Wider use of growth hormone in children and adolescents who have rheumatic disorders is not without risk, however, and growth hormone may lead to a flare of previously well-controlled SLE [30].

Children who have bronchial asthma, allergic rhinitis, and atopic dermatitis have a two- to five-times higher incidence of short stature, skeletal retardation, and delayed puberty. This limitation in growth probably is secondary to the severity and underlying mechanisms of their disorder. Local growth factor prostaglandin E_2, which is important in bone mineralization, is a messenger substance for both the immediate and late allergic reaction. Platelet-activating factor is one of the strongest mediators in the pathogenesis of allergic disorders, and it influences prostaglandin E_2 synthesis in osteoblasts [31]. Inhaled and nasal glucocorticoids rarely suppress adrenal function, although they may decrease prepubertal growth [32].

Children who have CF have reduced growth velocity and a delayed adolescent growth spurt [33]. This reduced growth rate may result from a combination of poor nutrition, pancreatic insufficiency, chronic inflammatory lung disease, and intestinal disease. Even with vigorous treatment of these problems, including dietary interventions to provide calories and fat-soluble vitamins in excess of usual recommended amounts [33], severe CF is associated with poor weight gain and slower growth [34]. Relative insulin deficiency rather than nutritional deprivation or poor clinical status may be implicated in the poor linear growth of children who have relatively stable lung disease [34].

Abnormal growth in CF also may be related to the primary dysfunction of a chloride channel regulated by cyclic-AMP. The gene for this chloride channel, *CFTR*, is found in the thalamus, hypothalamus, and amygdala of the brain, sites related to regulation of appetite, energy expenditure, and sexual maturation [33]. Inhibition of *CFTR* inhibits secretion of gonadotropin-releasing hormone in cell lines [33]. Failure of *CFTR* function may be related to inhibition of pubertal maturation as well as growth [33].

Twenty percent of all children in the 1993 National CF Patient Registry were below the fifth percentile for height or weight for age [35], 28% were below the tenth percentile for height, and 34% were below the tenth percentile for weight [36]. Growth hormone treatment enhances nutrition, linear growth, and weight gain in children who have CF [36], may improve height, weight, bone mineral content, and lean body mass in prepubertal children [37], and may reduce the number of hospitalizations with or without significantly changing pulmonary function, even in children receiving enteral nutritional supplementation [37,38]. Children homozygous for the Delta *F508* mutation, which is associated with the most severe disease, fail to normalize growth despite improved care [39].

Children who have CF often are treated with glucocorticoids, which can compound these growth problems. Attempts to mitigate the effects of steroids with alternate day therapy have yielded equivocal results, and although girls may regain their growth, boys have persistent growth impairment, even when the treatment is discontinued [40]. Focusing on reduced height alone as an important adverse effect of glucocorticoids may reflect cultural rather than medical imperatives [33]. Glucocorticoids also may compound the risk of diabetes, cataracts, and osteoporosis [33], which are not uncommon in CF.

The general consequences of malnutrition in CF may include growth failure, increased mortality, delayed puberty, decreased physical well being, and psychologic disorders [41]. Short stature and pubertal delay emphasize the differences between patients who have CF and their peers and have a greater impact on their quality of life than the longer-term issues of compromised survival [41,42]. Adjustment and self-esteem in patients who have CF are poorer than in peers, especially in girls [42]. With intensive, coordinated care in a CF center, outcome and growth may improve independent of improved pulmonary function and normalize in most children who have CF [39].

Growth itself is an important prognostic factor in survival of patients who have CF. Analysis of data from 19,000 patient records in the National Cystic Fibrosis Patient Registry showed that shorter patients are much more likely to die at a younger age than taller patients [43]. Short stature in CF may be a marker of more severe disease [43]. Ironically, the problem of worsening growth failure in children and adolescents who have CF is compounded by increased survival [41]. As patients live longer, and their clinical symptoms become more severe, nutritional status may worsen, and growth remains impaired [41]. It is important that linear growth be maximized through medical and nutritional intervention [43]. As patients who have CF age, bone mineralization is decreased, and rates of osteoporosis are significantly increased; adults who have late-stage CF are at high risk for fractures and severe kyphosis [44].

PSYCHOSOCIAL CONSIDERATIONS

Normative developmental tasks throughout childhood center on developing a sense of self and acquiring autonomy in all areas of life. When compared with their cohort in the general population, however, young adults who are chronically ill with a wide variety of disorders have lower academic and employment achievement, receive less vocational education and have less permanent employment [45], are more likely to be single [46], and have delayed independence [3]. Cohorts have not been followed long enough to establish whether this group "catches up" developmentally at a later point in adulthood, which might allow for survivors to make the transition from dependence to independence in their relationships and work.

Cross-sectional data on almost 100,000 children younger than 18 years in the 1992–1994 National Health Interview Survey showed that an estimated 6.5% of all children in the United States experienced some degree of disability (defined as a long-term reduction in ability to conduct social role activities such as school or play) because of a chronic condition [47]. The presence of a childhood disability is associated with elevated use of health care services, and these youth are four times as likely to be hospitalized and have eight times as many total hospital days as the general population. As these children have survived longer, physicians have become increasingly aware that the natural progression of pediatric disease and the consequences of treatment can adversely affect brain development and that compromises in cognitive abilities leading to mild impairments may have more permanent consequences in adolescence and adulthood [9]. Thus, childhood disability from chronic conditions significantly affects the educational and health care systems in the long term. Additionally, added caretaking demands and lost income for parents and the eventual detrimental impact of childhood disability on social and economic status in adulthood all take a toll [47].

The stage or severity of illness, including the degree of life threat, does not independently predict a person's adjustment to chronic illness. Low self-esteem in childhood, poor school attendance, and family factors all play significant roles. Older children, boys, children from poor families, and those from single-parent households have a significantly higher prevalence of disability even after multivariate analysis [47]. Medical illness may have some protective effects. For example, drug use, criminal convictions, and cigarette smoking are less common in young adults who have insulin-dependent diabetes mellitus than in their peers [48].

The high degree of variation in outcome measures such as restricted activity, days of school lost, severity of limitation, and use of medical services for different childhood conditions is notable and suggests that noncategorical approaches for studying chronic illness disability may not be adequate. Consideration of individual underlying conditions may be more relevant when developing health and social policies and improving outcomes of specific chronic conditions. This possibility also is supported by a literature review of the efficacy of psychologic interventions for chronic pediatric illnesses, which found 19 studies since 1980 that met criteria of external and internal validity for diabetes, CF, cancer, and sickle cell disease but overall showed a lack of evidence as to what sort of intervention is best for which patients [49]. Interventions need to be targeted individually, and the efficacy of different approaches needs to be assessed.

PSYCHIATRIC CONSEQUENCES

Investigations of psychiatric disorders in pediatric conditions have been limited by small and varied demographic samples, lack of consistent testing measurements, frequent subthreshold *Diagnostic and Statistical Manual of Mental Disorders,* fourth edition (DSM-IV) diagnoses, and lack of appropriate control groups. The full range of developmental and childhood psychiatric disorders, including adjustment disorder, major depression, anxiety, and delirium, are seen in children and adolescents who have chronic illness. Psychiatric disorders are most likely to be present when the chronic physical disorder involves the brain. Some aspects of treatment of life-threatening medical illness may be experienced as repeated trauma; the impact may not manifest during or immediately after treatment but rather may appear as long-term effects on affect modulation and interpersonal relationships [50].

Congenital Heart Disease

Depression is common in patients who have congenital heart disease and can exacerbate the physical consequences of the illness [51]. Children who have congenital heart disease may have more medical fear and general fear of the unknown, physiologic anxiety, depression, and delinquent behaviors than the general population [52]. Those who have cyanotic malformations may be at higher risk for these problems, which may be exacerbated further by maternal anxiety [52]. Adults who have more complex cyanotic disorders may have more problems with depression than those who have less severe lesions [53]. Slightly more than 36% of adults who have congenital heart disease meet DSM-IV criteria for a depressive episode or generalized anxiety disorder, and an additional 27% meet criteria for problematic emotional functioning [53]. Risk for either depression or anxiety is correlated significantly with medical severity [53]. Current research, however, demonstrates a wide range of psychiatric disturbances in adult survivors of congenital heart disease, and some studies demonstrate a lower prevalence of psychopathology [54]. Even when patients are found to have symptoms of psychiatric illness, they rarely receive psychiatric treatment [54,55]. Once surgery and hospitalizations are in the past, adult patients may strive to obtain a normal life, and, having survived a life-threatening illness, they may not worry about minor difficulties and ultimately achieve good social and vocational adjustment [54].

Cystic Fibrosis

As a group, adults who have CF do not demonstrate significant levels of depression, anxiety, or other psychopathology [56]. Psychologic and psychosocial functioning in patients who have CF is similar to that of healthy peers, at least until the disease becomes severe and the patient's physical and social activities become increasingly limited [57]. They then may have an increased risk for psychiatric problems, such as depression, and typically score poorly on physical functioning measures in quality-of-life assessments [57]. Coping styles have a large effect on quality of life, and compliance is a complicated problem for many patients [57]. Men may be at higher risk for depression and anxiety, and better lung function predicts less anxiety. A higher level of psychosocial support is a strong predictor of better psychologic functioning [56]. Major psychiatric illness also may occur in adults who have CF, and both bipolar disorder [58] and paranoia [59] have been reported.

Rheumatic Disorders

Pediatric rheumatic disorders are more common in girls than boys and affect about 200,000 children in the United States. Juvenile rheumatoid arthritis accounts for 75% to 85% of rheumatic diseases affecting children. These disorders are not curable, and the main goal of treatment is disease management, which includes reducing pain, controlling inflammation, maintaining function, and preventing deformities or persistent organ failure [60]. Rheumatologic disorders in pediatric patients typically are more severe clinically than the same disorders in adults and may have significant psychiatric and medical consequences. These conditions are treated with potent immunosuppressive medications, steroids, and immune modulators that also may be associated with psychiatric side effects. Psychiatric symptoms may be a reflection of an autoimmune process or related to the underlying vasculitis, or the psychiatric disorder may be unrelated and coincidental. Children who have rheumatologic disorders are at an increased risk for adjustment problems, particularly internalizing problems such as anxiety and depression, often seen in association with higher levels of family stress. Greater social support reduces the risk for these adjustment disorders [60]. Classmate and parental support seems to be the best predictor of adjustment [60]; and in contrast, poor body image and lack of satisfaction with social support are most predictive of poor psychosocial adjustment and function [61]. Parental functioning seems to play a role in determining the long-term effects of psychiatric complications of pediatric rheumatologic disorders, and parental distress and maternal depression are associated with more behavior problems in the ill child [62].

JIA is the most common rheumatologic disorder in childhood. Central nervous system (CNS) involvement is rare in JIA, but depressive and anxiety disorders are common and are attributed to social isolation, chronic pain, and deformity. Among adults who had long-standing JIA, who on average had 28 years of illness, 31.6% were anxious, 5.2% were depressed, and 21.1% had suffered previously from depression [61]. Pain intensity and level of anxiety were higher in this group of adults than in children and adolescents who had JIA [61]. Both physical and psychologic factors influence pain, and psychologic variables explain most of the variance in depression and anxiety in adults who had JIA [61].

As a patient enters adulthood, pain-coping strategies become an important predictor of pain, and higher levels of denial and dependence are detrimental to pain management [61]. The age of onset of disease may have an effect later in life on the effectiveness of learned coping strategies to avoid anxiety or depression; a later age of onset is associated with impaired self-identity and self-confidence and a greater sense of loss [61].

SLE is the prototypical generalized autoimmune disease, with variable clinical features affecting all organ systems. CNS involvement occurs in more than half of the children and adolescents who have SLE, usually early in the course of the disease, and typically includes both neurologic and psychiatric symptoms [63–65]. Cognitive, mood, and psychotic symptoms in CNS lupus may be related to an underlying vasculitis or may reflect the impact of antiphospholipid, antineuronal, antireceptor antibodies. Although there are numerous studies of psychiatric problems in adult patients who have SLE, and some studies describe mood, cognitive, and psychotic problems in pediatric patients who have SLE [66], there are no outcome studies of the long-term consequences of pediatric psychosocial dysfunction.

The presence of delirium, psychosis, confusion, depression, or mania in a patient who has SLE suggests primary CNS involvement. The diagnosis of CNS-SLE should be suspected when neuropsychiatric symptoms occur in patients known to have SLE and should be investigated in children and adolescents who have acute onset of delirium or profound psychiatric symptoms, with or without neurologic symptoms [66].

SLE is associated with both primary and secondary effects on psychosocial functioning. The prevalence rate of depressive symptoms in SLE is 30% [67]. Depression may be related to the effect of pain and fatigue on mood symptoms [68]. Psychosis, depression, anxiety, cognitive deficits, and emotional distress are seen frequently in patients who have SLE [69]. Depression and other neuropsychiatric symptoms in patients who have SLE are associated with increased risk for suicidal behavior [70]. Fortunately, in patients who have SLE, depression usually responds to antidepressant therapy [67].

Depression may predict cognitive dysfunction in patients who have SLE [71]. Emotional disturbances and problems with social functioning, personal discomfort in social situations, and depressed mood are more frequent in patients who have SLE with skin and joint abnormalities, confirming that psychosocial dysfunction may not only be a reflection of direct CNS involvement [72].

The pathogenesis of neuropsychiatric SLE has been attributed to autoantibody-mediated neural dysfunction, vasculopathy, and coagulopathy. Several autoantibodies have been reported in serum and cerebrospinal fluid, including antineuronal, antiribosomal P proteins, antiglial fibrillary acidic proteins, antiphospholipid, and antiendothelial antibodies [73]. Anti-Nedd5 antibodies have been found to be associated with psychosis in patients who have SLE [73]. Anti-N-methyl-D-aspartate receptor antibodies have been associated with neuropsychiatric symptoms in SLE, but their presence alone does not explain cognitive dysfunction, depression, or anxiety in patients who have SLE [74]. Anti-NR2a antibodies may be associated with depressed mood but may not be associated with cognitive dysfunction in patients who have SLE [75].

Antineuronal antibodies and abnormalities seen on a single-photon emission CT scan seem to be useful in diagnosing CNS-SLE in pediatric patients [66].

TRANSITION TO ADULT CARE

Adolescence is a complex period of transition from childhood to adulthood. Having a chronic illness adds to the complexity (Table 1). Issues of puberty, autonomy, personal identity, sexuality, education, and vocational choices become more difficult for an adolescent who also is coping with chronic illness. This period may be complicated further by medical setbacks, impaired physical or mental abilities, forced dependence, and perceived poor prognosis [76]. For adolescents who have a chronic illness, perception of their illness severity is related directly to their psychosocial well being [77]. A generation ago, few children who had severe chronic illness or disability survived to 21 years, and issues of transition from pediatric to adult health care were rarely considered [76]. Now more than 90% of children who have chronic or disabling conditions survive beyond their second decade, and more than 30% of young people 10 to 17 years old have a chronic condition [78].

The previously unanticipated problem of transitioning a pediatric patient who has congenital heart disease, malignancies, rheumatologic disorders, CF, or transplants to adult care is beginning to be addressed. There are two different approaches to planning for the transition of adolescents who have chronic medical problems to adult medical care. One approach is transfer to a specialized center with care focused on pediatric disorders in adults, such as with CF or congenital heart disease [79]. The other involves the transfer to adult specialists of patients who have had a pediatric onset of what is usually considered an adult disorder, such as IBD or a rheumatologic disorder [80]. Either way, the process of transition usually begins with a discussion of the planned transfer to adult care long (as much as a year or more) before it is anticipated to occur. Ideally, the process should be a guided educational and

Table 1
Differences between pediatric and adult care

Pediatric Care	Adult Care
Family oriented	Individual focused
Developmental aspects considered	Specifically focused on health
Coordinates with schools and social services	Less communication with social services or workplace
More help with treatment regimen	More accepting of treatment refusal
More trainee supervision	Less trainee supervision
Paternalistic	Shared treatment decisions

Data from Robertson L. When should young people with chronic rheumatic disease move from paediatric to adult-centred care? Best Pract Res Clin Rheumatol 2006;20(2):387–97.

therapeutic transition rather than an administrative event [81]. Transition can be viewed as a positive step as the patient graduates from a pediatric to adult program. It may be difficult for chronically ill adolescent patients to break ties with the pediatrician, to feel accepted by their peer group, and to plan realistically for the future [82], although parents and pediatricians typically are more concerned about the transition than are the patients and their adult physicians [83].

It often is difficult for pediatricians to let go of their patients, and the age limit of pediatric practice has been steadily increasing. In 1938, the American Academy of Pediatrics defined the limit of pediatric practice at 16 to 18 years. By 1972, this age limit had increased to 21 years. In 1990 the American Academy of Pediatrics stated that the services of a pediatrician may continue to be the optimal source of health care past the age of 21 years, which may have the effect of prolonging entry into adulthood for young individuals who have chronic diseases [83]. In 1989 the Surgeon General of the United States convened a multidisciplinary conference to address strategies for the implementation of medical care systems for growing youth with special needs, and a transition manual was published to aid health professionals in the transfer of chronically ill adolescents to adult care systems [84]. The British National Health Service has highlighted the importance of ensuring safe and effective transition from children's services into adulthood [84]. The American Academy of Pediatrics Committee on Children with Disabilities and Committee on Adolescence issued a policy statement addressing issues of transition in 1996 that remains the current standard [85].

Transfer is not the same as transition. Transfer occurs when information or people move from pediatric to adult care. Transition is a multifaceted process that addresses the psychosocial, educational, and vocational needs of adolescents as they move from child-oriented to adult-oriented care. Ideally, the patient should be provided a coordinated, uninterrupted care plan that is developmentally appropriate and comprehensive [86].

The primary barriers to effective transition are limitations in the health care system itself, related to funding and identification of appropriate resources, rather than family or adolescent resistance [78]. There is little agreement on the best methods or optimal time for transition from pediatric to adult care, but the process of transition can be improved by timely discussion among the patient and family and treatment team members in both the pediatric and adult settings [87]. There now are more than 1 million adults who have congenital heart defects living in the United States; under current guidelines these patients should be seen every 12 to 24 months by a cardiologist with specific expertise in congenital heart disease to monitor for potential serious complications in this population [79]. Unfortunately, more than a quarter of patients have no cardiac follow-up after they turn 18 years old and pediatric cardiac care is discontinued [79]. Some patients fail to get follow-up for more than 10 years and typically demonstrate a poor level of knowledge about their heart condition [88]. Failure to address transition properly during adolescence may result in an adult who cannot effectively be responsible for his/her own care [89].

Noncompliance with treatment, particularly prevalent in adolescents, requires attention to psychologic and social issues as well as medical factors [90]. The young person must have sufficient self-management skills to adapt to adult-oriented medical systems, and long-term social support may need to be established before the transfer is complete [87].

It is important that pediatric relationships are terminated appropriately as part of the transition process [91]. Pediatricians themselves can become barriers in the process of transitioning to adult care and may resist the transition process because they lack confidence in their adult colleagues [92]. Pediatric medical practice and adult medical practice represent two different medical subcultures [91]. Often there is lack of communication between internists and pediatricians, no common guidelines, and differences in the management of patients [93]. For example, endocrinologists treating adults use different tests to re-evaluate diagnosis and higher doses of medications such as growth hormone than pediatricians caring for adolescents [93].

A move toward a culture of personal responsibility for health care is crucial for the promotion of the maturing patient's independence [92]. The purpose of transition is to prepare the patient for the transfer to adult medicine by helping the patient gain an understanding of the clinical picture of the disease, treatment goals, and possibilities, and develop a personal responsibility for medication and diet [94]. A carefully planned transition to adult health care should improve self-reliance, enhance autonomy and independence, and support young people in attaining their maximum potential and meaningful adult lives [95].

SUMMARY

There are many challenges in coping with and adapting to life with a chronic disease, and increased survival cannot be assumed to be associated with increased quality of life. A recent systematic review shows there is wide variation in outcomes depending on the definitions and measurements used to estimate the prevalence of chronic health conditions, making the impact of disability on children's health and social functioning difficult to assess; various authors have called for an international consensus about the conceptual definition of chronic health conditions in childhood [96]. It frequently is difficult to determine if problems in psychosocial functioning are caused by the underlying illness, by treatment, or by the resultant effects of either illness or treatment on physical growth or cognitive development. Assessment and treatment of mental health should be an integral component of the comprehensive care of chronically ill children and adolescents. Transition of care is an important process that addresses significant changes from child-oriented to adult-oriented care. Adults who have chronic health conditions should continue to be evaluated periodically for late consequences of the childhood illness and early medical care, and attention should be paid to their ongoing psychosocial, psychiatric, educational, and vocational needs.

References

[1] CF Foundation 2005. Cystic Fibrosis Foundation, 50 years of progress, hope. Bethesda (MD): Cystic Fibrosis Foundation; 2005.

[2] American Academy of Pediatrics, Committee on Psychosocial Aspects of Child and Family Health. The new morbidity revisited: a renewed commitment to the psychosocial aspects of pediatric care. Pediatrics 2001;108(5):1227–30.

[3] Gledhill J, Rangel L, Garralda E. Surviving chronic physical illness: psychosocial outcome in adult life. Arch Dis Child 2000;83:104–10.

[4] Janse AJ, Uiterwaal CSPM, Genke RJBJ, et al. A difference in perception of quality of life in chronically ill children was found between parents and pediatricians. J Clin Epidemiol 2005;58:495–502.

[5] Knapp PK, Harris ES. Consultation-liaison in child psychiatry: a review of the past 10 years. Part I: clinical findings. J Am Acad Child Adolesc Psychiatry 1998;37(1):17–25.

[6] Stuber ML, Schneider S, Kassam-Adams N, et al. The medical traumatic stress toolkit. CNS Spectr 2006;11:137–42.

[7] Rutter M. Implications of resilience concepts for scientific understanding. Ann NY Acad Sci 2006;1094:1–12.

[8] Pao M, Ballard ED, Rosenstein DL. Growing up in the hospital. JAMA 2007;297:2752–5.

[9] Armstrong FD. Neurodevelopment and chronic illness: mechanisms of disease and treatment. Ment Retard Dev Disabil Res Rev 2006;12:168–73.

[10] Fitzgerald M, Beggs S. The neurobiology of pain: developmental aspects. Neuroscientist 2001;7(3):246–57.

[11] National Child Traumatic Stress Network. Medical events and traumatic stress in children and families. Available at: http://www.nctsnet.org/nccts/nav.do?pid=typ_mt. Accessed December 12, 2005.

[12] Patel L, Dixon M, David TJ. Growth and growth charts in cystic fibrosis. J R Soc Med 2003;96(Suppl 43):35–41.

[13] Voss LD. Short normal stature and psychosocial disadvantage: a critical review of the literature. J Pediatr Endocrinol Metab 2001;14(6):701–11.

[14] Hochberg Z. Mechanisms of steroid impairment of growth. Horm Res 2002;58(Suppl 1): 33–8.

[15] Mushtaq T, Ahmed SF. The impact of corticosteroids on growth and bone health. Arch Dis Child 2002;87(2):93–6.

[16] Saha M-T, Ruuska T, Laippala P, et al. Growth of prepubertal children with inflammatory bowel disease. J Pediatr Gastroenterol 1998;26(3):310–4.

[17] Newby EA, Sawczenko A, Thomas AG, et al. Interventions for growth failure in childhood Crohn's disease. Cochrane Database Syst Rev 2005;3:CD003873.

[18] Uchida K, Araki T, Toiyama Y, et al. Preoperative steroid-related complications in Japanese pediatric patients with ulcerative colitis. Dis Colon Rectum 2006;49(1):74–9.

[19] Ballinger A. Management of growth retardation in the young patient with Crohn's disease. Expert Opin Pharmacother 2002;3(1):1–7.

[20] Hung YT, Yang L-Y. Follow-up of linear growth of body height in children with nephritic syndrome. J Microbiol Immunol Infect 2006;39(5):422–5.

[21] Emma F, Sesto A, Rizzoni G. Long term linear growth of children with severe steroid-responsive nephrotic syndrome. Pediatr Nephrol 2003;18(8):783–8.

[22] Vester U, Schaefer A, Kranz B, et al. Development of growth and body mass index after pediatric renal transplantation. Pediatr Transplant 2005;9(4):445–9.

[23] Motoyama O, Hasegawa A, Ohara T, et al. A prospective trial of steroid withdrawal after renal transplantation treated with cyclosporine and mizoribine in children: results obtained between 1990 and 2003. Pediatr Transplant 2005;9(2):232–8.

[24] Grote FK, Van Suijlekom-Smit LWA, Mul D, et al. Growth hormone treatment in children with rheumatic disease, corticosteroid induced growth retardation and osteopenia. Arch Dis Child 2006;91(1):56–60.

[25] Bechtold S, Ripperger P, Bonfig W, et al. Bone mass development and bone metabolism in juvenile idiopathic arthritis: treatment with growth hormone for four years. J Rheumatol 2004;31(7):1407–12.

[26] Bechtold S, Ripperger P, Hafner R, et al. Growth hormone improves height in patients with juvenile idiopathic arthritis: 4 year data of a controlled study. J Pediatr 2003;143(4):512–9.

[27] Simon D, Lucidarme N, Prieur A-M, et al. Treatment of growth failure in juvenile chronic arthritis. Horm Res 2002;58(Suppl 1):28–32.

[28] Simon D, Fernando C, Czernichow P, et al. Linear growth and final height in patients with systemic juvenile idiopathic arthritis treated with longterm glucocorticoids. J Rheumatol 2002;9(6):1296–300.

[29] Simon D, Lucidarme N, Prieur A-M, et al. Linear growth in children suffering from juvenile idiopathic arthritis requiring steroid therapy: natural history and effects of growth hormone treatment on linear growth. J Pediatr Endocrinol 2001;14(Suppl 6):1483–6.

[30] Bae YS, Bae SC, Lee SW, et al. Lupus flare associated with growth hormone. Lupus 2001;10(6):448–50.

[31] Baum WF, Schneyer U, Lantzsch AM, et al. Delay of growth and development in children with bronchial asthma, atopic dermatitis and allergic rhinitis. Exp Clin Endocrinol Diabetes 2002;110(2):53–9.

[32] Sizonenko PC. Effects of inhaled or nasal glucocorticoids on aqdrenal function and growth. J Pediatr Endocrinol 2002;15(1):5–26.

[33] Davis PB, Kercsmar CM. Growth in children with chronic lung disease. N Engl J Med 2000;342(12):887–8.

[34] Ripa P, Robertson I, Dowley D, et al. The relationship between insulin, insulin-like growth factor axis and growth in children with cystic fibrosis. Clin Endocrinol 2002;56(3):383–9.

[35] Lai HC, Kosorok MR, Sondel SA, et al. Growth status in children with cystic fibrosis based on the National Cystic Fibrosis Patient Registry data: evaluation of various criteria used to identify malnutrition. J Pediatr 1998;132(3 Pt 1):478–85.

[36] Hardin DS, Sy JP. Effects of growth hormone treatment in children with cystic fibrosis: the National Cooperative Growth Study experience. J Pediatr 1997;131(1 Pt 2):S65–9.

[37] Hardin DS, Stratton R, Krramer JC, et al. Growth hormone improves weight velocity and height velocity in prepubertal children with cystic fibrosis. Horm Metab Res 1998;30(10):636–41.

[38] Hardin DS, Rice J, Ahn C, et al. Growth hormone treatment enhances nutrition and growth in children with cystic fibrosis receiving enteral nutrition. J Pediatr 2005;146:324–8.

[39] Keller BM, Aebischer CC, Kraemer R, et al. Growth in prepubertal children with cystic fibrosis, homozygous for the Delta F508 mutation. J Cyst Fibros 2003;2(2):76–83.

[40] Lai HC, FitzSimmons SC, Allen DB, et al. Risk of persistent growth impairment after alternate-day prednisone treatment in children with cystic fibrosis. N Engl J Med 2000;342(12):851–9.

[41] McNaughton SA, Stormont DA, Shepherd RW, et al. Growth failure in cystic fibrosis. J Paediatr Child Health 1999;35(1):86–92.

[42] Sawyer SM, Rosier MJ, Phelan PD, et al. The self-image of adolescents with cystic fibrosis. J Adolesc Health 1995;16(3):204–8.

[43] Beker LT, Russek-Cohen E, Fink RJ. Stature as a prognostic factor in cystic fibrosis. J Am Diet Assoc 2001;101(4):438–42.

[44] Aris RM, Renner JB, Winders AD, et al. Increased rate of fractures and severe kyphosis: sequelae of living into adulthood with cystic fibrosis. Ann Intern Med 1998;128(3):186–93.

[45] Kokkonen J. The social effects in adult life of chronic physical illness since childhood. Eur J Pediatr 1995;154:676–81.

[46] Pless IB, Cripps HA, Davies JMC, et al. Chronic physical illness in childhood: psychological and social effects in adolescence and adult life. Dev Med Child Neurol 1989;31:746–55.

[47] Newachek PW, Halfon N. Prevalence and impact of disabling chronic conditions in childhood. Am J Public Health 1998;88(4):610–7.

[48] Jacobson AM, Hauser ST, Willett JB, et al. Psychological adjustment to IDDM: 10-year follow-up of an onset cohort of child and adolescent patients. Diabetes Care 1997;20:811–8.

[49] Beale IL. Scholarly literature review: efficacy of psychological interventions for pediatric chronic illnesses. J Pediatr Psychol 2006;31(5):437–51.

[50] Stuber ML, Shemesh E, Saxe GN. Posttraumatic stress responses in children with life-threatening illnesses. Child Adolesc Psychiatr Clin N Am 2003;12:195–209.

[51] Lip GYH, Lane DA, Millane TA, et al. Psychological interventions for depression in adolescent and adult congenital heart disease. Cochrane Database Syst Rev 2003;3:CD004394.

[52] Gupta S, Giuffre RM, Crawford S, et al. Covert fears, anxiety and depression in congenital heart disease. Cardiol Young 1998;8(4):491–9.

[53] Bromberg JI, Beasley PJ, D'Angelo EJ, et al. Depression and anxiety in adults with congenital heart disease: a pilot study. Heart Lung 2003;32(2):105–10.

[54] Cox D, Lewis G, Stuart G, et al. A cross sectional study of the prevalence of psychopathology in adults with congenital heart disease. J Psychosom Res 2002;52(2):65–8.

[55] Horner T, Liberthson R, Jellinek MS. Psychosocial profile of adults with complex congenital heart disease. Mayo Clin Proc 2000;75(1):31–6.

[56] Anderson D, Flume PA, Hardy KK. Psychological functioning of adults with cystic fibrosis. Chest 2001;119(4):1079–84.

[57] Pfeffer PE, Pfeffer JM, Hodson ME. The psychosocial and psychiatric side of cystic fibrosis in adolescents and adults. J Cyst Fibros 2003;2:61–8.

[58] Turkel SB, Cafaro DR. Lithium treatment of a bipolar patient with cystic fibrosis. Am J Psychiatry 1992;149:574.

[59] Stepniak-Ziolkiewicz I, Pierzchala W. Cystic fibrosis and pregnancy. Wiad Lek 2002;55(5-6):346–50.

[60] von Weiss RT, Rapoff MA, Varni JW, et al. Daily hassles and social support as predictors of adjustment in children with pediatric rheumatic disease. J Pediatr Psychol 2002;27(2):155–65.

[61] Packham JC, Hall MA, Pimm TJ. Long-term follow-up of 246 adults with juvenile idiopathic arthritis: predictive factors for mood and pain. Rheumatology 2002;41(12):1444–9.

[62] Frank RG, Hagglund KH, Schopp LH, et al. Disease and family contributors to adaptation in juvenile rheumatoid arthritis and juvenile diabetes. Arthritis Care Res 1998;11(3):166–76.

[63] Rosenberg AM. Systemic lupus erythematosus in children. Springer Semin Immunopathol 1994;16:261–79.

[64] Silber TJ, Chatoor I, White PH. Psychiatric manifestations of SLE in children and adolescents. Clin Pediatr 1984;23:331–5.

[65] Steinlin MI, Blaser SI, Gilday DL, et al. Neurologic manifestations of pediatric systemic lupus erythematosus. Pediatr Neurol 1995;13:191–7.

[66] Turkel SB, Miller JH, Reiff A. Case series: neuropsychiatric symptoms with pediatric systemic lupus erythematosus. J Am Acad Child Adolesc Psychiatry 2001;40:282–5.

[67] Kawakatsu S, Wada T. Rheumatic disease and depression. Nippon Rinsho 2001;59(8):1578–82, [in Japanese].

[68] Hutchinson GA, Nehall JE, Simeon DT. Psychiatric disorders in systemic lupus erythematosus. West Indian Med J 1996;45(2):48–50.

[69] Denberg SD, Carbotte RM, Denburg JA. Psychological aspects of systemic lupus erythematosus: cognitive function, mood, and self report. J Rheumatol 1997;24:998–1003.

[70] Karassa FB, Magliano M, Isenberg DA. Suicide attempts in patients with systemic lupus erythematosus. Ann Rheum Dis 2003;62(1):58–60.

[71] Monastero R, Bettini P, Del Zotto E, et al. Prevalence and pattern of cognitive impairment in systemic lupus erythematosus patients with and without overt neuropsychiatric manifestations. J Neurol Sci 2001;184(1):33–9.

[72] Waterloo K, Omdal R, Husby G, et al. Emotional status in systemic lupus erythematosus. Scand J Rheumatol 1998;27(6):410–4.

[73] Valesini G, Alessandri C, Celestino D, et al. Anti-endothelial antibodies and neuropsychiatric systemic lupus erythematosus. Ann NY Acad Sci 2006;1069:118–28.

[74] Harrison MJ, Ravdin LD, Lockshin MD. Relationship between serum NR2a antibodies and cognitive dysfunction in systemic lupus erytehmatosus. Arthritis Rheum 2006;54(8):2515–22.

[75] Lapteva L, Nowak M, Yarboro CH, et al. Anti-N-methyl-D-aspartate receptor antibodies, cognitive dysfunction, and depression in systemic lupus erythematosus. Arthritis Rheum 2006;54(8):2505–14.

[76] Blum RW, Garell D, Hodgman CH, et al. Transition from child-centered to adult health care systems for adolescents with chronic conditions. J Adolesc Health 1993;14:570–6.

[77] Leung SS, Steinbeck KS, Kohn MR, et al. Chronic illness perception in adolescence: implications for the doctor-patient relationship. J Paediatr Child Health 1997;33(2):107–12.

[78] Scal P, Evans T, Blozis S, et al. Trends in transition from pediatric to adult health care services for young adults with chronic conditions. J Adolesc Health 1999;24:259–64.

[79] Reid GJ, Irvine MJ, McCrindle BW, et al. Prevalence and correlates of successful transfer from pediatric to adult health care among a cohort of young adults with complex congenital heart defects. Pediatrics 2004;113:197–205.

[80] Tucker LB, Cabral DA. Transition of the adolescent patient with rheumatic disease: issues to consider. Pediatr Clin North Am 2005;52:641–52.

[81] Viner R. Transition from paediatric to adult care: bridging the gaps or passing the buck? Arch Dis Child 1999;81:271–5.

[82] Conway SP. Transition from paediatric to adult-oriented care for adolescents with cystic fibrosis. Disabil Rehabil 1998;20(6):209–16.

[83] Schildlow DV, Fiel SB. Life beyond pediatrics: transition of chronically ill adolescents from pediatric to adult health care systems. Med Clin North Am 1990;74(5):1113–20.

[84] Child Health and Maternity Services Branch. Transition: getting it right for young people, improving the transition of young people with long term conditions from children's to adult health services. London: National Health Services; 2006. p. 1–46.

[85] Ziring PR, Brazdziunas D, Gonzalez de Pijem L, et al. Transition of care provided for adolescents with special health care needs. Pediatrics 1996;98(6):1203–6.

[86] Robertson L. When should young people with chronic rheumatic disease move from paediatric to adult-centred care? Best Pract Res Clin Rheumatol 2006;20(2):387–97.

[87] Watson AR. Transitioning adolescents from pediatric to adult dialysis units. Adv Perit Dial 1996;12:176–8.

[88] Dore A, de Guise P, Mercier L-A. Transition of care to adult congenital heart centres: what do patients know about their heart condition? Can J Cardiol 2002;18(2):141–6.

[89] Knauth A, Verstappen A, Reiss J, et al. Transition and transfer from pediatric to adult care of the young adult with complex congenital heart disease. Cardiol Clin 2006;24:619–29.

[90] Watson AR. Problems and pitfalls of transition from paediatric to adult renal care. Pediatr Nephrol 2005;20(2):113–7.

[91] Reiss JG, Gibson RW, Walker LR. Health care transition: youth, family and provider perspectives. Pediatrics 2005;115(5):1449–50.

[92] Fox A. Physicians as barriers to successful transitional care. Internat J Adolesc Med Health 2002;14(1):3–7.

[93] Volta C, Luppino T, Street ME, et al. Transition from pediatric to adult care of children with chronic endocrine diseases: a survey on the current modalities in Italy. J Endocrinol Invest 2003;26(2):157–62.

[94] Donckerwolcke RA, van Zeben-van der Aa DM. Transfer of the care for adolescents with chronic diseases: from pediatrics to specialists for adults. Ned Tijdschr Geneeskd 2002;146(25):1205–6.

[95] Rosen DS. Transition of young people with respiratory diseases to adult health care. Paediatr Respir Rev 2004;5(2):124–31.

[96] van der Lee JH, Mokkink LB, Grootenhuis MA, et al. Definitions and measurement of chronic health conditions in childhood: a systematic review. JAMA 2007;287:2741–51.

Psychiatr Clin N Am 30 (2007) 837–854

PSYCHIATRIC CLINICS
OF NORTH AMERICA

Psychiatric Issues in Toxic Exposures

James S. Brown, Jr., MD, MPH[a,b,*]

[a]Department of Psychiatry, Virginia Commonwealth University School of Medicine, Richmond, VA 23113, USA
[b]Clinical Services, Crossroads Community Services Board, 216 Bush River Drive, P.O. Drawer 248, Farmville, VA 23901, USA

C hemical toxins pose challenges to local, regional, and international mental health, especially in the world's increasingly global community. Although exposures to some chemicals in the United States are less common now than just a few decades ago, today's psychiatric literature recognizes that heavy metals, industrial chemicals, pesticides, and ionizing radiation remain threats in the twenty-first century. Weapons of mass destruction (WMD) have also emerged as potential causes of mass psychiatric casualties. To illustrate how frequently the media report potential toxic exposures of psychiatric importance, the author retrieved the following news from March to June, 2007:

1. The risk for regional nuclear war now exceeds the threat of global nuclear war. Regional nuclear war would kill millions, cause large numbers of radiation casualties, and lead to global environmental catastrophe [1].
2. Regional poisoning from naturally occurring arsenic in South Asia may be the largest mass poisoning in human history [2]. Observers report thousands of cases of arsenicosis and more than 120,000,000 people living in contaminated areas [2].
3. The US Food and Drug Administration recalled pet foods contaminated with melamine, a compound used in plastics [3]. Whether melamine entered the human food chain remains undecided at this writing, but the event demonstrates how pet injury in a chemical disaster would increase individual stress reactions.
4. The US Food and Drug Administration advised consumers to throw away toothpaste imported from China because the toothpaste may contain diethylene glycol [4].

Also emerging in the twenty-first century is the view that gene-environment interactions probably cause many chronic diseases. The Exposure Biology Program at the National Institutes of Health now envisions a personal biosensor designed to warn the wearer of so-called "environmental stressors," such as

*Corresponding author. P.O. Box 622, Midlothian, VA 23113.
E-mail address: jbrown2185@aol.com

0193-953X/07/$ – see front matter
doi:10.1016/j.psc.2007.07.004
© 2007 Elsevier Inc. All rights reserved.
psych.theclinics.com

pesticides and solvents [5]. Because certain pesticides and solvents also cause psychiatric illness, preventive strategies like personal biosensors might eventually have psychiatric applications. To assist psychiatrists in remaining acquainted with chemical injuries and their psychiatric aftermath from direct neurotoxicity or traumatic stress, this article focuses on certain chemicals or toxic exposures with the greatest potential for causing psychiatric injury in the twenty-first century. The author previously published an extensive review of this subject elsewhere [6]. Relying mostly on sources from the twenty-first century, this article updates the previous work and reinforces the importance of these issues to current psychiatric practice.

CHEMICAL EXPOSURES FROM WARFARE AND TERRORISM

Judging from recent events and the present threat of regional wars and terrorist attacks, psychiatrists should familiarize themselves with the psychiatric effects of chemical warfare and terrorism. Table 1 lists frequently encountered symptoms of military- or terrorist-related chemical exposures. In addition to chemical warfare in World War I and the Iran-Iraq War of 1980 to 1988, examples of military-related chemicals of psychiatric importance include herbicides, such as Agent Orange, used during the Vietnam War. Diabetes, heart disease, and other long-term health effects in exposed Vietnam War veterans

Table 1
Commonly reported psychiatric symptoms of military-related exposures

Symptom	Nerve gas[a]	Ionizing radiation	Agent orange	GWS
Mood lability	X			X
Anxiety	X		X	
Irritability	X		X	X
Depression	X	X		
Apathy	X			X
Agitation	X		X	
Suicidal	X		X	
Confusion	X			
Poor concentration	X	X		
Memory loss	X	X		X
Hallucinations	X	X		
Paranoia	X	X		
Dissociation	X			
Nightmares	X	X		
Insomnia	X		X	X
Excessive dreaming	X			
Fatigue	X	X	X	X
Poor appetite	X	X		
Change in libido	X		X	
Somatic complaints	X			X
Mental retardation	X			
Dementia	X			

Abbreviation: GWS, Gulf War syndrome.
[a]Includes related pesticides.

have been attributed to Agent Orange [7]. Investigators attribute the health problems from Agent Orange to dioxin, a contaminant of the herbicide. Whether dioxin has specific neurotoxic qualities remains unclear, but psychiatric symptoms have been reported with exposure (see Table 1) [8].

The Gulf War of 1990 to 1991 ended with large numbers of veterans developing so-called "Gulf War syndrome" (GWS), a nonspecific condition manifested by psychiatric and somatic symptoms purported to result from chemical exposures during the war. Extensive research performed since the war identified stress as the likely cause of GWS rather than any chemical or biologic exposures [9]. Proponents of the view that stress caused most cases of GWS attribute the syndrome to combat stress-related conditions similar to those resulting from other modern wars [9].

Recent developments in GWS research include the finding that Gulf War veterans have elevated rates of amyotrophic lateral sclerosis (ALS) [10–12]. Even though stress is the leading cause of most cases of GWS, chemical exposures did occur during the war, as shown by the confirmed exposure of thousands of troops during the war to subclinical levels of nerve gases released by the destruction of an ammunition dump in Khamisiyah, Iraq. Later studies found increased health problems and impaired neurobehavioral functioning in the exposed troops [13–15]. Although a wide disparity still exists among studies of GWS, clinicians should remain vigilant for neurologic illness in Gulf War veterans.

"Nerve gas" is the common name for at least four organophosphate chemical weapons. The primary nerve gases include tabun, soman, sarin, and VX. Terrorists used sarin in attacks in Japan in the 1990s [16]. All nerve gases, such as the chemically related organophosphate insecticides that are discussed in this article, exert their effects by inhibiting acetylcholinesterase and allowing synaptic accumulation of acetylcholine and continuous nervous stimulation [17]. The resulting widespread parasympathetic and sympathetic stimulation ends with multisystem organ failure. Table 1 lists the psychiatric symptoms in survivors of clinically recognized nerve gas poisoning (and related pesticides). Table 2 lists the *Diagnostic and Statistical Manual of Mental Disorders, Fourth Edition*, text revision (DSM-IV-TR) [18] psychiatric disorders resulting from organophosphate compounds. The mental effects of these chemicals, recognized more than 50 years ago [19], include mood and perceptual abnormalities, with changes in behavior and cognition.

Other chemical weapons include cyanide, chlorine, phosgene, mustard, arsenic compounds, and a compound called BZ. Arsenic and BZ have the greatest potential to cause psychiatric impairment as a result of direct neurotoxic effects. BZ, also known as 3-quinuclidinyl benzilate (QNB) or "Agent Buzz," is a hallucinogenic chemical developed by the United States as a psychiatric chemical weapon [20,21]. BZ has anticholinergic effects and lethality similar to atropine and can be absorbed through the lungs, skin, and gastrointestinal tract. Keeping in mind that atropine is a nerve gas antidote and that atropine overdoses with mental status changes can occur in mass toxicologic events [22], the

Table 2
Diagnostic and Statistical Manual of Mental Disorders, Fourth Edition, text revision diagnoses for chemical exposures

Diagnosis	NG	Lead[a]	Mercury	Solvents	CO
Substance-induced					
Delirium	X			X	X
Psychotic d/o	X			X	X
Persisting amnestic d/o	X	X	X	X	X
Anxiety d/o	X	X	X	X[b]	X
Mental retardation		X			
Symptoms of dementia		X	X		X
Inhalant intoxication				X	
Inhalant-induced					
Intoxication delirium				X	
Persisting dementia				X	
Psychotic d/o				X	
Mood d/o				X	
Anxiety d/o				X	
Inhalant-related d/o not otherwise specified				X	

Abbreviations: CO, carbon monoxide; d/o, disorder; NG, nerve gas and related organophosphate pesticides.
[a]Includes organic and inorganic lead.
[b]Specifically for solvent anesthetics.
Data from American Psychiatric Association. Diagnostic and statistical manual of mental disorders. 4th edition. Text revision. Washington (DC): American Psychiatric Association; 2000.

diagnosis of BZ poisoning in a chemical attack should be considered if victims present with hallucinations and an anticholinergic syndrome [21].

Chemical weapons are WMD and weapons of terror. Recent reviews highlight the importance of early recognition and management of behavioral responses to terror induced by WMD [23–26]. One review emphasizes three phases of response to a WMD attack: immediate, intermediate, and long-term [23]. These phases correlate with similar phases described for technologic and natural disasters. The typical response begins with intense emotions or fight-or-flight reactions, followed by an intermediate phase with autonomic arousal leading to longer term somatic stress and psychiatric illnesses. Long-term reactions range from mourning to psychiatric disability, with losses of the sense of community among survivors. Recent studies describe survivors of chemical weapons exposures after the Japanese terrorist attacks in the 1990s [27] and the Iran-Iraq war in the 1980s [28].

Psychiatric management of victims of any potential or known toxic event should include monitoring for mass hysteria or mass psychogenic illness. Mass hysteria usually consists of rapidly spreading psychologic reactions to perceived but usually not true exposures, often exaggerated by media reports. The caveat "usually not true" is necessary because some psychogenic reactions occur in response to real exposures affecting small numbers of victims. The most recent occurrences of probable mass hysteria resulted from diverse exposures, including drinking sodas, watching television cartoons, and vaccinations [29,30].

IONIZING RADIATION

Forms of ionizing radiation, including x-rays, gamma radiation, and atomic particles, damage living cells at the molecular level [31]. In the brain, this damage leads to mental changes, although the stress alone from perceived or actual exposure to ionizing radiation can also result in psychiatric impairment (see Table 1). Sources of ionizing radiation that cause psychiatric sequelae include therapeutic radiation, nuclear accidents like the one at Chernobyl, and nuclear bombs at Hiroshima and Nagasaki, Japan in World War II. Table 2 lists the DSM-IV-TR [18] psychiatric disorders that can result from ionizing radiation.

Cranial radiation therapy (CRT), although often necessary for cancer survival, increases risk for cognitive and other psychiatric changes, especially in children [32–34]. Irradiation of fetuses can cause mental retardation. To prevent mental retardation from in utero exposure completely, the recommended maximum total radiation dose for a fetus is 5 mSv (0.5 rem), or less than 0.5 mSv (0.05 rem) in any single month [31]. For comparison, a diagnostic x-ray dose delivers approximately 0.39 mSv [31]. Not all CRT causes measurable neurobehavioral changes, and in some cases, improvement in cognitive function results from CRT depending on the location and type of tumor and the type and dose of radiation received [6,35–37]. Diagnosis and treatment of depression during CRT help to maintain the patient's quality of life [38,39].

CRT can also cause radiation necrosis of the brain. In these instances, mood alterations, cognitive changes, and psychosis can develop over a period of months after exposure. This reaction differs from the so-called "cerebral" form of the acute radiation syndrome that results from an exposure of at least 50 Sv (5 rem). In the cerebral form of acute radiation syndrome, nausea and vomiting develop quickly and progress rapidly to loss of consciousness and death within 48 hours [31].

The long-term physiologic effect of noninjurious ionizing radiation on mental functioning is not clearly defined. In Gulf War veterans with bodily retained fragments of depleted uranium from exploded ammunition, subtle changes in central nervous system function have been observed [40,41]. Although this suggests that radiation from retained uranium may increase risk for later dementia, studies of nuclear bomb survivors in Japan did not correlate radiation exposure with dementia [42–44]. One nested case-control study of female nuclear weapons workers did find increased risk for death from dementia associated with total lifetime radiation exposure, however [45]. Most long-term studies of radiation survivors conclude that survivors are at risk for mood disorders, especially anxiety, as a response to concern about the possible effects of radiation exposure [46–48].

Stress and posttraumatic responses to radiation identical to those described for WMD and technologic disasters typically occur after nuclear accidents and attacks. The fear of ionizing radiation when little or no radiation is present can also induce psychiatric symptoms and illness [6]. A so-called "dirty bomb" containing depleted uranium instead of nuclear weapons–grade material in a large city would likely cause widespread fear and traumatic stress symptoms and behaviors. Common names for these responses include "A-bomb neurosis," "radiation response syndrome," and "radiophobia" [49,50]. Radiophobia remains a concern for occupational, military, and accidental radiation exposures [51–56].

INSECTICIDES

Insecticides of the greatest psychiatric importance include chlorinated hydrocarbons like dichlorodiphenyltrichloroethane (DDT) and anticholinesterases, with the latter represented by the organophosphates (eg, parathion) and carbamates. The internationally dispersed geographic locations of clinical reports of the psychiatric effects of insecticides reflect the global variation of laws controlling the use of insecticides. In the United States, early uses of chlorinated hydrocarbons resulted in numerous reports of psychiatric morbidity before most of these chemicals were removed from the market. Many chemicals banned in the United States are still used in certain other countries, however, where researchers continue to describe impaired human neurodevelopment from domestically banned chemicals like DDT and dichlorodiphenyldichloroethylene (DDE) [57–59]. Clinically symptomatic exposures to anticholinesterase pesticides have the same psychiatric effects as the anticholinesterase chemical weapons discussed previously (see Tables 1 and 2). Recent literature on the mental effects of long-term or low-dose exposures to anticholinesterase pesticides remains controversial [60–64].

NEUROTOXIC METALS

Despite advances in environmental awareness and public health measures to combat metal exposures, these poisonings continue to cause psychiatric illness. Using Medline, the author retrieved more than 60 clinical reports of the psychiatric symptoms caused by exposure to mercury or lead published since 2002. This number did not include studies hypothesizing that metal poisoning causes autism, a theory that has received considerable attention during the past several years. The neurotoxic metals of greatest notoriety and importance to clinical practice today are aluminum [65], arsenic [66], lead [67], manganese [68], mercury [69], and thallium [70,71]. Not all studies correlate low-level heavy metal exposure, such as mercury from dental amalgam or certain other routes, with adverse psychiatric outcomes [72,73]. Table 3 summarizes frequently reported psychiatric symptoms from the most commonly encountered neurotoxic metals. Table 2 shows the psychiatric disorders that the DSM-IV-TR attributes to various metal exposures [18].

Some neurotoxic metal exposures result from unpredictable circumstances, such as the arsenic poisoning in Asia described previously. The literature on arsenic poisoning reflects how metal poisonings can arise from improper disposal of chemicals or chemical weapons. In 2000, Japanese researchers

Table 3
Commonly reported psychiatric symptoms of heavy metal exposure

Symptom	Aluminum	Arsenic	Lead[a]	Manganese	Mercury	Thallium	Tin
Mood lability	X		X	X	X		
Depression	X		X		X	X	X
Anxiety	X	X	X	X	X	X	
Irritability	X	X			X	X	X
Mania		X			X		X
Agitation	X	X	X	X	X	X	X
Violence	X		X		X	X	X
Personality change	X	X	X	X	X	X	X
Shyness/social withdrawal					X		
Bizarre behavior	X	X					
Laughing/crying				X			
Suicidal	X	X	X		X		
Homicidal	X				X		
Memory loss	X	X	X	X	X	X	X
Poor concentration	X	X	X	X	X	X	X
Confusion	X		X			X	X
Hallucinations	X	X	X	X		X	X
Paranoia	X	X	X	X		X	X
Insomnia	X		X	X		X	X
Developmental delay			X			X	X
Mental retardation			X		X	X	

[a] Inorganic and organic lead.

identified residents of an apartment building in Kamisu, Japan using water from a well contaminated with diphenylarsinic acid (DPAA), a degradation product of arsenical chemical weapons produced by Japan during World War II [74]. Poisoned adults presented with severe cerebellar symptoms, and children developed mental retardation with cerebral atrophy.

Health effects from arsenic-contaminated drinking water also occur in the United States [75]. The diverse sources of arsenic exposure in the United States range from arsenic-treated wood debris from Hurricane Katrina [76] to herbal supplements [77]. One case report attributes arsenic toxicosis with memory loss and skin rash to daily "herbal kelp" consumption [77]. Chronic arsenic exposure frequently causes neurologic deficits with skin rash or melanosis [78].

Opinion remains divided over the role of metals, notably aluminum, in the pathogenesis of Alzheimer's disease [79]. Little doubt exists that aluminum causes so-called "dialysis dementia" (DD). DD, first described in the 1970s, developed in patients on dialysis who were dialyzed with tap water with high aluminum content or received large amounts of phosphate-binding antacids containing aluminum. DD became an infrequent complication of dialysis after dialysis centers reduced aluminum exposure, but case reports still describe sporadic cases of dementia from other water-related exposures to aluminum [6,65]. The current prevailing opinion holds that aluminum exposure does not cause

Alzheimer's dementia but might play a role in the development or progression of the disease [79,80].

Childhood lead poisoning continues to pose serious public health problems, especially in inner-city areas, where populations at risk live in dwellings containing leaded paint [81,82]. Classic symptoms of lead poisoning, organic and inorganic, include gastrointestinal complaints and neurologic abnormalities [6]. Other signs, such as gingival lead lines, basophilic stippling of red blood cells, and anemia, are more indicative of inorganic lead poisoning. The most recent opinion regarding tolerable lead levels in children is that injury can likely occur at low lead levels (ie, levels less than 10 µg/dL [81,83]. Adult lead poisoning continues to result from occupational or environmental exposures to lead-based products [84]. Globalization and the subsequently rising quantities of contaminated imported goods from countries without strong environmental regulations have been blamed for at least one community outbreak of lead poisoning in California [85]. Other imported sources of lead poisoning include low-cost jewelry [86].

The earliest descriptions of manganese poisoning, originally called "manganese madness" in Chilean manganese miners in the early twentieth century, included symptoms of uncontrollable laughing or crying with euphoria, agitation, and other manic or psychotic symptoms. Even today, manganese poisoning has been reported with similar symptoms, notably in welders and foundry workers [68,87,88]. In these cases, MRI often identifies manganese deposition in the brain [68].

Mercury poisoning with psychiatric sequelae results from exposures to inorganic and organic mercury. Mercury has caused outbreaks of poisoning when improperly disposed of or used as a medicine, pesticide, or paint ingredient [6]. The expression from Lewis Carroll's *Alice in Wonderland,* "mad as a hatter," is a reference to erethism, a condition caused by mercury poisoning of hatters who used mercury to prepare fur for making hats [6]. Classic descriptions of erethism consisted of excessive embarrassment, irritability, depression, and anxiety. Clinicians should remain aware of continued ethnic folk medicine uses of elemental mercury in which mercury is injected subcutaneously or otherwise to "ward off evil," to "increase strength," or to perform various forms of spiritual healing [6,89].

As with many other toxins discussed in this article, there have been an increasing number of reports of mercury poisoning from international sources [90–92]. Consumption of fish has been associated with elevated mercury exposure and psychiatric or neuropsychologic symptoms [71], but the health benefits of eating fish seem to outweigh the risks for mercury exposure, with the exception that pregnant women, nursing mothers, or persons who eat large quantities of fish should limit their intake of high- mercury-containing species [93].

Thallium, cadmium, and tin are neurotoxic metals for which clinical reports are infrequent and poisoning is presumed less common. Thallium poisoning, long known for adverse psychiatric outcomes, still occurs from accidental exposures and homicide or suicide [70,94]. Thallium poisoning should be suspected in patients who have various psychiatric complaints accompanied by alopecia, painful neuropathy, and gastrointestinal disturbances. Cadmium poisoning occurs primarily in industrial environments, and the few reports of psychologic manifestations of exposure are limited to descriptions of neuropsychologic deficits [95,96].

Tin, especially organotin, has neurotoxic properties that cause psychiatric illness with neurologic abnormalities [6]. Psychiatric toxicity from organotin exposure has not been reported since the 1980s, but there has been recent speculation that organic tin compounds can disrupt endocrine function [97,98].

AUTISM, METALS, AND OTHER CHEMICAL EXPOSURES

Theories that autism is caused by toxic exposure have gained considerable popularity [99]. Heavy metals were considered as possible culprits [100,101], but it has been suggested that autistic children might have high blood lead levels not because lead causes autism but because autistic children ingest lead through pica and other eating habits [102]. As a chemical cause of autism, most of the focus has been on thimerosal, an organic mercury-containing preservative in children's vaccines. Rigorous epidemiologic studies in the United States, Great Britain, Denmark, and Sweden have found no evidence to support a link between thimerosal and autism [103–107]. Despite the lack of evidence, the belief in such a link remains in vogue and in litigation. Other hypotheses linking solvents or pesticides to autism have been proposed but lack an evidence base [108–110].

SOLVENTS

Solvents comprise a large category of chemicals with an established reputation for causing psychiatric impairment from exposure. Carbon disulfide (CD) exposure in the nineteenth-century rubber industry resulted in suicides of factory workers secondary to CD-induced psychosis and mania in the workplace [111]. No question exists about the neurotoxicity and psychiatric importance of numerous solvents, including CD, trichloroethylene, methyl chloride, toluene, ethylene oxide, mixtures like gasoline, and several others. The magnitude and duration of solvent exposure necessary to cause psychiatric problems remain controversial, however [6]. Table 4 lists the commonly reported symptoms from solvent exposures, including abused inhalants, which are often solvents [112–116]. Table 2 lists the DSM-IV-TR [18] psychiatric disorders attributed to solvent or inhalant exposure or abuse.

Inhalation or "huffing" of solvents and other inhalants has become a serious but underrecognized public health problem responsible for considerable morbidity and mortality [6,117,118]. Abused inhalants that contain solvents include cleaning fluids, gasoline, paints and glues, personal hygiene products, refrigerants, deodorants, and numerous other commercial products [6]. Physical signs of solvent inhalation range from physical depositions in or around airways to measurable levels of chemicals in tissue autopsy [6,118]. Inhalant abusers have

Table 4
Commonly reported symptoms of exposure to selected solvents and inhalants

Symptom	CD	TCE	MC	BEN	STY	TOL	XYL	EO	M
Mood lability	X	X	X			X	X		X
Anxiety	X	X	X	X				X	X
Irritability	X	X	X		X	X		X	X
Depression	X	X	X		X	X		X	X
Mania	X	X	X						
Bizarre behavior	X								
Agitation	X	X	X						
Suicidal	X	X							
Homicidal	X	X							
Confusion	X	X							
Poor concentration	X	X	X		X	X		X	X
Memory loss	X	X	X		X	X	X	X	X
Hallucinations	X	X						X	
Paranoia	X	X							
Insomnia	X	X	X	X	X	X	X		X

Abbreviations: BEN, benzene; CD, carbon disulfide; EO, ethylene oxide; M (mixtures); MC, methyl chloride; STY, styrene; TCE, trichloroethylene; TOL, toluene; XYL, xylene.

high prevalences of psychiatric disorders [113], and many have MRI/CT brain abnormalities, including diffuse white matter abnormalities, brain atrophy, and basal ganglia abnormalities [6].

Abuse of solvents may include methanol or isopropanol [119–121]. Nonintentional exposures to these particular chemicals have also caused large outbreaks [122] and individual accidental poisonings [123], sometimes in combination with ethylene glycol [124] or other solvents [120]. Often lethal, these poisonings may present with metabolic anion gap acidosis, visual changes, neuropathy, Parkinson's syndrome, and abnormal CT and MRI findings [121,122,124–126].

Reports of solvent exposures causing psychiatric symptoms highlight the increasing occupational exposure to these chemicals in other nations. Cases of CD poisoning became rare in American medical literature by the twenty-first century but then appeared from South Korea, Yugoslavia, Taiwan, and Italy [127–130]. Other solvents for which there are recent reports of psychiatric illness from other countries include mixed solvents [131,132], toluene [133], and 1-bromopropane [134].

TOXIC GASES

Toxic gases of psychiatric importance not already discussed previously include carbon monoxide (CO) and hydrogen sulfide (HS). CO poisoning occurs in suicidal and accidental circumstances. CO poisoning frequently involves inadequately vented kerosene heaters and woodstoves. New to the twenty-first century have been epidemics of CO poisoning from improper use of portable electrical generators after power losses from hurricanes [135–138]. Therefore,

Table 5
Commonly reported symptoms of exposure to toxic gases

Symptom	CO	HS
Irritability	X	X
Depression	X	X
Anxiety	X	X
Agitation	X	X
Mania	X	X
Violence	X	X
Homicidal	X	
Memory loss	X	X
Poor concentration	X	X
Dementia	X	X
Delirium	X	
Delusions	X	X
Hallucinations	X	X
Paranoia	X	
Insomnia	X	X
Other changes	X	X

psychiatrists should have an elevated index of suspicion for the possibility of neuropsychiatric toxicity from CO poisoning whenever there are major power outages. Table 5 lists the psychiatric symptoms attributed to these gases in the United States and elsewhere [139–142]. CO-poisoned victims must be monitored for delayed neuropsychiatric toxicity, also known as postinterval syndrome, presenting with severe psychiatric symptoms, sometimes including homicidal and suicidal behavior [143–146]. Brain CT and MRI often reveal cerebral atrophy, periventricular white matter degeneration, and bilateral low-density areas in the basal ganglia [6]. Treatment of CO poisoning may include hyperbaric oxygen, which may be able to reverse neuropsychiatric deficits [6].

Table 6
Helpful tests for psychiatric evaluation of selected chemical exposures

Test	Nerve gases[a]	Heavy metals	Solvents	CO
Complete blood cell count	X	X	X	X
Electrolytes	X	X	X	X
Liver/renal function	X	X	X	X
Urinalysis	X	X	X	X
Urine pesticide screen	X			
Neurologic examination	X	X	X	X
Neuropsychologic testing	X	X	X	X
Electroencephalogram	X	X	X	X
Urinary/blood heavy metal screen		X		
MRI		X[b]	X	X
Carboxyhemoglobin				X

[a] Includes organophosphate pesticides and related compounds.
[b] Especially for manganese and mercury.

GENERAL CLINICAL APPROACH AND SUMMARY

Clinical tests can assist the psychiatric diagnosis of chemically exposed individuals. Table 6 lists suggested tests for further assessment. In summary, psychiatrists and other mental health providers may encounter a wide range of victims in the acute recovery and triage of a chemical disaster or attack and should consider the following:

1. Some victims have psychiatric injury from direct neurotoxic injury.
2. Even when no chemical is present, fear of chemical exposure can induce psychiatric symptoms or illness in some victims.
3. In a mass chemical accident or attack, especially with a neurotoxic agent, the clinician might encounter at least five categories of acute psychiatric casualties
   a. Victims with neurotoxic injury
   b. Victims with acute stress
   c. Victims with neurotoxic injury and acute stress
   d. Victims with preexisting mental illnesses exacerbated by neurotoxic injury or acute stress
   e. Victims of mass hysteria

References

[1] Toon OB, Robock A, Turco RP, et al. Consequences of regional-scale nuclear conflicts. Science 2007;315:1224–5.

[2] Bhattacharjee Y. A sluggish response to humanity's biggest mass poisoning [news]. Science 2007;315:1659–61.

[3] U.S. Food and Drug Administration. Testimony by Stephen F. Sundlof before the Senate Agriculture, Rural Development, and Related Agencies Appropiations Subcommittee, April 12, 2007. Available at: http://www.fda.gov/ola/2007/petfood041207.html. Accessed August 27, 2007.

[4] U.S. Food and Drug Administration. FDA advises consumers to avoid toothpaste from China containing harmful chemical. Available at: http://www.fda.gov/bbs/topics/NEWS/2007/NEW01646.html. Accessed August 27, 2007.

[5] Schwartz D, Collins F. Environmental biology and human disease (policy forum). Science 2007;695–6.

[6] Brown JS Jr. Environmental and chemical toxins and psychiatric illness. Washington, DC: American Psychiatric Publishing; 2002.

[7] Kang HK, Dalager NA, Needham LL, et al. Health status of Army Chemical Corps Vietnam veterans who sprayed defoliant in Vietnam. Am J Ind Med 2006;49(11):875–84.

[8] Michalek JE, Barrett DH, Morris RD, et al. Serum dioxin and psychological functioning in U.S. Air Force veterans of the Vietnam war. Mil Med 2003;168(2):153–9.

[9] Engel CC, Hyams KC, Scott K. Managing future Gulf War syndromes: international lessons and new models of care. Philos Trans R Soc Lond B Biol Sci 2006;361(1468):707–20.

[10] Horner RD, Kamins KG, Feussner JR, et al. Occurrence of amyotrophic lateral sclerosis among Gulf War veterans. Neurology 2003;61(6):742–9.

[11] Haley RW. Excess incidence of ALS in young Gulf War veterans. Neurology 2003;61(6):750–6.

[12] Weisskopf MG, O'Reilly EJ, McCullough ML, et al. Prospective study of military service and mortality from ALS. Neurology 2005;64(1):32–7.

[13] Proctor SP, Heaton KJ, Heeren T, et al. Effects of sarin and cyclosarin exposure during the 1991 Gulf War on neurobehavioral functioning in US army veterans. Neurotoxicology 2006;27(6):931–9.

[14] Bullman TA, Mahan CM, Kang HK, et al. Mortality in US Army Gulf War veterans exposed to 1991 Khamisiyah chemical munitions destruction. Am J Public Health 2005;95(8): 1382–8.

[15] Smith TC, Gray GC, Weir JC, et al. Gulf War veterans and Iraqi nerve agents at Khamisiyah: postwar hospitalization data revisited. Am J Epidemiol 2003;158(5): 457–67.

[16] Okumura T, Takasu N, Ishimatsu S, et al. Report on 640 victims of the Tokyo subway sarin attack. Ann Emerg Med 1996;28:129–35.

[17] Ecobichon DJ. Toxic effects of pesticides. In: Klaassen CD, editor. Casarett and Doull's toxicology: the basic science of poisons. New York: McGraw-Hill; 1996. p. 643–89.

[18] American Psychiatric Association. Diagnostic and statistical manual of mental disorders. 4th edition. Text revision. Washington, DC: American Psychiatric Association; 2000.

[19] Holmes JH, Gaon M. Observations on acute and multiple exposure to anticholinesterase agents. Trans Am Clin Climatol Assoc 1956;68:86–103.

[20] Sidell FR. What to do in case of an unthinkable chemical warfare attack or accident. Postgrad Med 1990;88:70–84.

[21] Holstege CP, Baylor M. CBRNE-Incapacitating Agents, 3-Quinuclidinyl Benzelate. Available at: http://www.emedicine.com/emerg/topic912.htm. Accessed August 27, 2007.

[22] Leiba A, Goldberg A, Hourvitz A, et al. Who should worry for the "worried well"? Analysis of mild casualties center drills in non-conventional scenarios. Prehospital Disaster Med 2006;21(6):441–4.

[23] Lacy TJ, Benedek DM. Terrorism and weapons of mass destruction: managing the behavioral reaction in primary care. South Med J 2003;96(4):394–9.

[24] Romano JA Jr, King JM. Psychological casualties resulting from chemical and biological weapons. Mil Med 2001;166(Suppl 12):21–2.

[25] Ritchie EC, Friedman M, Watson P, et al. Mass violence and early mental health intervention: a proposed application of best practice guidelines to chemical, biological, and radiological attacks. Mil Med 2004;169(8):575–9.

[26] DiGiovanni C Jr. The spectrum of human reactions to terrorist attacks with weapons of mass destruction: early management considerations. Prehospital Disaster Med 2003;18(3): 253–7.

[27] Yanagisawa N, Morita H, Nakajima T. Sarin experiences in Japan: acute toxicity and long-term effects. J Neurol Sci 2006;249(1):76–85.

[28] Hashemian F, Khoshnood K, Desai MM, et al. Anxiety, depression, and posttraumatic stress in Iranian survivors of chemical warfare. JAMA 2006;296(5):560–6.

[29] Kharabshe S, Al-Otoum H, Clements J, et al. Mass psychogenic illness following tetanus-diphtheria toxoid vaccination in Jordan. Bull World Health Organ 2001;79(8):764–70.

[30] Radford B, Bartholomew R. Pokemon contagion: photosensitive epilepsy or mass psychogenic illness? South Med J 2001;94(2):197–204.

[31] Upton AC. Ionizing radiation. In: Wallace RB, editor. Public health and preventive medicine. Stamford (CT): Appleton & Lange; 1998. p. 619–26.

[32] Anderson VA, Godber T, Smibert E, et al. Impairments of attention following treatment with cranial irradiation and chemotherapy in children. J Clin Exp Neuropsychol 2004;26(5): 684–97.

[33] Vannatta K, Gerhardt CA, Wells RJ, et al. Intensity of CNS treatment for pediatric cancer: prediction of social outcomes in survivors. Pediatr Blood Cancer 2006;49(5):716–22.

[34] Cole PD, Kamen BA. Delayed neurotoxicity associated with therapy for children with acute lymphoblastic leukemia. Ment Retard Dev Disabil Res Rev 2006;12(3):174–83.

[35] Brown PD, Buckner JC, O'Fallon JR, et al. Effects of radiotherapy on cognitive function in patients with low-grade glioma measured by the Folstein mini-mental state examination. J Clin Oncol 2003;21(13):2519–24.

[36] Torres IJ, Mundt AJ, Sweeney PJ, et al. A longitudinal neuropsychological study of partial brain radiation in adults with brain tumors. Neurology 2003;60(7):1113–8.

[37] Lam LC, Leung SF, Chan YL. Progress of memory function after radiation therapy in patients with nasopharyngeal carcinoma. J Neuropsychiatry Clin Neurosci 2003;15(1):90–7.

[38] Kohda R, Otsubo T, Kuwakado Y, et al. Prospective studies on mental status and quality of life in patients with head and neck cancer treated by radiation. Psychooncology 2005;14(4):331–6.

[39] Hahn CA, Dunn R, Halperin EC. Routine screening for depression in radiation oncology patients. Am J Clin Oncol 2004;27(5):497–9.

[40] McDiarmid MA, Keogh JP, Hooper FJ, et al. Health effects of depleted uranium on exposed Gulf War veterans. Environ Res 2000;82(2):168–80.

[41] McDiarmid MA, Hooper FJ, Squibb K, et al. Health effects and biological monitoring results of Gulf War veterans exposed to depleted uranium. Mil Med 2002;167(Suppl 2): 123–4.

[42] Yamada M, Kasagi F, Sasaki H, et al. Association between dementia and midlife risk factors: the Radiation Effects Research Foundation Adult Health Study. J Am Geriatr Soc 2003;51(3):410–4.

[43] Yamada M, Sasaki H, Kasagi F, et al. Study of cognitive function among the Adult Health Study (AHS) population in Hiroshima and Nagasaki. Radiat Res 2002;158(2):236–40.

[44] Yamada M, Sasaki H, Mimori Y, et al. Prevalence and risks of dementia in the Japanese population: RERF's adult health study Hiroshima subjects. Radiation Effects Research Foundation. J Am Geriatr Soc 1999;47(2):189–95.

[45] Sibley RF, Moscato BS, Wilkinson GS, et al. Nested case-control study of external ionizing radiation dose and mortality from dementia within a pooled cohort of female nuclear weapons workers. Am J Ind Med 2003;44(4):351–8.

[46] Kawano N, Hirabayashi K, Matsuo M, et al. Human suffering effects of nuclear tests at Semipalatinsk, Kazakhstan: established on the basis of questionnaire surveys. J Radiat Res (Tokyo) 2006;47(Suppl A):A209–17.

[47] Yamada M, Izumi S. Psychiatric sequelae in atomic bomb survivors in Hiroshima and Nagasaki two decades after the explosion. Soc Psychiatry Psychiatr Epidemiol 2002;37(9): 409–15.

[48] Honda S, Shibata Y, Mine M, et al. Mental health conditions among atomic bomb survivors in Nagasaki. Psychiatry Clin Neurosci 2002;56(5):575–83.

[49] [no authors listed] Radiophobia: a new psychological syndrome. West J Surg Obstet Gynecol 1951;59(11):viii–x.

[50] Myslobodsky M. The origin of radiophobias. Perspect Biol Med 2001;44(4):543–55.

[51] Takamura N, Kryshenko N, Masyakin V, et al. Chernobyl-induced radiophobias and the incidence of tuberculosis. Lancet 2000;356(9225):257.

[52] Pastel RH. Radiophobia: long-term psychological consequences of Chernobyl. Mil Med 2002;167(Suppl 2):134–6.

[53] Dawson SE, Madsen GE. American Indian uranium millworkers: a study of the perceived effects of occupational exposure. J Health Soc Policy 1995;7(2):19–31.

[54] Morita N, Takamura N, Ashizawa K, et al. Measurement of the whole-body 137Cs in residents around the Chernobyl nuclear power plant. Radiat Prot Dosimetry 2005;113(3): 326–9.

[55] Pastel RH, Mulvaney J. Fear of radiation in U.S. military medical personnel. Mil Med 2001;166(Suppl 12):80–2.

[56] Foster RP, Goldstein MF. Chernobyl disaster sequelae in recent immigrants to the United States from the former Soviet Union (FSU). J Immigr Minor Health 2007;9(2):115–24.

[57] Eskenazi B, Marks AR, Bradman A, et al. In utero exposure to dichlorodiphenyltrichloroethane (DDT) and dichlorodiphenyldichloroethylene (DDE) and neurodevelopment among young Mexican American children. Pediatrics 2006;118(1):233–41.

[58] Ribas-Fito N, Cardo E, Sala M, et al. Breastfeeding, exposure to organochlorine compounds, and neurodevelopment in infants. Pediatrics 2003;111(5 Pt 1):e580–5.

[59] Dorner G, Plagemann A. DDT in human milk and mental capacities in children at school age: an additional view on PISA 2000. Neuro Endocrinol Lett 2002;23(5–6): 427–31.

[60] Solomon C, Poole J, Palmer KT, et al. Neuropsychiatric symptoms in past users of sheep dip and other pesticides. Occup Environ Med 2006;64(4):259–66.

[61] Ruckart PZ, Kakolewski K, Bove FJ, et al. Long-term neurobehavioral health effects of methyl parathion exposure in children in Mississippi and Ohio. Environ Health Perspect 2004;112(1):46–51.

[62] Salvi RM, Lara DR, Ghisolfi ES, et al. Neuropsychiatric evaluation in subjects chronically exposed to organophosphate pesticides. Toxicol Sci 2003;72(2):267–71.

[63] Rauh VA, Garfinkel R, Perera FP, et al. Impact of prenatal chlorpyrifos exposure on neuro-development in the first 3 years of life among inner-city children. Pediatrics 2006;118(6): e1845–59.

[64] Roldan-Tapia L, Parron T, Sanchez-Santed F. Neuropsychological effects of long-term expo-sure to organophosphate pesticides. Neurotoxicol Teratol 2005;27(2):259–66.

[65] Exley C, Esiri MM. Severe cerebral congophilic angiopathy coincident with increased brain aluminium in a resident of Camelford, Cornwall, UK. J Neurol Neurosurg Psychiatry 2006;77(7):877–9.

[66] Wasserman GA, Liu X, Parvez F, et al. Water arsenic exposure and intellectual function in 6-year-old children in Araihazar, Bangladesh. Environ Health Perspect 2007;115(2): 285–9.

[67] Opler MG, Brown AS, Graziano J, et al. Prenatal lead exposure, delta-aminolevulinic acid, and schizophrenia. Environ Health Perspect 2004;112(5):548–52.

[68] Bowler RM, Koller W, Schulz PE. Parkinsonism due to manganism in a welder: neurolog-ical and neuropsychological sequelae. Neurotoxicology 2006;27(3):327–32.

[69] Haas NS, Shih R, Gochfeld M. A patient with postoperative mercury contamination of the peritoneum. J Toxicol Clin Toxicol 2003;41(2):175–80.

[70] Rusyniak DE, Furbee RB, Kirk MA. Thallium and arsenic poisoning in a small midwestern town. Ann Emerg Med 2002;39(3):307–11.

[71] Knobeloch L, Steenport D, Schrank C, et al. Methylmercury exposure in Wisconsin: a case study series. Environ Res 2006;101(1):113–22.

[72] DeRouen TA, Martin MD, Leroux BG, et al. Neurobehavioral effects of dental amalgam in children: a randomized clinical trial. JAMA 2006;295(15):1784–92.

[73] Weil M, Bressler J, Parsons P, et al. Blood mercury levels and neurobehavioral function. JAMA 2005;293(15):1875–82.

[74] Ishii K, Tamaoka A, Otsuka F, et al. Diphenylarsinic acid poisoning from chemical weapons in Kamisu, Japan. Ann Neurol 2004;56(5):741–5.

[75] Knobeloch LM, Zierold KM, Anderson HA. Association of arsenic-contaminated drinking-water with prevalence of skin cancer in Wisconsin's Fox River Valley. J Health Popul Nutr 2006;24(2):206–13.

[76] Dubey B, Solo-Gabriele HM, Townsendt TG. Quantities of arsenic-treated wood in demo-lition debris generated by Hurricane Katrina. Environ Sci Technol 2007;41(5):1533–6.

[77] Amster E, Tiwary A, Schenker MB. Case report: potential arsenic toxicosis secondary to herbal kelp supplement. Environ Health Perspect 2007;115(4):606–8.

[78] Mukherjee SC, Saha KC, Pati S, et al. Murshidabad—one of the nine groundwater arsenic-affected districts of West Bengal, India. Part II: dermatological, neurological, and obstetric findings. Clin Toxicol (Phila) 2005;43(7):835–48.

[79] Shcherbatykh I, Carpenter DO. The role of metals in the etiology of Alzheimer's disease. J Alzheimers Dis 2007;11(2):191–205.

[80] Perl DP, Moalem S. Aluminum and Alzheimer's disease, a personal perspective after 25 years. J Alzheimers Dis 2006;9(Suppl 3):291–300.

[81] Chiodo LM, Jacobson SW, Jacobson JL. Neurodevelopmental effects of postnatal lead exposure at very low levels. Neurotoxicol Teratol 2004;26(3):359–71.

[82] Reyes NL, Wong LY, MacRoy PM, et al. Identifying housing that poisons: a critical step in eliminating childhood lead poisoning. J Public Health Manag Pract 2006;12(6): 563–9.

[83] Woolf AD, Goldman R, Bellinger DC. Update on the clinical management of childhood lead poisoning. Pediatr Clin North Am 2007;54(2):271–94.

[84] Anderson HA, Islam KM. Trends in occupational and adult lead exposure in Wisconsin 1988–2005. WMJ 2006;105(2):21–5.

[85] Handley MA, Hall C, Sanford E, et al. Globalization, binational communities, and imported food risks: results of an outbreak investigation of lead poisoning in Monterey County, California. Am J Public Health 2007;97(5):900–6.

[86] Weidenhamer JD, Clement ML. Widespread lead contamination of imported low-cost jewelry in the US. Chemosphere 2007;67(5):961–5.

[87] Bouchard M, Mergler D, Baldwin M, et al. Neuropsychiatric symptoms and past manganese exposure in a ferro-alloy plant. Neurotoxicology 2006;28(2):290–7.

[88] Bowler RM, Roels HA, Nakagawa S, et al. Dose-effect relationships between manganese exposure and neurological, neuropsychological and pulmonary function in confined space bridge welders. Occup Environ Med 2007;64(3):167–77.

[89] Pradad VL. Subcutaneous injection of mercury: "warding off evil." Environ Health Perspect 2004;112(13):1326–8.

[90] Abbasiou P, Zaman T. A child with elemental mercury poisoning and unusual brain MRI findings. Clin Toxicol (Phila) 2006;44(1):85–8.

[91] Bose-O'Reilly S, Drasch G, Beinhoff C, et al. The Mt. Diwata study on the Philippines 2000—treatment of mercury intoxicated inhabitants of a gold mining area with DMPS (2,3-dimercapto-1-propane-sulfonic acid, Dimaval). Sci Total Environ 2003;307(1–3):71–82.

[92] Counter SA, Buchanan LH, Ortega F. Neurocognitive screening of mercury-exposed children of Andean gold miners. Int J Occup Med Environ Health 2006;12(3): 209–14.

[93] Mozaffarian D, Rimm EB. Fish intake, contaminants, and human health: evaluating the risks and benefits. JAMA 2006;296(15):1885–99.

[94] Jha S, Kumar R, Kumar R. Thallium poisoning presenting as paresthesias, paresis, psychosis and pain in abdomen. J Assoc Physicians India 2006;54:53–5.

[95] Viaene MK, Masschelein R, Leenders J, et al. Neurobehavioral effects of occupational exposure to cadmium: a cross sectional epidemiological study. Occup Environ Med 2000;57(1):19–27.

[96] Hart RP, Rose CS, Hamer RM. Neuropsychological effects of occupational exposure to cadmium. J Clin Exp Neuropsychol 1989;11(6):933–43.

[97] Nakanishi T, Nishikawa J, Tanaka K. Molecular targets of organotin compounds in endocrine disruption: do organotin compounds function as aromatase inhibitors in mammals? Environ Sci 2006;13(2):89–100.

[98] Santos MM, Micael J, Carvalho AP, et al. Estrogens counteract the masculinizing effect of tributyltin in zebrafish. Comp Biochem Physiol C Toxicol Pharmacol 2006;142(1–2): 151–5.

[99] Grandjean P, Landrigan PJ. Developmental neurotoxicity of industrial chemicals. Lancet 2006;368(9553):2167–78.

[100] Shearer TR, Larson K, Neuschwander J, et al. Minerals in the hair and nutrient intake of autistic children. J Autism Dev Disord 1982;12(1):25–34.

[101] Jackson MJ, Garrod PJ. Plasma zinc, copper, and amino acid levels in the blood of autistic children. J Autism Child Schizophr 1978;8(2):203–8.

[102] Cohen DJ, Johnson WT, Caparulo BK. Pica and elevated blood lead level in autistic and atypical children. Am J Dis Child 1976;130(1):47–8.

[103] Heron J, Golding J, ALSPAC Study Team. Thimerosal exposure in infants and developmental disorders: a prospective cohort study in the United Kingdom does not support a causal association. Pediatrics 2004;114(3):577–83.

[104] Madsen KM, Lauritsen MB, Pedersen CB, et al. Thimerosal and the occurrence of autism: negative ecological evidence from Danish population-based data. Pediatrics 2003; 112(3 Pt 1):604–6.

[105] Andrews N, Miller E, Grant A, et al. Thimerosal exposure in infants and developmental disorders: a retrospective cohort study in the United Kingdom does not support a causal association. Pediatrics 2004;114(3):584–91.

[106] Smeeth L, Cook C, Fombonne E, et al. MMR vaccination and pervasive developmental disorders: a case-control study. Lancet 2004;364(9438):963–9.

[107] Parker SK, Schwartz B, Todd J, et al. Thimerosal-containing vaccines and autistic spectrum disorder: a critical review of published original data. Pediatrics 2004;114(3):793–804.

[108] Adams JB, Holloway CE, George F, et al. Analyses of toxic metals and essential minerals in the hair of Arizona children with autism and associated conditions, and their mothers. Pediatrics 2006;110(3):193–209.

[109] D'Amelio M, Ricci I, Sacco R, et al. Paraoxonase gene variants are associated with autism in North America, but not in Italy: possible regional specificity in gene-environment interactions. Mol Psychiatry 2005;10(11):1006–16.

[110] Windham GC, Zhang L, Gunier R, et al. Autism spectrum disorders in relation to distribution of hazardous air pollutants in the San Francisco Bay area. Environ Health Perspect 2006;114(9):1438–44.

[111] Hartman DE. Neuropsychological toxicology of solvents. Neuropsychological toxicology. identification and assessment of human neurotoxic syndromes. New York: Pergamon Press; 1988. p. 108–59.

[112] Fornazzari L, Pollanen MS, Myers V, et al. Solvent abuse-related toluene leukoencephalopathy. J Clin Forensic Med 2003;10(2):93–5.

[113] Wu LT, Howard MO. Psychiatric disorders in inhalant users: results from the national epidemiologic survey on alcohol and related conditions. Drug Alcohol Depend 2007;88(2–3): 146–55.

[114] Finch CK, Lobo BL. Acute inhalant-induced neurotoxicity with delayed recovery. Ann Pharmacother 2005;39(1):169–71.

[115] Miller PW, Mycyk MB, Leikin JB, et al. An unusual presentation of inhalant abuse with dissociative amnesia. Vet Hum Toxicol 2002;44(1):17–9.

[116] Cairney S, Maruff P, Burns CB, et al. Neurological and cognitive recovery following abstinence from petrol sniffing. Neuropsychopharmacology 2005;30(5):1019–27.

[117] Williams JF, Storck M, Academy of Pediatrics Committee on Substance Abuse, et al. Inhalant abuse. Pediatrics 2007;119(5):1009–117.

[118] Hahn T, Avella J, Lehrer M. A motor vehicle accident fatality involving the inhalation of 1, 1-difluoroethane. J Anal Toxicol 2006;30(8):638–42.

[119] Bebarta VS, Heard K, Dart RC. Inhalational abuse of methanol products: elevated methanol and formate levels without vision loss. Am J Emerg Med 2006;24(6):725–8.

[120] Frenia ML, Schauben JL. Methanol inhalation toxicity. Ann Emerg Med 1993;22(12): 1919–23.

[121] LoVecchio F, Sawyers B, Thole D, et al. Outcomes following abuse of methanol-containing carburetor cleaners. Hum Exp Toxicol 2004;23(10):473–5.

[122] Hovda KE, Hunderi OH, Tafjord AB, et al. Methanol outbreak in Norway 2002–2004: epidemiology, clinical features and prognostic signs. J Intern Med 2005;258(2): 181–90.

[123] Stremski E, Hennes H. Accidental isopropanol ingestion in children. Pediatr Emerg Care 2000;16(4):238–40.

[124] Reddy NJ, Lewis LD, Gardner TB, et al. Two cases of rapid onset Parkinson's syndrome following toxic ingestion of ethylene glycol and methanol. Clin Pharmacol Ther 2007;81(1): 114–21.

[125] Alfred S, Coleman P, Harris D, et al. Delayed neurologic sequelae resulting from epidemic diethylene glycol poisoning. Clin Toxicol 2005;43(3):155–9.

[126] Blanco M, Cadado R, Vazquez F, et al. CT and MR imaging findings in methanol intoxication. AJNR Am J Neuroradiol 2006;27(2):452–4.

[127] Fonte R, Edallo A, Candura SM. Cerebellar atrophy as a delayed manifestation of chronic carbon disulfide poisoning. Ind Health 2003;41(1):43–7.

[128] Ku MC, Huang CC, Kuo HC, et al. Diffuse white matter lesions in carbon disulfide intoxication: microangiopathy or demyelination. Eur Neurol 2003;50(4):220–4.

[129] Krstev S, Perunicic B, Farkic B, et al. Neuropsychiatric effects in workers with occupational exposure to carbon disulfide. J Occup Health 2003;45(2):81–7.

[130] Cho SK, Kim RH, Yim SH, et al. Long-term neuropsychiatric effects and MRI findings in patients with CS2 poisoning. Acta Neurol Scand 2002;106(5):269–75.

[131] Schofield PW, Gibson R, Tavener M, et al. Neuropsychological health in F-111 maintenance workers. Neurotoxicology 2006;27(5):852–60.

[132] Kaukiainen A, Riala R, Martikainen R, et al. Solvent-related health effects among construction painters with decreasing exposure. Am J Ind Med 2004;46(6):627–36.

[133] Lee YL, Pai MC, Chen JH, et al. Central neurological abnormalities and multiple chemical sensitivity caused by chronic toluene exposure. Occup Med 2003;53(7):479–82.

[134] Ichihara G, Li W, Shibata E, et al. Neurologic abnormalities in workers of a 1-bromopropane factory. Environ Health Perspect 2004;112(13):1319–25.

[135] Centers for Disease Control and Prevention (CDC). Carbon monoxide poisonings after two major hurricanes—Alabama and Texas. August-October 2005. MMWR Morb Mortal Wkly Rep 2006;55(9):236–9.

[136] Hampson NB, Stock AL. Storm-related carbon monoxide poisoning: lessons learned from recent epidemics. Undersea Hyperb Med 2006;33(4):257–63.

[137] Centers for Disease Control and Prevention (CDC). Carbon monoxide poisoning after Hurricane Katrina—Alabama, Louisiana, and Mississippi, August–September 2005. MMWR Morb Mortal Wkly Rep 2005;54(39):996–8.

[138] Van Sickle D, Chertow DS, Schulte JM, et al. Carbon monxide poisoning in Florida during the 2004 hurricane season. Am J Prev Med 2007;32(4):340–6.

[139] Hirsch AR. Hydrogen sulfide exposure without loss of consciousness: chronic effects in four cases. Toxicol Ind Health 2002;18(2):51–61.

[140] Nam B, Kim H, Choi Y, et al. Neurologic sequela of hydrogen sulfide poisoning. Ind Health 2004;42(1):83–7.

[141] Erdogan MS, Islam SS, Chaudhari A, et al. Occupational carbon monoxide poisoning among West Virginia workers' compensation claims: diagnosis, treatment duration, and utilization. J Occup Environ Med 2004;46(6):577–83.

[142] Prockop LD. Carbon monoxide brain toxicity: clinical, magnetic resonance imaging, magnetic resonance spectroscopy, and neuropsychological effects in 9 people. J Neuroimaging 2005;15(2):144–9.

[143] Vacchiano G, Torino R. Carbon-monoxide poisoning, behavioral changes and suicide: an unusual industrial accident. J Clin Forensic Med 2001;8(2):86–92.

[144] Ku BD, Shin HY, Kim EJ, et al. Secondary mania in a patient with delayed anoxic encephalopathy after carbon monoxide intoxication. J Clin Neurosci 2006;13(8):860–2.

[145] Asian S, Karcioglu O, Bilge F, et al. Post-interval syndrome after carbon monoxide poisoning. Vet Hum Toxicol 2004;46(4):183–5.

[146] Lam SP, Fong SY, Kwok A, et al. Delayed neuropsychiatric impairment after carbon monoxide poisoning from burning charcoal. Hong Kong Med J 2004;10(6):428–31.

Psychiatr Clin N Am 30 (2007) 855–863

PSYCHIATRIC CLINICS
OF NORTH AMERICA

INDEX

Note: Page numbers of article titles are in **boldface** type.

0193-953X/07/$ – see front matter
doi:10.1016/S0193-953X(07)00105-0
© 2007 Elsevier Inc. All rights reserved.
psych.theclinics.com

United States Postal Service

Statement of Ownership, Management, and Circulation
(All Periodicals Publications Except Requestor Publications)

1. Publication Title	2. Publication Number	3. Filing Date
Psychiatric Clinics of North America	0 0 0 7 7 0 3	9/14/07

4. Issue Frequency	5. Number of Issues Published Annually	6. Annual Subscription Price
Mar, Jun, Sep, Dec	4	$194.00

7. Complete Mailing Address of Known Office of Publication (*Not printer*) (*Street, city, county, state, and ZIP+4*)

Elsevier Inc.
360 Park Avenue South
New York, NY 10010-1710

Contact Person: Stephen Bushing
Telephone (*Include area code*): 215-239-3688

8. Complete Mailing Address of Headquarters or General Business Office of Publisher (*Not printer*)

Elsevier Inc., 360 Park Avenue South, New York, NY 10010-1710

9. Full Names and Complete Mailing Addresses of Publisher, Editor, and Managing Editor (*Do not leave blank*)

Publisher (*Name and complete mailing address*)

John Schrefer, Elsevier, Inc., 1600 John F. Kennedy Blvd. Suite 1800, Philadelphia, PA 19103-2899

Editor (*Name and complete mailing address*)

Sarah Barth, Elsevier, Inc., 1600 John F. Kennedy Blvd. Suite 1800, Philadelphia, PA 19103-2899

Managing Editor (*Name and complete mailing address*)

Catherine Bewick, Elsevier, Inc., 1600 John F. Kennedy Blvd. Suite 1800, Philadelphia, PA 19103-2899

10. Owner (*Do not leave blank. If the publication is owned by a corporation, give the name and address of the corporation immediately followed by the names and addresses of all stockholders owning or holding 1 percent or more of the total amount of stock. If not owned by a corporation, give the names and addresses of the individual owners. If owned by a partnership or other unincorporated firm, give its name and address as well as those of each individual owner. If the publication is published by a nonprofit organization, give its name and address.*)

Full Name	Complete Mailing Address
Wholly owned subsidiary of	4520 East-West Highway
Reed/Elsevier, US holdings	Bethesda, MD 20814

11. Known Bondholders, Mortgagees, and Other Security Holders Owning or Holding 1 Percent or More of Total Amount of Bonds, Mortgages, or Other Securities. If none, check box ☐ None

Full Name	Complete Mailing Address
N/A	

12. Tax Status (*For completion by nonprofit organizations authorized to mail at nonprofit rates*) (*Check one*)
The purpose, function, and nonprofit status of this organization and the exempt status for federal income tax purposes:
☑ Has Not Changed During Preceding 12 Months
☐ Has Changed During Preceding 12 Months (*Publisher must submit explanation of change with this statement*)

PS Form 3526, September 2006 (Page 1 of 3 (Instructions Page 3)) PSN 7530-01-000-9931 PRIVACY NOTICE: See our Privacy policy in www.usps.com

---

13. Publication Title	14. Issue Date for Circulation Data Below
Psychiatric Clinics of North America	September 2007

15. Extent and Nature of Circulation			Average No. Copies Each Issue During Preceding 12 Months	No. Copies of Single Issue Published Nearest to Filing Date
a. Total Number of Copies (*Net press run*)			2300	2200
b. Paid Circulation (By Mail and Outside the Mail)	(1)	Mailed Outside-County Paid Subscriptions Stated on PS Form 3541. (*Include paid distribution above nominal rate, advertiser's proof copies, and exchange copies*)	1226	1144
	(2)	Mailed In-County Paid Subscriptions Stated on PS Form 3541 (*Include paid distribution above nominal rate, advertiser's proof copies, and exchange copies*)		
	(3)	Paid Distribution Outside the Mails Including Sales Through Dealers and Carriers, Street Vendors, Counter Sales, and Other Paid Distribution Outside USPS®	392	397
	(4)	Paid Distribution by Other Classes Mailed Through the USPS (e.g. First-Class Mail®)		
c. Total Paid Distribution (*Sum of 15b (1), (2), (3), and (4)*)		▲	1618	1541
d. Free or Nominal Rate Distribution (By Mail and Outside the Mail)	(1)	Free or Nominal Rate Outside-County Copies Included on PS Form 3541	80	63
	(2)	Free or Nominal Rate In-County Copies Included on PS Form 3541		
	(3)	Free or Nominal Rate Copies Mailed at Other Classes Mailed Through the USPS (e.g. First-Class Mail)		
	(4)	Free or Nominal Rate Distribution Outside the Mail (Carriers or other means)		
e. Total Free or Nominal Rate Distribution (*Sum of 15d (1), (2), (3) and (4)*)		▲	80	63
f. Total Distribution (*Sum of 15c and 15e*)		▲	1698	1604
g. Copies not Distributed (*See instructions to publishers #4 (page 43)*)		▲	602	596
h. Total (*Sum of 15f and g*)		▲	2300	2200
i. Percent Paid (*15c divided by 15f times 100*)		▲	95.29%	96.07%

16. Publication of Statement of Ownership

☐ If the publication is a general publication, publication of this statement is required. Will be printed in the **December 2007** issue of this publication.
☐ Publication not required

17. Signature and Title of Editor, Publisher, Business Manager, or Owner		Date
[signature] Anne Fanucci – Executive Director of Subscription Services		September 14, 2007

I certify that all information furnished on this form is true and complete. I understand that anyone who furnishes false or misleading information on this form or who omits material or information requested on the form may be subject to criminal sanctions (including fines and imprisonment) and/or civil sanctions (including civil penalties).